Immunoassays for Veterinary and Food Analysis—1

Based on the Proceedings of the Second International Symposium on 'Advances in Immunoassays for Veterinary and Food Analysis', held at the University of Surrey, Guildford, UK, 15–17 July 1986. The Symposium was organised jointly by M. N. Clifford, R. Jackman, B. A. Morris and J. A. Morris for the Departments of Biochemistry of the MAFF Central Veterinary Laboratory, Weybridge and the University of Surrey, Guildford.

The meeting was sponsored by the following organisations, whose support is gratefully acknowledged:

Amersham International plc
Coralab Research
Dako (UK) Ltd
Dynatech Laboratories Ltd
Grand Metropolitan Biotechnology Ltd
(Biokits Ltd)
Guildhay Antisera Ltd
May & Baker (Diagnostics) Ltd
Rhône Poulenc (UK) Ltd

Immunoassays for Veterinary and Food Analysis—1

Edited by

B. A. MORRIS

M. N. CLIFFORD

Department of Biochemistry, University of Surrey, Guildford, UK

and

R. JACKMAN

Department of Biochemistry, Ministry of Agriculture, Fisheries and Food, Central Veterinary Laboratory, New Haw, Weybridge, UK

ELSEVIER APPLIED SCIENCE
LONDON and NEW YORK

ELSEVIER APPLIED SCIENCE PUBLISHERS LTD
Crown House, Linton Road, Barking, Essex IG11 8JU, England

Sole Distributor in the USA and Canada
ELSEVIER SCIENCE PUBLISHING CO., INC.
52 Vanderbilt Avenue, New York, NY 10017, USA

WITH 35 TABLES AND 131 ILLUSTRATIONS

British Library Cataloguing in Publication Data

International Symposium on Advances in Immunoassays for Veterinary and Food Analysis. *(2nd:1986:Guildford)*
Immunoassays for veterinary and food analysis: [based on the proceedings of the Second International Symposium on Advances in Immunoassays for Veterinary and Food Analysis held at the University of Surrey, Guildford, UK on 15–17 July, 1986].

1. Food—Analysis 2. Immunoassay 3. Animals —Diseases 4. Immunoassay
I. Title II. Morris, B. A. III. Clifford, M. N.
IV. Jackman, R.
664'.07 TX545

ISBN 1-85166-138-7

Library of Congress CIP Data applied for

Printed in Great Britain by Galliard (Printers) Ltd, Great Yarmouth

To Our Families

Foreword

The food chain is a continuum which starts with soil, seeds, plants and animals and ends up with food and drink that is prepared and ready for consumers' health and enjoyment. Immunoassay techniques are now being used at many points in this chain: for the diagnosis and surveillance of disease in both plants and animals; for the monitoring and control of chemical and other residues in food derived from plant and animal sources. There is no break point between the responsibilities of the plant and animal pathologist on the one hand and the food technologist, on the other. Hence this joint symposium which brought together the various groups having a direct interest in the development of improved cost-effective immunoassay techniques for use at one or other point in the food chain. I mention the need for the techniques to be cost-effective because in the public sector, as in the private, there is the ever present but latterly increasing emphasis on the need to reduce the costs of disease monitoring and control procedures. Immunoassay methods appear very promising in this respect as well as in their technical characteristics. We all look forward to further developments which meet both the technical and cost requirements. In the meantime it is good to have a record of the recent advances in this fast-moving field of scientific endeavour.

R. L. Bell
Director General of the Agricultural Development and Advisory Service and Chief Scientific Adviser, Ministry of Agriculture, Fisheries and Food, London.

Food scientists and technologists, faced with increasing demands for precise analytical data, have perforce become accustomed to contemplating and sometimes adopting new methods of analysis. The proceedings of the 1983 Symposium 'Immunoassays in Food Analysis', published early in 1985, provided the means whereby immunoassay methods could be brought conveniently to their attention and contributed significantly to the willingness of the food industry to accept rather than just contemplate such methods. This volume, the proceedings of the 1986 Symposium, 'Advances in Immunoassays for Veterinary and Food Analysis', records advances of practical significance, not only to specialised, but also to routine analyses and reinforces the points originally advanced—immunoassays couple great versatility, sensitivity and specificity with impressively low equipment, reagent and sample preparation costs and relatively high sample throughput. Application of these considerations and operating laboratory experience in the various sectors of the food industry will directly influence further progress in this field. This book and the preceding companion volume are essential reading for all food scientists and technologists whose remits encompass analysis or interaction with analysts.

W. D. B. HAMILTON
Director, Scientific Affairs, Kellog Co. and
President, Institute of Food Science and Technology.

Preface

In the three years since the first symposium on Immunoassays in Food Analysis was held, there have been many major developments in the subject, both in methodological improvements and areas of application, confirming our prediction that interest in these topics would continue to grow rapidly. The intervening years have also seen the appearance of the first commercial kits for measuring these food analytes. It was therefore felt appropriate to hold a second meeting to review these latest developments.

It was also evident that the boundary between food and veterinary analysis was disappearing, producing a single area of activity. In any case, the distinctions between muscle and meat, plants for human consumption and animal feeding stuffs are largely philosophical. As a result of discussions between the Departments of Biochemistry at the University of Surrey and the Central Veterinary Laboratory, it was decided to hold a joint meeting to cover the application of immunoassays to both veterinary and food analysis. These proceedings are based upon that meeting which was held in July 1986 at the University of Surrey.

It was a truly international event with over 170 participants from twelve different countries. A pre-symposium workshop allowed workers new to the field to acquire a firm grasp of the basic principles involved. The symposium itself provided a forum for veterinary scientists, food scientists, analysts and managers to exchange ideas amongst themselves, as well as with the kit manufacturers and suppliers of specialised immunological reagents, to facilitate further exploitation of these rapidly developing fields.

We should like to thank all the speakers, chairmen, poster presenters and those participants who contributed to the discussion for their enthusiasm and for making it such a successful meeting. We should particularly like to thank Dr John Morris of the Central Veterinary Laboratory for his initiative and help as one of the joint organisers of the meeting; Professor Kit Hitchcock and Mr Andy Crimes for organising the pre-symposium demonstration of ELISA; Mrs Mary Lewis, our Conference Secretary, for once again dealing so efficiently with the administration; all our colleagues at Weybridge and Guildford for their enthusiastic help and encouragement, especially Mr Tony Dell and Mr Roger Levey for their help with the organisation of the trade exhibition; the commercial organisations listed on the frontispiece for their generous financial support of the meeting; the staff of Elsevier Applied Science Publishers for all their help and advice in preparing these proceedings for publication; lastly, but by no means least, our wives and families for their forbearance and unstinting support during the preparations for the meeting and the editing of these proceedings.

All contributions have been critically refereed and edited for content and style. We hope that this book will be read as a companion volume to that reporting the first symposium, since we made no attempt to repeat the topics covered in that first volume. The lack of a paper on a topic particularly dear to a reader's heart neither implies that we are unaware of the application nor that we consider it unimportant and we would welcome their contribution to the third symposium. We are confident that the present volume will be as catalytic as the first in encouraging further the exploitation of immunoassay in veterinary and food analysis.

B. A. Morris
M. N. Clifford
R. Jackman

Contents

Session IV. Problems and Strategies in Immunoassay Application (Chairman: Professor C. H. S. Hitchcock, Unilever Ltd, Bedford, UK)

Session V. Novel Antibody-based Alternatives to Immunoassays (Chairman: B. A. Morris, Department of Biochemistry, University of Surrey, Guildford, UK)

Poster Presentations

List of Contributors and Poster Presenters

M. Abad
Idetek Inc., 1057 Sneath Lane, San Bruno, California 94066, USA

J. C. Allen
North East Wales Institute, Deeside Industrial Park, Deeside, Clwyd CH5 4BR, UK

D. Allison
Idetek Inc., 1057 Sneath lane, San Bruno, California 94066, USA

D. B. Archer
AFRC Institute of Food Research, Norwich Laboratory, Colney Lane, Norwich NR4 7UA, UK

S.-E. Birkeland
Department of Dairy and Food Industries, Agricultural University of Norway, PO Box 36, N-1432 Ås-NLH, Norway

C. D. H. Boarer
MAFF Central Veterinary Laboratory, Woodham Lane, New Haw, Weybridge, Surrey KT15 3NB, UK

S. Bramham
AFRC Institute of Food Research, Norwich Laboratory, Colney Lane, Norwich NR4 7UA, UK

T. Brock
Idetek Inc., 1057 Sneath lane, San Bruno, California 94066, USA

R. A. CALVERLEY
Analytichem International, PO Box 234, Cambridge CB2 1PE, UK

A. A. G. CANDLISH
Division of Immunology, Department of Bioscience and Biotechnology, University of Strathclyde, Todd Centre, 31 Taylor Street, Glasgow G4 0NR, UK

H. W.-S. CHAN
AFRC Institute of Food Research, Norwich Laboratory, Colney Lane, Norwich NR4 7UA, UK

J. CLAYTON
Division of Clinical Biochemistry, Department of Biochemistry, University of Surrey, Guildford, Surrey GU2 5XH, UK

M. N. CLIFFORD
Division of Nutrition and Food Science, Department of Biochemistry, University of Surrey, Guildford, Surrey GU2 5XH, UK

N. T. CROSBY
Department of Trade and Industry, Laboratory of the Government Chemist, Cornwall House, Waterloo Road, London SE1 8XY, UK

R. L. DARLEY
Department of Biochemistry, University of Surrey, Guildford, Surrey GU2 5XH, UK

J. H. M. DAVINA
Research Institute for Animal Production 'Schoonoord', PO Box 501, 3700 AM Zeist, The Netherlands

D. L. FAILLA
Department of Clinical Pathology, School of Veterinary Medicine, University of California, Davis, California 95616, USA

M. T. FOX
Department of Microbiology and Parasitology, Royal Veterinary College, Royal College Street, London NW1 0TU, UK

K. W. FREEBAIRN
Department of Trade and Industry, Laboratory of the Government Chemist, Cornwall House, Waterloo Road, London SE1 8XY, UK

D. GERRELLI
Department of Microbiology and Parasitology, Royal Veterinary College, Royal College Street, London NW1 0TU, UK

P. A. GIBBS
Applied Microbiology Section, Leatherhead Food Research Association, Randalls Road, Leatherhead, Surrey KT22 7RY, UK

I. A. GOODBRAND
Division of Immunology, Department of Bioscience and Biotechnology, University of Strathclyde, Todd Centre, 31 Taylor Street, Glasgow G4 0NR, UK

S. L. GORHAM
Virginia-Maryland Regional College of Veterinary Medicine, University of Maryland, College Park, Maryland 20742, USA

Y. GOTOH
Faculty of Pharmaceutical Sciences, Nagasaki University, Nagasaki 852, Japan

B. J. GOULD
Department of Biochemistry, University of Surrey, Guildford, Surrey GU2 5XH, UK

N. M. GRIFFITHS
Meat Legislation Advisory Service, Meat and Livestock Commission, PO Box 44, Queensway House, Bletchley, Milton Keynes MK2 2KF, UK

G. V. GROOM
NEQAS Unit, Tenovus Institute for Cancer Research, Heath Park, Cardiff CF4 4XX, UK

D. J. GROVES
Division of Clinical Biochemistry, Department of Biochemistry, University of Surrey, Guildford, Surrey GU2 5XH, UK

P. HAMBLETON

Public Health Laboratory Service, Centre for Applied Microbiology and Research, Porton Down, Salisbury, Wiltshire SP4 0JG, UK

M. H. HARVEY

Department of Chemical Pathology, Lewisham Group Laboratory, Lewisham Hospital, London SE13 6LH, UK

R. M. HATFIELD

Division of Clinical Biochemistry, Department of Biochemistry, University of Surrey, Guildford, Surrey GU2 5XH, UK

R. R. HENRY

Division of Clinical Biochemistry, Department of Biochemistry, University of Surrey, Guildford, Surrey GU2 5XH, UK

C. H. S. HITCHCOCK

Unilever Ltd, Colworth House, Sharnbrook, Bedford MK44 1LQ, UK

R. JACKMAN

MAFF Central Veterinary Laboratory, Woodham Lane, New Haw, Weybridge, Surrey KT15 3NB, UK

D. E. JACOBS

Department of Microbiology and Parasitology, The Royal Veterinary College, Royal College Street, London NW1 0TU, UK

L. JANG

Idetek Inc., 1057 Sneath Lane, San Bruno, California 94066, USA

S. L. JONES

AFRC Institute of Food Research, Bristol Laboratory, Langford, Bristol BS18 7DY, UK

A. S. KANG

AFRC Institute of Food Research, Norwich Laboratory, Colney Lane, Norwich NR4 7UA, UK

H. A. KEMP

AFRC Institute of Food Research, Norwich Laboratory, Colney Lane, Norwich NR4 7UA, UK

T. KINOUE

Faculty of Pharmaceutical Sciences, Nagasaki University, Nagasaki 852, Japan

T. KITAGAWA

Department of Microbiological Chemistry, Faculty of Pharmaceutical Sciences, Nagasaki University, Nagasaki 852, Japan

Y. KOHRI

Faculty of Pharmaceutical Sciences, Nagasaki University, Nagasaki 852, Japan

W. KOOPS

Research Institute for Animal Production 'Schoonoord', PO Box 501, 3700 AM Zeist, The Netherlands

E. KRESS-ROGERS

Leatherhead Food Research Association, Randalls Road, Leatherhead, Surrey KT22 7RY, UK

J. LANDON

Department of Chemical Pathology, St Bartholomew's Hospital, London EC1A 7BE, UK

I. D. LUMLEY

Department of Trade and Industry, Laboratory of the Government Chemist, Cornwall House, Waterloo Road, London SE1 8XY, UK

M. MCMILLAN

Department of Chemical Pathology, Lewisham Group Laboratory, Lewisham Hospital, London SE13 6LH, UK

N. M. MACKENZIE

Royal Veterinary College, Royal College Street, London NW1 0TU, UK

E. T. MALLINSON

Virginia-Maryland Regional College of Veterinary Medicine, University of Maryland, College Park, Maryland 20742, USA

V. MARKS
Department of Biochemistry, University of Surrey, Guildford, Surrey GU2 5XH, UK

W. W. MARQUARDT
Virginia-Maryland Regional College of Veterinary Medicine, University of Maryland, College Park, Maryland 20742, USA

J. MELLING
Public Health Laboratory Service, Centre for Applied Microbiology and Research, Porton Down, Salisbury, Wiltshire SP4 0JG, UK

E. N. C. MILLS
AFRC Institute for Food Research, Norwich Laboratory, Colney Lane, Norwich NR4 7UA, UK

N. K. MODI
Porton International Ltd, 29 Chesham Place, London SW1X 8HB, UK

M. R. A. MORGAN
AFRC Institute for Food Research, Norwich Laboratory, Colney Lane, Norwich NR4 7UA, UK

B. A. MORRIS
Division of Clinical Biochemistry, Department of Biochemistry, University of Surrey, Guildford, Surrey GU2 5XH, UK

M. E. MOUNT
Department of Clinical Pathology, School of Veterinary Medicine, University of California, Davis, California 95616, USA

A. B. J. NIX
Department of Mathematical Statistics and Operational Research, University College, Cardiff CF1 1AL, UK

A. NOLAN
MAFF Central Veterinary Laboratory, Woodham Lane, New Haw, Weybridge, Surrey KT15 3NB, UK

W. Ohtani
Faculty of Pharmaceutical Sciences, Nagasaki University, Nagasaki 852, Japan

D. G. Oliver
Idetek Inc., 1057 Sneath Lane, San Bruno, California 94066, USA

S. Opie
Campden Food Preservation Research Association, Chipping Campden, Glos. GL55 6LD, UK

I. Patel
Department of Trade and Industry, Laboratory of the Government Chemist, Cornwall House, Waterloo Road, London SE1 8XY, UK

P. D. Patel
Biopolymers Section, Leatherhead Food Research Association, Randalls Road, Leatherhead, Surrey KT22 7RY, UK

R. L. S. Patterson
AFRC Institute of Food Research, Bristol Laboratory, Langford, Bristol BS18 7DY, UK

J. J. Pembroke-Hattersley
MAFF Central Veterinary Laboratory, Woodham Lane, New Haw, Weybridge, Surrey KT15 3NB, UK

A. C. Pinder
AFRC Institute of Food Research, Norwich Laboratory, Colney Lane, Norwich NR4 7UA, UK

S. R. Pitt
Department of Microbiology and Parasitology, The Royal Veterinary College, Royal College Street, London NW1 0TU, UK

B. Roberts
Division of Nutrition and Food Science, Department of Biochemistry, University of Surrey, Guildford, Surrey GU2 5XH, UK

A. Robertson
Campden Food Preservation Research Association, Chipping Campden, Glos. GL55 6LD, UK

P. L. ROEDER

MAFF Central Veterinary Laboratory, Woodham Lane, New Haw, Weybridge, Surrey KT15 3NB, UK

J. SARGEANT

Lord Rank Research Centre, High Wycombe, Bucks., UK. Present address: *Beeches Biotech, Beeches Farm, Buckland St Mary, Chard, Somerset, UK*

C. C. SHONE

Public Health Laboratory Service, Centre for Applied Microbiology and Research, Porton Down, Salisbury, Wiltshire SP4 0JG, UK

P. SINGH

Idetek Inc., 1057 Sneath Lane, San Bruno, California 94066, USA

J. E. SMITH

Division of Immunology, Department of Bioscience and Biotechnology, University of Strathclyde, Todd Centre, 31 Taylor Street, Glasgow G4 0NR, UK

D. B. SNYDER

Virginia-Maryland Regional College of Veterinary Medicine, University of Maryland, College Park, Maryland 20742, USA

T. SØRHAUG

Department of Dairy and Food Industries, Agricultural University of Norway, PO Box 36, N-1432 Ås-NLH, Norway

C. J. STANLEY

Department of Trade and Industry, Laboratory of the Government Chemist, Cornwall House, Waterloo Road, London SE1 8XY, UK

L. STEPANIAK

Department of Dairy and Food Industries, Agricultural University of Norway, PO Box 36, N-1432 Ås-NLH, Norway

W. H. STIMSON

Division of Immunology, Department of Bioscience and Biotechnology, University of Strathclyde, The Todd Centre, 31 Taylor Street, Glasgow G4 0NR, UK

S. M. Thamsborg
Institute of Internal Medicine, Royal Veterinary and Agricultural University, Bülowsvej 13, DK-1870 Frederiksberg C, Denmark

C. J. Thorns
MAFF Central Veterinary Laboratory, Woodham Lane, New Haw, Weybridge, Surrey KT15 3NB, UK

A. P. F. Turner
Cranfield Biotechnology Centre, Cranfield Institute of Technology, Cranfield, Bedford MK43 0AL, UK

K. Uchihara
Faculty of Pharmaceutical Sciences, Nagasaki University, Nagasaki 852, Japan

D. Upadhyaya
Campden Food Preservation Research Association, Chipping Campden, Glos. GL55 6LD, UK

G. Vagias
Department of Dairy and Food Industries, Agricultural University of Norway, PO Box 36, N-1432 Ås-NLH, Norway

N. Vail
Idetek Inc., 1057 Sneath Lane, San Bruno, California 94066, USA

D. F. M. van de Wiel
Research Institute for Animal Production 'Schoonoord', PO Box 501, 3700 AM Zeist, The Netherlands

C. van Peteghem
Laboratorium voor Bromatologie, Faculteit van de Farmaceutische Wentenschappen, Rijksuniversiteit-Gent, Harelbekestraat 72, B-9000 Gent, Belgium

C. M. Ward
AFRC Institute of Food Research, Norwich Laboratory, Colney Lane, Norwich NR4 7UA, UK

W. A. Watson

MAFF Central Veterinary Laboratory, Woodham Lane, New Haw, Weybridge, Surrey KT15 3NB, UK

S. Wie

Environmental Diagnostics Inc., Burlington, North Carolina, USA

A. P. Wilkinson

AFRC Institute of Food Research, Norwich Laboratory, Colney Lane, Norwich NR4 7UA, UK

H. Windemann

Institut für Biochemie, Universität Bern, Freiestrasse 3, 3012 Bern, Switzerland

List of Abbreviations

A	Absorbance
Ab	Antibody
Ab_1	Primary or first antibody
Ab_2	Second or double antibody
ABTS	2,2′-Azinobis(3-ethylbenzothiazoline-6-sulphonic acid)
Ag	Antigen
AMP	Adenosine 5′-monophosphate
AP	Alkaline phosphatase
ATP	Adenosine 5′-triphosphate
BSA	Bovine serum albumin
CELIA	Competitive enzyme-linked immunosorbent assay
c.f.	Confer (compare)
DEAE	Diethylaminoethyl
DMSO	Dimethylsulphoxide
EIA	Enzyme immunoassay
ELISA	Enzyme-linked immunosorbent assay
EMIT	Enzyme mediated immunoassay technique
FCS	Foetal calf serum
FITC	Fluorescein isothiocyanate
HPLC	High pressure liquid chromatography
HRP	Horseradish peroxidase
IELIA	Inhibition enzyme-linked immunoassay
IEMA	Immunoenzymometric assay
IgG	Immunoglobulin G
KLH	Keyhole limpet haemocyanin
LC	Liquid chromatography

Mab	Monoclonal antibody
NMR	Nuclear magnetic resonance
NSB	Non-specific binding
OPD	*o*-Phenylenediamine
PAGE	Polyacrylamide gel electrophoresis
PBS	Phosphate-buffered saline
PBST	Phosphate-buffered saline-Tween
PVC	Polyvinyl chloride
q.v.	*quod vide* (which see)
RIA	Radioimmunoassay
RT	Room temperature
SDS	Sodium dodecyl sulphate
TLC	Thin layer chromatography
Tris	Tris(hydroxymethyl)aminomethane

Glossary

(compiled by B. A. Morris (1985);
revised by B. A. Morris, M. N. Clifford and R. Jackman)

Affinity.† The energy with which the combining sites of an antibody bind its specific antigen. It is essentially the same as the association constant (K_A) in physical chemistry with

$$K_A = \frac{[AgAb]}{[Ab][Ag]} \text{ in litres/mole,}$$

where [AgAb], [Ab] and [Ag] are the molar concentrations of the antigen–antibody complex, free antibody and free antigen respectively (cf. Avidity). The dissociation constant (K_D) is given by the relationship

$$K_D = \frac{1}{K_A}$$

and has the dimensions of moles/litre.

Analyte. The substance in a test sample whose quantity is to be determined or presence detected.

Antibody or immunoglobulin. A binding protein which is synthesised by the immune system of an animal in response to either the invasion of a foreign organism or the injection of an immunogen. May be divided into a number of different classes, the principal one usually employed in an immunoassay being immunoglobulin G, IgG (MW 160 000) (cf. Antiserum).

Antigen. A substance that will react with its specific antibody. (cf. Hapten, Immunogen).

Antigen-free matrix. Matrix (q.v.) from which the antigen has been

* Denotes revised definition.
† Denotes new definition.

selectively removed e.g. by an immunosorbent, for the purpose of diluting the standards.

Antigenic determinant. Feature of an antigen which defines the recognition pattern of an antibody (cf. Epitope, Idiotopes).

Antiserum.* Serum containing polyclonal antibodies (q.v.) to an antigen (q.v.)

Avidity.* The mean affinity of a polyclonal antiserum (q.v.).

Bias. A systematic error in the assay system.

Bound fraction. The portion of the incubation mixture which contains the antigen–antibody complex (cf. Free fraction).

Carrier protein. A large molecular weight protein to which haptens (q.v.) are covalently linked in order to elicit an immune response to the latter (c.f. Coating conjugate).

Classical immunoassay. The original immunoassay concept, first reported by Yalow & Berson, is a limited reagent immunoassay (q.v.) in which antigen (the analyte) and labelled antigen compete for a fixed, but limited, number of antibody binding sites (cf. Immunometric assay).

Coating conjugate.† A protein or peptide to which hapten (q.v.) has been covalently linked and which is used for coating the wells of a microtitration plate (q.v.) in an ELISA (q.v.) (cf. Carrier protein).

Competitive ELISA.* A limited reagent form of enzyme-linked immunosorbent assay, in which either: (1) the antigen in a test sample or standard solution competes with enzyme-labelled antigen for the limited binding sites on the immobilised antibody; or (2) the antigen in a test sample or standard competes with immobilised antigen for a limited number of binding sites on the enzyme-labelled antibody (cf. Non-competitive ELISA).

Cross-reaction. Ability of substances, other than the antigen, to bind to the antibody, and the ability of substances other than the antibody to bind the antigen. Such substances, if present in a test sample, may compete with the antigen for the binding site, thus leading to an erroneous potency estimate. These substances may be natural precursors of the antigen (or a binding protein), degradation products (from *in vivo* or *in vitro* degradation) or other substances that carry on their surface a molecular configuration similar to the antigenic determinants on the antigen being measured.

Delayed addition immunoassay.* A limited reagent immunoassay in which the antigen (in the test sample or standard) is incubated for a period prior to the addition of labelled antigen. If the antibody is of sufficiently high affinity (q.v.), this form of assay may increase sensitivity, compared with the more usual assay procedure in which all three reactants are incubated together for the same length of time.

Detection limit. The smallest amount or concentration of analyte which, with a stated confidence (commonly two standard deviations, or expressed as confidence or fiducal limits), can be distinguished from zero. This value depends on the precision of the measurements of zero dose solution and of the specimen (cf. Sensitivity).

Direct ELISA.† An ELISA (q.v.) in which quantitation is achieved by means of either an enzyme-labelled primary antibody (q.v.) or enzyme-labelled antigen (q.v.) (cf. Indirect ELISA).

Disequilibrium (or non-equilibrium) immunoassay. An immunoassay in which the reaction between antigen and antibody is stopped before equilibrium has been reached. Frequently used in continuous flow automated immunoassay systems which enable exact reproducible timing between reagent addition and the separation step (cf. Equilibrium immunoassay).

Dynamic or working range.† The range of analyte (q.v.) concentration over which precision is acceptable.

Enzyme immunoassay. Sometimes referred to as *Enzymoimmunoassay*. An assay procedure based on the reversible and non-covalent binding of an antigen by a specific antibody, in which one of the reactants is labelled with an enzyme.

Enzyme-linked immunosorbent assay (ELISA). An enzyme immunoassay (q.v.) in which one of the reactants is adsorbed on the surface of the wells of a microtitration plate (q.v.).

Enzyme mediated immunoassay technique (EMIT). A homogeneous enzyme immunoassay (q.v.) for haptens (q.v.) in which the enzyme is linked to the hapten in such a way that the enzyme activity is altered when the hapten combines with its antibody. The activity may be enhanced or, more usually, reduced. EMIT is the registered trade mark of the Syva Corp., USA.

Epitope.† An antigenic determinant (q.v.) of a conventional, non-immunoglobulin, antigen (cf. Idiotopes).

Equilibrium immunoassay. An immunoassay in which the assay components in the incubation mixture are allowed to react until the concentration of each reactant has ceased to change with time, i.e. equilibrium has been attained (cf. Delayed addition immunoassay; Disequilibrium immunoassay).

Excess reagent immunoassay. An immunoassay in which the antibody is present in excess, as in immunometric assays (q.v.) (cf. Limited reagent immunoassay).

F_{ab} fragment.† The fragment containing the antigen combining site after digestion of an immunoglobulin molecule with papain.

$F_{(ab')_2}$ fragment.† The fragment containing the antigen combining site after digestion of an immunoglobulin molecule with pepsin; consists of two F_{ab} fragments (q.v.) joined by the hinge region.

F_c fragment.† The species-specific region of an immunoglobulin remaining after digestion and removal of the antigen combining sites with either papain or pepsin.

First or primary antibody. An antibody reacting specifically with the antigen being measured (cf. Second antibody).

Fluoroimmunoassay. A classical immunoassay (q.v.) in which the antigen is labelled with a fluorophore for use as the tracer.

Free fraction. The portion of the incubation mixture which, after phase separation (q.v.), does not contain the antigen–antibody complex (cf. Bound fraction). It may be free antigen, as in classical immunoassay (q.v.), or free antibody, as in immunometric assay (q.v.).

Hapten. An antigen (q.v.) which is not usually immunogenic (q.v.) but which becomes so when coupled to a larger molecule, usually a protein.

Heterogeneous immunoassay. An immunoassay in which it is necessary to separate the antigen–antibody complex (bound fraction q.v.) from the free reactants, usually antigen, prior to measuring the quantity of label in either the bound or free phases/fractions (cf. Homogeneous immunoassay).

Homogeneous immunoassay. An immunoassay in which it is not necessary to separate the antigen–antibody complex from the free reactants prior to end point measurement (cf. Heterogeneous immunoassay).

Hook effect. A phenomenon associated with the standard curve of a competitive immunoassay (q.v.) in which increasing the concentration of antigen from zero level initially produces an *increase* in binding of the labelled antigen before resulting in a fall in binding, i.e. a 'hooked' curve; problem may be overcome by using the antiserum at a higher dilution.

Idiotopes.† Antigenic determinants (q.v.) on the conformational structures of one set of antibodies which distinguish it from those of other sets (cf. Epitope).

Idiotype.† The collection of idiotopes (q.v.) on each immunoglobulin (q.v.) molecule.

Immunoassay. An assay procedure based on the reversible and non-covalent binding of an antigen by antibody using a labelled form of one or the other to quantify the system. Can be used to detect or quantify either antigens or antibodies.

Immunogen. A substance that, when injected into a suitable animal, stimulates the production of antibody or antibodies that can combine with the same substance as an antigen (q.v.).

Immunometric assay. A non-competitive excess reagent immunoassay (q.v.) based on the reversible and non-covalent binding of an antigen by excess specific antibody (or antibodies) labelled with a tracer molecule. An immunoassay using labelled antibodies instead of labelled antigens to quantitate the assay (see Sandwich or two-site immunometric assays).

Immunoreactivity. The ability of a specified antigen to combine with its antibody, or a specified antibody to combine with its antigen.

Inaccuracy. The numerical difference between the average of a series of estimates and the true or accepted value.

Indirect ELISA.† An ELISA (q.v.) in which quantitation is achieved by means of an enzyme-labelled second antibody (q.v.) (cf. Direct ELISA).

Label. The substance attached to one of the assay reactants for the purpose of determining the proportion of that reactant which has formed an antigen–antibody complex, by yielding a perceptible signal.

Labelled antigen. A form of the specified antigen to which a label (q.v.) has been attached covalently.

Limited reagent immunoassay. An immunoassay in which the amount of antibody added is insufficient to bind all the labelled antigen in the reaction mixture (cf. Excess reagent immunoassay).

Luminoimmunoassay. A classical immunoassay (q.v.) in which the antigen is labelled with either a bioluminescent or chemiluminescent molecule for use as the tracer.

Matrix. Substances other than the analyte (q.v.) which are present in the sample or sample extract (cf. Antigen-free matrix).

Microtitration plate. A disposable plastic tray, containing 96 wells, which is used to hold the incubates in ELISA.

Misclassification. The extent to which the free, i.e. non-bound, reactants are present in the bound fraction and vice versa after phase separation (q.v.).

Monoclonal antibodies. Antibodies derived from a single clone of lymphocytes, produced by a hybridoma as a result of fusion of a sensitised lymphocyte with a myeloma cell (cf. Polyclonal antibodies).

Multivalent antigen. An antigen with two or more antigenic determinants (q.v.).

Non-competitive ELISA. An excess reagent form of enzyme-linked immunosorbent assay (cf. Competitive ELISA).

Non-equilibrium immunoassay. See disequilibrium immunoassay.

Non-specific binding (NSB). The fraction of labelled material apparently present in the bound fraction for reasons other than specific binding to the binding site of an antibody.

Parallelism. The extent to which the dose-response curves of two substances are identical, except for displacement along the dose axis of one relative to the other. If the curves are curvilinear, this condition is described as 'generalised parallelism'. It is one test of identity of two preparations, e.g. analyte and standard.

Phase separation. Procedure by which the free fraction is separated from the bound fraction prior to measurement of the amount of labelled reactant present in one or the other fraction.

Polyclonal antibodies. Antibodies to a given antigen which are present in an antiserum (q.v.) and which are derived from several clones of lymphocytes produced in a single animal as the result of an injection of immunogen (cf. Monoclonal antibodies).

Precision/imprecision. The closeness of agreement between the results obtained by applying a given procedure several times under prescribed conditions.

As precision has no numerical value, the term imprecision, to which a numerical value can be assigned, may be preferable in some contexts.

Imprecision consists of variability among replicate analyses of the same material, and is usually expressed as the standard deviation, or variance or coefficient of variation.

Precision profile. Graphical representation of the precision, or more correctly, the imprecision, of measurements obtained with an assay system over a range of dose levels of the analyte.

Such profiles are of value in assessing the reliance that can be placed on an assay estimate at a particular dose level, because the precision in immunoassays may vary considerably with analyte concentration.

Primary antibody.† An antibody reacting with the analyte (q.v.) when this is an antigen (q.v.) (cf. Second antibody).

Radioimmunoassay. A classical immunoassay (q.v.) in which the antigen is labelled with a radionucleide for use as a tracer.

Ruggedness. Characteristic of an assay system which makes the results obtained unaffected by changes in the assay reagents and procedures.

In practice, non-ruggedness is manifested by poor precision, poor inter-assay variability and poor inter-laboratory agreement.

Sandwich or two-site assay. An immunometric assay (q.v.) using two different antibodies, each recognising a separate antigenic determinant (q.v.) on the analyte molecule, one of the antibodies being immobilised on a solid support and the other being labelled with a tracer molecule. By sequential incubations, the analyte is sandwiched between the two antibodies. This assay system is inherently more specific than classical immunoassay (q.v.) since two separate antigenic determinants on the analyte are recognised simultaneously. Its use is obviously restricted to the measurement of multivalent antigens (q.v.).

Second or double antibody. An antibody raised against the immunoglobulins (usually IgG) of the species in which the first antibody (q.v.) was raised.

Sensitivity. The ability of a method to distinguish significantly between small differences in concentration of analyte (cf. Detection limit).

Specificity.* Of an antibody for a particular antigen is the degree to which it is not influenced by substances of similar structure and composition.

Titre. The final dilution of an antiserum or purified antibody preparation which binds a specified fraction (commonly 50%) or a specified amount of a stated quantity of the labelled antigen: usually expressed numerically as the reciprocal of the dilution.

Tracer. See Label.

Two-site immunometric assay. See Sandwich assay.

REFERENCES

MORRIS, B. A. (1985) In: *Immunoassays in Food Analysis*, B. A. Morris & M. N. Clifford, (eds.), Elsevier Applied Science Publishers, London, pp. xv–xxi.

SÖNKSEN, P. H. (1974) In: Radioimmunoassay and Saturation Analysis. *British Medical Bulletin*, **30**, 103.

WHO Expert Committee on Biological Standardisation (1981) Requirements for Immunoassay Kits. World Health Organisation Technical Report, Series No. 658, WHO, Geneva.

SESSION I

Recent Developments in Immunoassay Design

1

Opportunities and Incentives for Developing Food Immunoassays

C. H. S. HITCHCOCK

Unilever Research, Colworth Laboratory, Sharnbrook, Bedford, UK

INTRODUCTION

As food technology becomes more sophisticated, food products more complex and consumers more concerned about the composition of the food they eat, the problems facing the food analyst become more difficult. Classical proximate analysis still provides basic data in terms of protein, fat, carbohydrate, mineral and water content. More detailed data are obtained by traditional chemical and biochemical methods; for instance, the determination of vitamins, fatty acids, amino acids, steroids, sugars and metals. In addition, the safety of foodstuffs can be monitored by special techniques designed to detect traces of chemicals such as mycotoxins, pesticides, drugs, polycyclic hydrocarbons, halogenated compounds and solvents.

In this country, over a hundred years ago (1860), food analysis was recognised as a distinct discipline of social value with the establishment of the Public Analysts by the Adulteration Act. Since then, the techniques of analytical chemistry have evolved, slowly becoming more powerful, more elaborate and more costly. By the time a method has been initiated, tested, optimised, standardised and established, it is understandable that it tends to be preferred to a newer method unless distinct advantages can be demonstrated. Also food analysts tend to be conservative because their methods become ossified in codes of practice, agreed regulations and legislation.

When determinations of new analytes are required, they tend to be approached by traditional chromatography, the objective being to isolate the analyte; if necessary, high-resolution equipment coupled with complementary methods such as mass spectroscopy may be invoked to improve resolution or sensitivity. The emphasis here is on the efficiency of the separation method; often non-specific end point detection allows determination of several analytes in the same sample extract. Immunoassay represents the reverse of this approach: here the immunoreagent (antibody) is so specific that the analyte (antigen) may even be determined *in situ* without isolation. This approach is very attractive, particularly now that clinical biochemists have established enzyme-labelled and other non-isotopic immunoassay techniques.

The specificity and avidity of well-designed antibody–antigen interactions can result in a specific and sensitive analytical technique, which may also have other advantages for the food analyst (Hitchcock, 1984; Morgan, 1985). The sensitivity often allows dilution of the sample extract, thus minimising matrix interference. The use of solid-phased antibodies has the further advantage that they can immunosorb and concentrate the analyte in the sample before analysis. Immunoassay is a relatively rapid and robust procedure which can be automated if necessary, using equipment that is already commercially available. It can be designed either as a cheap qualitative screening method or as a reliable quantitative procedure.

FOOD ANALYTES

Opportunities

The range of analytes amenable to immunoassay is limited only by their immunogenicity. Such analytes therefore include macromolecules (e.g. proteins) which can be intrinsically immunogenic and smaller molecules (e.g. steroids) which may be made immunogenic by covalent linkage to a suitable macromolecule. Haptens of minimum molecular weight are typified by aromatics (e.g. nitrobenzene), chlorocompounds (e.g. DDT) and apparently innocuous compounds such as tripeptides (e.g. Glu–His–Pro) and bis-succinylcholine, against all of which antibodies have been raised. The food analyst should therefore be able to apply immunoassays to the measurement of a wide variety of analytes as listed in Table 1.

For the first time, a generally applicable quantitative method is available to give a detailed analysis of the individual proteins in a food product. While total crude protein will doubtless continue to be determined by the Kjeldahl nitrogen method, the validity of the conversion factors employed is being increasingly questioned. Moreover, the final figure can only correspond to the total protein from all sources together with any non-protein nitrogen in the sample (e.g. peptides, nucleic acids, urea).

Table 1
Potential Analytes for Food Immunoassay

Analytes	*References*
1. Trace components	Morgan (1985)[a]
Residues, contaminants and endogenous components at ppb and ppt levels as haptens, potentially in all food systems	
1.1 Mycotoxins	Pestka & Chu (1984),[a] Groopman *et al.* (1984)[a]
Ochratoxin A_1	Morgan *et al.* (1983*b*), Lee & Chu (1984)
Aflatoxin B_1	Fan & Chu (1984), Candlish *et al.* (1985)
Aflatoxin M_1	Fremy & Chu (1984), Hu *et al.* (1984), Martlbauer & Terplan (1985), Jackman (1985)
Sterigmatocystin	Morgan *et al.* (1986)
Deoxynivalenol	Kemp *et al.* (1986)
T-2 toxin	Gendloff *et al.* (1984), Hunter *et al.* (1985)
1.2 Bacterial toxins	Patel (1985)[a]
Clostridium	Shone *et al.* (1985), Bartholomew *et al.* (1985)
Staphylococcus	Fey *et al.* (1984)
Escherichia	Thompson *et al.* (1984), Sack *et al.* (1980)
Vibrio	Sack *et al.* (1980)
1.3 Anabolic agents	Heitzman (1984),[a] Warwick *et al.* (1985)[a]
Diethylstilboestrol	Arnstadt (1981), Gridley *et al.* (1983), Vogt (1985)
Hexoestrol	Harwood *et al.* (1980)
Trenbolone	Heitzman & Harwood (1977)
Zeranol	
Dienoestrol	
Oestradiol	
1.4 Antibiotics	
Chloramphenicol	Arnold *et al.* (1984), Arnold & Somogyi (1985)
Penicillin	Rohner *et al.* (1985)
1.5 Antinutrients	
Solanine	Morgan *et al.* (1983*a*)
Trypsin inhibitor	
1.6 Vitamins	
B_{12}	Richardson *et al.* (1978)
D	Belsey *et al.* (1974), Wood (1983), Reinhardt *et al.* (1984)
1.7 Plant hormones	
Indole acetic acid	Weiler *et al.* (1981)
Gibberellins	Atzorn & Weiler (1983*a*), Atzorn & Weiler (1983*b*)
Abscisic acid	Weiler (1982)

(*continued*)

Table 1—*contd.*

Analytes	*References*
1.8 Other analytes	
Paraquat	Niewola *et al.* (1983)
Limonin	Jourdan *et al.* (1984)
Quassin	Robins *et al.* (1984*a*), Robins *et al.* (1984*b*)
Amyloglucosidase	Vaag (1985)
Pesticides	
Drugs	
Hormones	
2. Food proteins	Hitchcock (1984)[a]
Major proteinaceous ingredients in raw, cooked, sterilised and dried food products	
2.1 Meat	Griffiths & Billington (1984)
Myosin	Everett *et al.* (1983)
Collagen	Robins (1982), Dusemund & Barrach (1982)
Species-specific	Hitchcock & Crimes (1985),[a] Kangethe *et al.* (1982), Whittaker *et al.* (1983), Manz (1983), Patterson *et al.* (1984), Jones & Patterson (1985), Manz (1985), Patterson & Spencer (1985), Jones & Patterson (1986)
2.2 Soya	Hitchcock *et al.* (1981), Crimes *et al.* (1984), Olsman *et al.* (1985), Ravestein & Driedonks (1986)
2.3 Milk	Teufel & Sacher (1982), Staak & Kampe (1982), Lefier & Collin (1982)
2.4 Wheat	Windemann (1982), Skerritt & Smith (1985), Skerritt (1985), Skerritt *et al.* (1985)
2.5 Other analytes	
Egg	
Bean	
Pea	
Potato	
Blood	
Fungal protein	
Bacterial protein	

[a] Overviews.

Immunoassays can also be applied to the determination of natural endogenous toxicants, exogenous chemical residues and adventitious contaminants that might be introduced into the food chain. These substances are typically found at minute levels (10^{-6} or 10^{-9} g/g) and specific, sensitive screening methods are needed to replace cumbersome traditional chemical and microbiological techniques currently used.

Immunoassays have already established themselves as powerful aids to all branches of biochemical research; for example, the localisation and determination of low levels of abscisic acid in the leaves of stressed plants, so that future varieties for cloning can be selected at the nursery stage by a simple diagnostic test.

Problems

Immunoassays present many opportunities but significant difficulties limit their immediate exploitation. The availability of appropriate antisera or monoclonal antibodies is a prerequisite; however, they are not always readily available and have to be specially developed. They must be of sufficient titre, specificity and avidity, and a large batch of uniform material will be necessary to ensure consistent results over long periods of time in different laboratories. When immunoassays are standardised by collaborative testing and later accepted as official methods, the immunoreagents must be specified in the same way as any other analytical reagents. The generation of monoclonal antibodies is therefore recommended due to their uniform consistency; however, polyclonal antisera may sometimes have advantages.

Another difficulty lies in the nature of the samples that must be analysed. While clinical procedures are mainly confined to the examination of body fluids such as blood, urine and bile in the native state, food is often processed under conditions which alter the conformation of macromolecules and so transform their immunoreactivity. The solid food matrix is often a complex denatured mixture including animal and vegetable tissues from which the analyte must be extracted in consistent yield. The extract may also contain variable amounts of components which interfere with immunochemical interactions and so affect the validity of the assay. The vegetable components of some foods and animal feeds represent a potential source of interference; for example, phenols such as tannins, and surfactants such as saponins, interact non-specifically with proteins and therefore represent a possible analytical problem. Active enzymes and enzyme inhibitors may interfere in the end point determination. Other components of the food matrix may impede extraction of the analyte, especially if this is present at low levels. With some analytes, particularly those of low molecular weight, the extraction protocol can involve organic solvents. A procedure must therefore be developed to provide an aqueous or aqueous/alcoholic solution containing the maximum yield of analyte for immunoassay with the minimum of interference.

If the analyte is a protein, the manufacturing process may have converted it into an insoluble heat-denatured agglomerate. Organic solvents may be used to remove fat and water from the sample and the protein extracted into denaturants such as aqueous urea, guanidine hydrochloride, sodium dodecylsulphate, etc., containing a reducing agent such as mercapto-ethanol, dithiothreitol, etc. Such a procedure may solubilise the analyte whether or not it had been originally heat-denatured during the manufacture of the food. However, this aqueous solution cannot be analysed directly because the denaturants disrupt the antibody–antigen interaction on which the immunoassay depends. Before analysis, the denaturant must be effectively removed by dialysis or more conveniently by dilution, thus allowing the soluble random coils of the protein molecules to fold into a 'renatured' (but not necessarily native) state. This renatured protein can now interact with corresponding antisera, and can therefore be determined by immunoassay. Antisera to native protein have been found to be suitable for the assay of heat-denatured protein that has been renatured (Hitchcock *et al.*, 1981). Severe heat denaturation (especially above 100°C) causes some chemical change that cannot be reversed by renaturation, and this is probably why the observed response in the immunoassay to severely heated proteins is somewhat less than that of the fully renatured form. This reduced response may be overcome by raising antisera to the severely heated material.

The specificity of immunoassays is an essential element in their application, but ultraspecificity can be counterproductive in the determination of food proteins. Soya protein ingredients, for example, are all of somewhat different protein composition owing to natural biological variation of the plant; moreover, subsequent processing into flours, defatted flours, concentrates, isolates and extruded texturates can modify the structure of the proteins as well as their relative proportions. The soya-containing food product that is to be analysed has often been processed again under different conditions; the analyst is then interested in the total level of modified protein that originated in the soya bean as distinct from the protein from other ingredients such as meat, milk, wheat, potato and microbiological sources. The specificity of the antibody should therefore include a defined range of soya protein epitopes and exclude all non-soya epitopes; ideally the response of each soya protein should be similar so that varietal changes in composition do not affect the overall response, which should also be unaffected by processing. The use of an ultraspecific monoclonal antibody could therefore bring disadvantages, for if the response depends solely on the level of a single epitope, this might not always be quantitatively representative of the whole protein mixture and moreover might be masked or altered by the processing. Polyclonal antisera containing a variety of antibody clones to various soya proteins would seem to be a more logical basis for the particular assay. In any case, cross-reactions with non-soya proteins, particularly with vegetable proteins of similar structure (e.g. from other legumes), need to be avoided or removed by adsorption.

Economics

Whereas the scientific incentive to develop food immunoassay procedures is high, the economic incentives are more problematic. Medical diagnosis has always been an attractive field because the market for new clinical immunoassay kits is large. Each individual liable to suffer a particular clinical condition can be regarded as a potential customer; development and exploitation of kits designed to assay key metabolites in the hospital, surgery or home have been rapid and competitive. The expansion of the market for clinical testing by immunoassay has been predicted to increase from some thirty million dollars a decade ago to three thousand million dollars by 1990. The corresponding market in the food area is small in comparison; nevertheless there is a significant number of commercial and regulatory laboratories which would adopt convenient food immunoassays if they were available. Potential world expenditure on food immunoassay evidently provides adequate incentive for widespread commercial interest: for instance, figures published by Biotech (USA) suggest that fifty million dollars is spent annually on testing for the presence of aflatoxins (Li, 1985). In this country, there are about fifty public analysts' laboratories and several government food laboratories which monitor the output of a range of large and small food companies, manufacturers and retailers. All of these would be expected to make continuous use of immunoassays for effective routine procedures in quality assurance and quality control functions. Even some of the many smaller concerns which do not now undertake sophisticated analyses themselves might consider it worthwhile if offered convenient immunoassay methodology. Alternatively, increased analytical data for the food industry might be provided by the private analytical laboratories offering this service; similar contract analysis is increasingly available in the clinical field.

The annual worldwide numbers of analyses by immunoassay that would be undertaken for any particular analyte is very difficult to estimate, but it could be confidently expected to increase in response to consumer pressure. More informative labelling of food is currently being demanded by the consumer lobby and this could generate an increased demand for analyses. Nutritional labelling makes quantitative claims that must be justifiable, and the cost of quality assurance must be taken into account when considering the economics of the commercial advantages of this type of labelling. The demand for this information may arise voluntarily either from individual food companies seeking market advantage or from an agreed industrial code of practice. It may even become mandatory in the form of government regulations or embodied into law. In any case, the quality of food is checked by the industry concerned and by control authorities which will both require the appropriate methodology.

Since analytical data are sometimes limited by the expense of obtaining them, timely development of suitable immunoassays may satisfy an existing demand in such laboratories. In addition, the availability of cost-effective assays will generate an increase in this demand.

The demand would be even greater if a particular immunoassay were an approved or official standard method. Before this could happen, it would have to be demonstrated that the immunoassay was quantitatively acceptable and superior overall to the current approved method (if any). Validation would involve an inter-laboratory collaborative study for which guidelines are published by the Association of Official Analytical Chemists (AOAC) (Horwitz, 1984). Briefly, the recommended sequence of events is as follows: development of methodology; application to determination of analyte in standards, real samples and spiked samples; optimisation in one laboratory; preparation of a detailed written protocol; pilot study in a few additional laboratories; formal collaborative study of the methodology in at least five laboratories establishing the inter-laboratory analytical parameters (e.g. yield, accuracy, precision) by statistical analysis; and publication of the method with all the data for approval.

FOOD IMMUNOASSAY PROCEDURES

Several different procedures are available for exploiting the antibody–antigen interaction. Robust immunodiffusion methods are occasionally used, especially for analysis in the factory, at the dockside or elsewhere outside the well-equipped analytical laboratory. The identification of meat species is an area where rapid classical precipitin methods have given way to simple immunodiffusion (e.g. by the ORBIT on-site rapid beef-identification test procedure). Such precipitation techniques are not desirable for quantitative assays; ELISAs are therefore altogether more attractive and are currently the most popular immunological methods of analysis. It is here that useful advances are being made. Numerous ELISA formats are available; all represent a compromise between convenience of operation and cost of development. The overall speed of such determination is one factor to be considered, but it must be borne in mind that in food analysis the preparation of the sample is often much more time-consuming than the analytical procedure itself. There is therefore an advantage in choosing a format that will accommodate simply-prepared sample extracts.

The food analyst often resorts to a microscopical examination of a food sample, since this can allow rapid subjective conclusions about the nature of its components. The examination of stained sections is also very useful in cases where the stains can distinguish between the ingredients present. Immunocytochemistry has a role to play if identification of specific chemical epitopes is necessary. Appropriate antibodies covalently linked to fluorescent or enzyme labels can be used to locate the corresponding ingredients; this qualitative technique, developed for fundamental research in cellular biology, will doubtless be applied for the direct examination of food samples when justified (see Robertson *et al.*, Chapter 14).

Perhaps the ultimate objective of the food analyst, and one he is often asked to achieve, is instantaneous analysis by means of a direct read-out sensor. In particular, this would enable food processes to be controlled on-line, by using the analytical data to adjust the process continuously to a pre-set norm. The simple pH meter based on a specific electrode typifies the approach, but hitherto it has been difficult to develop practicable electrodes to undertake more sophisticated analysis. However, the development of the field-effect transistor (FET) and other novel devices has opened new opportunities for analytical methodology and process control since they are sensors which convert signals from their immediate chemical environment directly into electrical signals (see Kress-Rogers & Turner, Chapter 19). Specificity can be imposed on these systems by, for example, an interaction with an enzyme or immunoreagent at the tiny active surface of the device. Similarly, specific optical sensors may be designed in which light interacts with an immunoreagent immobilised on to a light guide and exposed to the sample. Such electronic and optical immunosensors hold promise not only for the analysis of food but also for process control.

ACKNOWLEDGEMENTS

Contributions to this review from M. N. Clifford, A. Crimes, R. Holbrook, L. Jones, B. A. Morris, P. Porter, W. Sidwell and M. Smith are gratefully acknowledged.

REFERENCES

ARNOLD, D. & SOMOGYI, A. (1985) Trace analysis of chloramphenicol residues in eggs, milk and meat: comparison of gas chromatography and radioimmunoassay. *Journal of the Association of Official Analytical Chemists*, **68**, 984–990.

ARNOLD, D., VOM BERG, D., BOERTZ, A. K., MALLICK, U. & SOMOGYI, A. (1984) Radioimmunological determination of chloramphenicol residues in musculature, milk and eggs. *Archiv für Lebensmittelhygiene*, **35**, 131–136.

ARNSTADT, K. I. (1981) Enzyme immunoassay for the estrogenic stilbene derivative diethylstilbestrol. *Zeitschrift für Lebensmittel Untersuchung und Forschung*, **173**, 255–260.

ATZORN, R. & WEILER, E. W. (1983*a*) Radioimmunoassays for the gibberellins A_1, A_3, A_4, A_7, A_9 and A_{20}. *Planta*, **159**, 1–6.

ATZORN, R. & WEILER, E. W. (1983*b*) Quantitation of gibberellins A_3, A_4 and A_7 by ultra-sensitive solid-phase immunoassays. *Planta*, **159**, 7–11.

BARTHOLOMEW, B. A., STRINGER, M. F., WATSON, G. N. & GILBERT, R. J. (1985) Development and application of an enzyme-linked immunosorbent assay for *Clostridium perfringens* type A enterotoxin. *Journal of Clinical Pathology*, **38**, 222–228.

BELSEY, R. E., DE LUCA, H. F. & POTTS, J. T. (1974) A rapid assay for 25-hydroxyvitamin D_3 without preparative chromatography. *Journal of Clinical Endocrinology and Metabolism*, **38**, 1046–1051.

CANDLISH, A. A. G., STIMSON, W. H. & SMITH, J. E. (1985) A monoclonal antibody to aflatoxin B_1: detection of the mycotoxin by enzyme immunoassay. *Letters in Applied Microbiology*, **1**, 57–61.

CRIMES, A. A., HITCHCOCK, C. H. S. & WOOD, R. (1984) Determination of soya protein in meat products by an enzyme-linked immunosorbent assay procedure: collaborative study. *Journal of the Association of Public Analysts*, **22**, 59–78.

DUSEMUND, B. & BARRACH, H. J. (1982) Double-antibody enzyme-linked immunosorbent microassay for quantification of collagen types I and II. *Journal of Immunochemical Methods*, **50**, 255–268.

EVERETT, A. W., PRIOR, G., CLARK, W. A. & ZAK, R. (1983) Quantitation of myosin in muscle (RIA). *Analytical Biochemistry*, **130**, 102–107.

FAN, T. S. L. & CHU, F. S. (1984) Indirect ELISA for detection of aflatoxin B_1 in corn and peanut butter. *Journal of Food Protection*, **47**, 263–266.

FEY, H., PFISTER, H. & RUEGG, O. (1984) Comparative evaluation of different enzyme-linked immunosorbent assay systems for the detection of staphylococcal enterotoxins A, B, C, and D. *Journal of Clinical Microbiology*, **19**, 34–38.

FREMY, J. M. & CHU, F. S. (1984) Direct ELISA for determining aflatoxin M_1 at picogram levels in dairy products. *Journal of the Association of Official Analytical Chemists*, **67**, 1098–1101.

GENDLOFF, E. H., PESTKA, J. J., SWANSON, S. P. & HART, L. P. (1984) Detection of T-2 toxin in *Fusarium sporotrichioides*-infected corn by ELISA. *Applied and Environmental Microbiology*, **47**, 1161–1163.

GRIDLEY, J. C., ALLEN, E. H. & SHIMODA, W. (1983) Radioimmunoassay for diethylstilbestrol and the monoglucuronide metabolite in bovine liver. *Journal of Agricultural and Food Chemistry*, **31**, 292.

GRIFFITHS, N. M. & BILLINGTON, M. J. (1984) The use of an enzyme-linked immunosorbent assay procedure for the determination of meat in compound meat products. *Journal of the Science of Food and Agriculture*, **35**, 909–914.

GROOPMAN, J. D., TRUDEL, L. J., DONAHUE, P. R., MARSHAK-ROTHSTEIN, A. & WOGAN, G. N. (1984) High-affinity monoclonal antibodies for aflatoxins and their application to solid-phase immunoassays. *Proceedings of the National Academy of Sciences, USA*, **81**, 7728–7731.

HARWOOD, D. J., HEITZMAN, R. J. & JOUQUEY, A. (1980) A radioimmunoassay method for the measurement of residues of the anabolic agent hexestrol in tissues of cattle and sheep. *Journal of Veterinary and Pharmacological Therapy*, **3**, 245–254.

HEITZMAN, R. J. (1984) Immunoassay techniques for measuring veterinary drug residues in farm animals, meat and meat products. In: *Analysis of Food Contaminants*, Gilbert, J. (ed.), Elsevier Applied Science Publishers, London and New York, pp. 73–115.

HEITZMAN, R. J. & HARWOOD, D. J. (1977) Residue levels of trenbolone and oestradiol-17β in plasma and tissues of steers implanted with anabolic steroid preparations. *British Veterinary Journal*, **133**, 564–571.

HITCHCOCK, C. H. S. (1984) Immunological methods. In: *Control of Food Quality and Food Analysis*, Birch, G. G. & Parker, K. J. (eds), Elsevier Applied Science, London, pp. 117–133.

HITCHCOCK, C. H. S. & CRIMES, A. A. (1985) Methodology for meat species identification. *Meat Science*, **15**, 215–224.

HITCHCOCK, C. H. S., BAILEY, F. J., CRIMES, A. A., DEAN, D. A. G. & DAVIS, P. J. (1981) Determination of soya proteins in food using an enzyme-linked immunosorbent assay procedure. *Journal of the Science of Food and Agriculture*, **32**, 157–165.

HORWITZ, W. (1984) Report of the committee on collaborative interlaboratory studies. *Journal of the Association of Official Analytical Chemists*, **67**, 432–440.

HU, W. J., WOYCHIK, N. & CHU, F. S. (1984) ELISA of picogram quantities of aflatoxin M_1 in urine and milk. *Journal of Food Protection*, **47**, 126–127.

HUNTER, K. W., BRIMFIELD, A. A., MILLER, M., FINKELMAN, F. D. & CHU, F. S. (1985) Preparation and characterisation of monoclonal antibodies to the tricothecene mycotoxin T-2. *Applied and Environmental Microbiology*, **49**, 168–172.

JACKMAN, R. (1985) Determination of aflatoxins by ELISA with special reference to aflatoxin M_1 in raw milk. *Journal of the Science of Food and Agriculture*, **36**, 685–698.

JONES, S. J. & PATTERSON, R. L. S. (1985) Double-antibody ELISA for detection of trace amounts of pig meat in raw meat mixtures. *Meat Science*, **15**, 1–13.

JONES, S. J. & PATTERSON, R. L. S. (1986) A modified indirect ELISA procedure for raw meat speciation using crude anti-species antisera and stabilised immunoreagents. *Journal of the Science of Food and Agriculture*, **37**, 767–775.

JOURDAN, P. S., MANSELL, R. L., OLIVER, D. G. & WEILER, E. W. (1984) Competitive solid-phase enzyme-linked immunoassay for the quantification of limonin in citrus. *Analytical Biochemistry*, **138**, 19–24.

KANGETHE, E. K., JONES, S. J. & PATTERSON, R. L. S. (1982) Identification of the species origin of fresh meat using an enzyme-linked immunosorbent assay procedure. *Meat Science*, **7**, 229–240.

KEMP, H. A., MILLS, E. N. C. & MORGAN, M. R. A. (1986) Enzyme-linked immunosorbent assay of 3-acetyl-deoxynivalenol applied to rice. *Journal of the Science of Food and Agriculture*, **37**, 888–894.

LEE, S. C. & CHU, F. S. (1984) ELISA of ochratoxin A in wheat. *Journal of the Association of Official Analytical Chemists*, **67**, 45–49.

LEFIER, D. & COLLIN, J. C. (1982) Enzyme-linked immunosorbent assay of bovine kappa-caseins. *Le Lait*, **62**, 541–548.

LI, T. (1985) Biotech Research announces first aflatoxin detection kit using enzyme immunoassay technology. Press release, April 9, 1985, Robert Marston & Associates, Inc., 485 Madison Avenue, New York, NY 10022.

MANZ, J. (1983) Detecting heat-denatured muscle protein by means of enzyme-linked immunosorbent assay: determining kangaroo muscle proteins. *Fleischwirtschaft*, **63**, 1767.

MANZ, J. (1985) Detecting heat-denatured muscle proteins by means of ELISA. *Fleischwirtschaft*, **65**, 497–499.

MARTLBAUER, E. & TERPLAN, G. (1985) A highly sensitive heterologous enzyme immunoassay for aflatoxin M_1 in milk and powdered milk. *Archiv für Lebensmittelhygiene*, **36**, 58.

MORGAN, M. R. A. (1985) Newer techniques in food analysis—immunoassays and their application to small molecules. *Journal of the Association of Public Analysts*, **23**, 59–63.

MORGAN, M. R. A., MCNERNEY, R., MATTHEW, J. A., COXON, D. T. & CHAN, H. W. S. (1983*a*) An enzyme-linked immunosorbent assay for total glycoalkaloids in potato tubers. *Journal of the Science of Food and Agriculture*, **34**, 593–598.

MORGAN, M. R. A., MCNERNEY, R. & CHAN, H. W. S. (1983*b*) The enzyme-linked immunosorbent assay of ochratoxin A in barley. *Journal of the Association of Official Analytical Chemists*, **66**, 1481–1484.

MORGAN, M. R. A., KANG, A. S. & CHAN, H. W. S. (1986) Production of antisera against sterigmatocystin hemiacetal and its potential use in an enzyme-linked immunosorbent assay. *Journal of the Science of Food and Agriculture*, **37**, 873–880.

NIEWOLA, Z., WALSH, S. T. & DAVIES, G. E. (1983) ELISA for paraquat. *International Journal of Immunopharmacology*, **5**, 211–218.

OLSMAN, W. J., DOBBELAERE, S. & HITCHCOCK, C. H. S. (1985) The performance of an SDS-PAGE and an ELISA method for the quantitative analysis of soya protein in meat products: an international collaborative study. *Journal of the Science of Food and Agriculture*, **36**, 499–507.

PATEL, P. D. (1985) Application of enzyme immunoassay techniques for the estimation of staphylococcal enterotoxins in food. In: *Immunoassays in Food*

Analysis, Morris, B. A. & Clifford, M. N. (eds), Elsevier Applied Science, London, pp. 141–155.

PATTERSON, R. M. & SPENCER, T. L. (1985) Differentiation of raw meat from phylogenetically related species by enzyme-linked immunosorbent assay. *Meat Science*, **15**, 119–123.

PATTERSON, R. M., WHITTAKER, R. G. & SPENCER, T. L. (1984) Species identification of raw meat by an improved enzyme-linked immunosorbent assay. *Journal of the Science of Food and Agriculture*, **35**, 1018.

PESTKA, J. J. & CHU, F. S. (1984) ELISA of mycotoxins. *Journal of Food Protection*, **47**, 305–308.

RAVESTEIN, P. & DRIEDONKS, R. A. (1986) Quantitative immunoassay for soya protein in raw and sterilized meat products. *Journal of Food Technology*, **21**, 19–32.

REINHARDT, T. A., HORST, R. L., ORF, J. W. & HOLLIS, B. W. (1984) A microassay for 1,25-dihydroxyvitamin D: application to clinical studies. *Journal of Clinical Endocrinology and Metabolism*, **58**, 91.

RICHARDSON, P. J., FAVELL, D. J., GIDLEY, G. C. & JONES, G. H. (1978) Application of a commercial radioassay test kit to the determination of vitamin B_{12} in food. *Analyst*, **103**, 865–868.

ROBINS, S. P. (1982) An enzyme-linked immunosorbent assay for the collagen cross-link pyridinoline. *Biochemical Journal*, **207**, 617–620.

ROBINS, R. J., MORGAN, M. R. A., RHODES, M. J. C. & FURZE, J. M. (1984*a*). Determination of quassin in picogram quantities by an enzyme-linked immunosorbent assay. *Phytochemistry*, **23**, 1119–1123.

ROBINS, R. J., MORGAN, M. R. A., RHODES, M. J. C. & FURZE, J. M. (1984*b*) An enzyme-linked immunosorbent assay for quassin and closely related metabolites. *Analytical Biochemistry*, **136**, 145–156.

ROHNER, P., SCHALLIBAUM, M. & NICOLET, J. (1985) Detection of Penicillin G and its benzylpenicilloyl derivatives in cow milk and serum by means of an ELISA. *Journal of Food Protection*, **48**, 59–62.

SACK, D. A., HUDA, S., NEOGI, P. K. B., DANIEL, R. R. & SPIRA, W. M. (1980) Microtiter ganglioside enzyme-linked immunosorbent assay for *Vibrio* and *Escherichia coli* heat-labile enterotoxins and antitoxin. *Journal of Clinical Microbiology*, **11**, 35–40.

SHONE, C., WILTON-SMITH, P., APPLETON, N., HAMBLETON, P., MODI, N., GATLEY, J. & MELLING, J. (1985) Monoclonal antibody-based immunoassay for type A *Clostridium botulinum* toxin is comparable to the mouse bioassay. *Applied and Environmental Microbiology*, **50**, 63–67.

SKERRITT, J. H. (1985) A sensitive monoclonal-antibody-based test for gluten detection: quantitative immunoassay. *Journal of the Science of Food and Agriculture*, **36**, 987–994.

SKERRITT, J. H. & SMITH, R. A. (1985) A sensitive monoclonal-antibody-based test for gluten detection: studies with cooked or processed foods. *Journal of the Science of Food and Agriculture*, **36**, 980–986.

SKERRITT, J. H., DIMENT, J. A. & WRIGLEY, C. W. (1985) A sensitive monoclonal-antibody-based test for gluten detection: choice of primary and secondary antibodies. *Journal of the Science of Food and Agriculture*, **36**, 995–1003.

STAAK, C. & KAMPE, U. (1982) Quantitation of hydrolysed milk protein in sausage by measuring the consumption of antibodies using the enzyme-linked immunosorbent assay. *Fleischwirtschaft*, **62**, 1477–1478.

Teufel, P. & Sacher, V. (1982) Determination of milk protein in meat products by ELISA. *Fleischwirtschaft*, **62**, 1474–1476.

Thompson, M. R., Brandwein, H., Labine-Racke, M. & Giannella, R. A. (1984) Simple and reliable enzyme-linked immunosorbent assay with monoclonal antibodies for detection of *Escherichia coli* heat-stable enterotoxins. *Journal of Clinical Microbiology*, **20**, 59–64.

Vaag, P. (1985) An enzyme-linked immunosorbent assay for amyloglucosidase in beer. In: *Immunoassays in Food Analysis*, Morris, B. A. & Clifford, M. N. (eds), Elsevier Applied Science, London, pp. 125–139.

Vogt, K. (1985) Simplified reassurance of the radioimmunological detection of diethylstilbestrol in canned meat and animal excreta. *Archiv für Lebensmittelhygiene*, **36**, 3.

Warwick, M. J., Bates, M. L. & Shearer, G. (1985) The use of immunoassay for monitoring anabolic hormones in meat. In: *Immunoassays in Food Analysis*, Morris, B. A. & Clifford, M. N. (eds), Elsevier Applied Science, London, pp. 169–186.

Weiler, E. W. (1982) An enzyme immunoassay for *cis*-(+)-abscisic acid. *Physiologia Plantarum*, **54**, 510–514.

Weiler, E. W., Jourdan, P. S. & Conrad, W. (1981) Levels of indole-3-acetic acid in intact and decapitated coleoptiles as determined by a specific and highly sensitive solid-phase enzyme immunoassay. *Planta*, **153**, 561–571.

Whittaker, R. G., Spencer, T. L. & Copland, J. W. (1983) An enzyme-linked immunosorbent assay for meat species determination. *Journal of the Science of Food and Agriculture*, **34**, 1143–1148.

Windemann, H. (1982) Enzyme-linked immunosorbent assay for wheat alpha-gliadin and whole gliadin. *Biochimica Biophysica Acta*, **709**, 110–121.

Wood, W. G. (1983) A simple competitive binding assay for serum 25-hydroxyvitamin D metabolites. *Aerztliche Laboratorium*, **29**, 352–356.

2

Opportunities and Incentives for Developing Veterinary Immunoassays

B. A. MORRIS

Department of Biochemistry, University of Surrey, Guildford, UK

The first veterinary immunoassays were extensions of the hormonal assays used in human clinical medicine. These were principally concerned with the measurement of the reproductive hormones, reflecting the different emphasis of the animal livestock industry. Since then the immunoassay technique, especially the ELISA, has been applied to many other areas of veterinary medicine, in particular that concerned with the diagnosis and control of infectious diseases (Wardley & Crowther, 1982). Today, besides being an aid to livestock management and disease prevention, it is increasingly being used by government agencies for the detection of veterinary residues, e.g. prohibited growth promoters (Bates *et al.*, 1985), as well as toxic contaminants, such as mycotoxins (Jackman, 1985). This paper will consider the recent developments in immunoassay technology and the opportunities they offer in the animal health field.

The ELISA is undoubtedly the most widely used form of immunoassay in veterinary science on account of its simplicity and suitability as a screening method. It is extensively used in the identification of bacterial and viral diseases, where its superiority over the immunoprecipitation methods has now been conclusively demonstrated. Not only is the result available more quickly, but the ELISA is able to detect the onset of a particular infection much earlier than the traditional immunodiffusion methods, often before clinical symptoms are apparent. This is because the ELISA is able to detect non-precipitating antibodies, which are the first antibodies to be produced in response to an invading pathogen. These antibodies are not detected by immunoprecipitation methods.

The choice of immunogen, with which to produce the anti-species' second antibody, is of critical importance. The use of an IgG preparation, purified by DEAE ion-exchange chromatography, will produce second antibodies which will not recognise IgM. A much better second antibody for this purpose would be produced if a crude immunoglobulin preparation, produced, for example, by ammonium sulphate fractionation, were used as the immunogen.

The ability of an ELISA to detect low levels or early signs of infection depends on the detection limit of the particular assay being used. Besides the precision of the measurement, the assay characteristic most likely to affect the detection limit is the level of NSB. The use of a detergent, such as Tween 20, in the wash buffer and the blocking of free binding sites which remain after coating the wells of the microtitration plate will do much to reduce the level of NSB in the assay and thus improve its detection limit. However, one of the most dramatic improvements in detection limit was achieved by the use of affinity-purified antibodies, especially enzyme-labelled second antibodies (Ishikawa *et al.*, 1982). These authors improved the performance of their assays still further by using only the F_{ab} fragments of their specific antibodies, which increased the detection limit by up to 120 times.

Other practical approaches for increasing the sensitivity of EIAs are considered by Gould elsewhere in this volume (see Gould, Chapter 5). In human medicine, chemiluminescent and fluorescent labels are rapidly replacing radiolabels, often with increased sensitivity, and it remains to be seen what impact these detection systems will have on veterinary science.

Another area of intensive development over the past few years has been that of monoclonal antibodies. Not only do they provide a theoretically unlimited supply of a reagent of constant characteristics, but the fact that each clone recognises a single epitope has enabled individual strains of a particular virus or bacterium to be identified. Because they are non-precipitating antibodies, they cannot be employed in immunoprecipitation methods and consequently immunoassay is the technique of choice for their use.

Until recently, one disadvantage of these monoclonal antibodies has been that both cell lines were of murine origin, and mice are not renowned for producing antibodies of high affinity. With the development of more rapid assay systems, especially in the test strip and dry state chemistry formats, there was an even greater need for reagent antibodies of higher and higher affinity, to shorten the assay time.

Sheep, on the other hand, have long been recognised for their ability to produce antibodies of greater affinity than those of mice and rabbits (Morris, 1985). Unfortunately, a suitable ovine myeloma cell line was not available previously to act as the immortal fusion partner in fusions involving ovine lymphocytes. Furthermore, interspecies fusions between murine myeloma cells and lymphocytes from other species having different chromosome numbers tend to produce unstable hybridomas which may cease to produce antibody due to loss of essential chromosomes. One way of overcoming this problem was developed by Ostberg & Pursch (1983) for producing human monoclonal antibodies. It involved the creation of a heteromyeloma cell line by fusing human lymphocytes with a murine myeloma cell line and sensitising the resulting hybridomas which had ceased to secrete antibody to selective media. This heteromyeloma was then re-fused with further human lymphocytes to produce a stable hetero-hybridoma secreting human antibodies. This strategy has been used by Tucker and her co-workers at Babraham (Tucker *et al.*, 1984) to produce bovine monoclonal antibodies to the Forssman antigen. It has now been used extensively at the University of Surrey, Department of Biochemistry, to produce both ovine and bovine monoclonal antibodies to the gonadal steroid hormones, using peripheral blood lymphocytes from sensitised donor animals (Groves *et al.*, 1987*a*,*b*; and p. 279, this volume).

Produced in this way, ovine monoclonal antibodies have a number of advantages over their murine counterparts. Providing that a suitable immunisation schedule is followed, ovine monoclonal antibodies have a much higher affinity, frequently having a K_D of 10^{-11}M or greater. Peripheral blood lymphocytes can be used from existing polyclonal antibody-producing animals, known to be producing good antisera, without loss of the donor. In addition, the same donor animal can be used repeatedly.

Another development in immunoassay technology has been the change in the way in which the assays can now be performed. In our hospitals, clinical biochemistry is moving nearer the patient, with the development of rapid, simple systems which can be used on the ward and in the casualty and intensive care departments, by non-scientific staff to provide the information they need in the shortest time possible. This trend is just being seen in the veterinary field with the shift to on-site testing where simple kits are used by semi- or non-skilled personnel. This has been made possible by the development of rapid assay systems using dry state chemistry and dipstick technology. An excellent illustration of this is the development of milk progesterone kits that can be used by the farmer and stockman in the milking parlour to detect oestrus and subsequently confirm pregnancy (Drew, 1986; see Davina *et al.*, p. 289, this volume).

The current trend is for pharmaceutical manufacturers to supply a package consisting of a diagnostic kit for the detection of a particular infection, and a vaccine or drug for therapeutic treatment of infected individuals. In the USA, a series of rapid immunoassay test cards has recently been introduced for farm use. The cards, about the size of a credit card, have the appropriate antigen immobilised on a small area of absorbent cellulose. The latter successively absorbs the liquid phases of the sample, wash solution, enzyme-labelled second antibody and substrate, leaving a coloured spot if antibodies to the specific pathogen are present. These test card formats can also be used by meat inspectors in the abattoir or factory to check for veterinary residues (see Mount *et al.*, p. 301, this volume).

There are several factors which are providing the incentives for these technological developments. The first is that as profit margins in agriculture have become reduced, there is an even greater incentive on the farmers' part for more efficient livestock production. The benefits apply equally well to both healthy and sick animals. An illustration of this, with healthy animals, is the use of the milk progesterone assay to reduce the calving to conception interval by identifying the onset of oestrus. The second factor is that now many infectious diseases can be recognised at an earlier stage using immunoassay techniques as opposed to the more lengthy and expensive culture methods. Infected individuals can be identified and eradication programmes implemented on a much more cost-effective basis, as is happening with Aujeszky's disease (pseudorabies) (Banks, 1983). Finally, immunoassays are increasingly being used in law enforcement situations, not only by individual governments, but also by the European Economic Community (E.E.C.) and international agencies. The recent E.E.C. ban on synthetic and natural growth promoters in livestock production is an excellent illustration of this (E.E.C., 1985).

Immunoassay is thus poised to make an even greater contribution to animal livestock production in the years ahead, and the extent to which it does so will depend on the support which this area of application receives from industry, especially the diagnostic kit manufacturers.

REFERENCES

BANKS, M. (1983) Rapid ELISA for Aujeszky's disease eradication. *Veterinary Record*, **113**, 94–95.

BATES, M. L., WARWICK, M. J. & SHEARER, G. (1985) Determination of synthetic growth promoters in bile. *Food Additives & Contaminants*, **2**, 37–46.

DREW, B. (1986) Farm practice—milk progesterone testing as an aid to cow fertility management. In: *In practice*, *Veterinary Record Supplement*, **8**, 17–20.

E.E.C. (1985) Council directive prohibiting the use in livestock farming of certain substances having a hormonal action. 85/358/EEC.

GROVES, D. J., MORRIS, B. A., TAN, K., DE SILVA, M. & CLAYTON, J. (1987*a*) Production of an ovine monoclonal antibody to testosterone by an interspecies fusion. *Hybridoma*, **6**, 71–76.

GROVES, D. J., MORRIS, B. A. & CLAYTON, J. (1987*b*) Preparation of a bovine monoclonal antibody to testosterone by interspecies fusion. *Research in Veterinary Science*, **43**, 253–256.

ISHIKAWA, E., IMAGAWA, M., YOSHITAKE, S., NIITSU, Y., URUSHIZAKI, I., INADA, M., IMURA, H., KANAZAWA, R., TACHIBANA, S., NAKAZAWA, N. & OGAWA, H. (1982) Major factors limiting sensitivity of sandwich enzyme immunoassay for ferritin, immunoglobulin E and thyroid stimulating hormone. *Annals of Clinical Biochemistry*, **19**, 379–384.

JACKMAN, R. (1985) Determination of aflatoxins by enzyme-linked immunosorbent assay with special reference to aflatoxin M_1 in raw milk. *Journal of the Science of Food and Agriculture*, **36**, 685–698.

MORRIS, B. A. (1985) Principles of immunoassay. In: *Immunoassays in Food Analysis*, Morris, B. A. & Clifford, M. N. (eds), Elsevier Applied Science Publishers, London, pp. 21–51.

OSTBERG, L. & PURSCH, E. (1983) Human × (mouse × human) hybridomas stably producing human antibodies. *Hybridoma*, **2**, 361–367.

TUCKER, E. M., DAIN, A. R., CLARKE, S. W. & DONKER, A. (1984) Specific bovine monoclonal antibody produced by a re-fused mouse/calf hybridoma. *Hybridoma*, **3**, 171–176.

WARDLEY, R. C. & CROWTHER, J. R. (1982) *The ELISA: Enzyme-linked Immunosorbent Assay in Veterinary Research and Diagnosis*, Martinus Nijhoff, The Hague.

[illegible] (19[illegible]). [illegible] as [illegible] ... [illegible] *Enzyme* [illegible] ... [illegible] ... [illegible]

[illegible] ... Fabricated ... [illegible] ... *Hybridoma*, 6, [illegible]

[illegible] ... (1987). [illegible] ... *Research* [illegible] ... 35, [illegible]

[illegible] ... S. [illegible] ... N. & [illegible] H. (19[illegible]). Major factors [illegible] ... [illegible]

[illegible]

[illegible]

[illegible]

[illegible]

3

Practical Developments in ELISA Methodology

R. JACKMAN

Central Veterinary Laboratory, New Haw, Weybridge, Surrey, UK

INTRODUCTION

The last few years have seen a considerable increase in the range, type, design and application of ELISAs. Many have been adaptations and refinements of existing techniques designed to increase sensitivity or decrease assay time while others have introduced ingenious novel protocols. So far few of these have had any real impact on the analytical scene. This paper deals with hapten ELISAs, primarily those applicable to the veterinary and food analysis fields.

ELISA METHODOLOGY

However novel or refined these recent developments have been, no one can disregard or replace the basic requirements for good, workable immunoassays, especially with regard to the quality of antibody, purity of conjugates and validation of assay performance. The use of high quality reagents has been advocated for many years in journals and textbooks, but the realisation and acceptance of their importance is more recent. It is therefore reasonable to stress these requirements, even in a paper concerning advances in methodology.

IMMUNOGEN

Several factors require consideration for the production of high affinity antibodies, not least being the quality of the immunogen. Many workers adopt standard synthetic procedures when preparing either a reactive derivative of the hapten, or when conjugating this to the carrier protein, and frequently assume the formation of a single product after each step. This is not necessarily so (see Morgan, Chapter 18). The development of more selective heterobifunctional cross-linking reagents, such as the maleimidohydroxysuccinimide esters to be described later (see Kitagawa *et al.*, Chapter 4), offer the ability to produce a far more strictly defined immunogen, especially when used with highly purified or selectively modified carrier proteins. Other such reagents used for conjugation include maleimide acid or benzoyl chloride (Monji *et al.*, 1980), succinimidyl (4-iodoacetyl) aminobenzoate (Weltman *et al.*, 1983), succinimidyl 3-(2-pyridyldithio) propionate (Masuko *et al.*, 1982) and the many photoreactive aryl azides (Ji & Ji, 1982). Purification of immunogen should also ensure the elimination of hapten adsorbed to the carrier protein, which may remain if dialysis is the only technique employed to separate the prepared conjugate from reactants.

Use of purified immunogen, especially at low doses, increases the chances of stimulating clones of cells producing high affinity antibody (Kim & Siskind, 1974). Polyclonal antiserum will still contain a number of different populations of antibodies and consideration may be given to selection of particular populations with desirable properties, usually by affinity chromatography. In this laboratory an immunoglobulin preparation extracted from chickens' eggs was separated into three distinct fractions exhibiting different affinities using a column of immobilised aflatoxin–caproic acid on AH-sepharose. Elutions were made with acidified water (pH 4–5), 2M glycine (pH 2·2) and 6M guanidine. The major benefit of this procedure was the observation that the fraction eluted with 2M glycine was considerably less affected by sample matrix problems when used in an ELISA for aflatoxin in milk.

Mixed populations of high and low affinity antibodies may also cause a 'hook' effect (Joel *et al.*, 1974). This phenomenon occurs when antigen binding decreases with increased antigen concentration and is due to increased competition by high levels of antigen for the binding sites of low affinity antibodies. Such an effect may also be observed due to changes in antibody affinity when bound to solid phase (Parsons, 1981) and is caused by negative cooperativity between closely packed antibody molecules (Anido, 1984).

ANTIBODY

For sensitive, rapid and reproducible immunoassays, antibody affinity as measured by its association constant (K_a), or average association constant

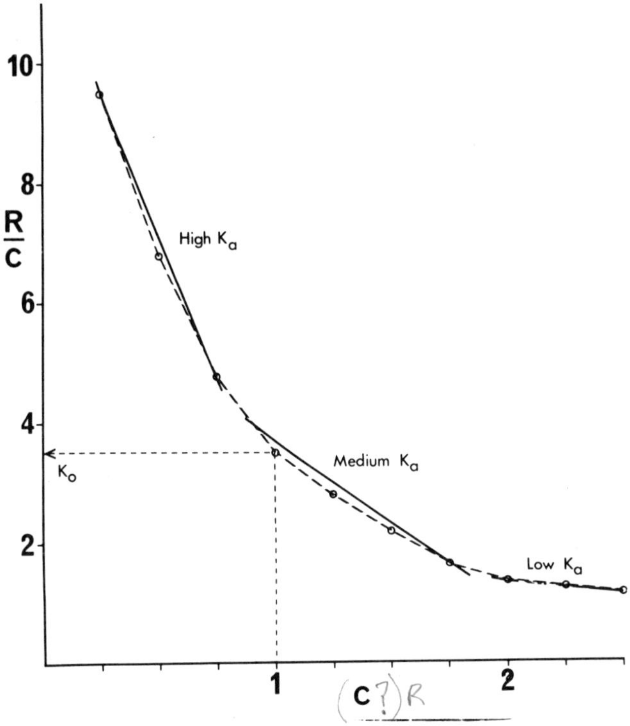

Fig. 1. Graphic plot of a Scatchard treatment of observed data points (– – –) showing division into three natural subpopulations of antibody with differing affinities (——) 3M. R, ratio, bound/total antibody; C, unbound hapten (mol/litre $\times 10^{-6}$).

(K_0) calculated from extrapolations of Scatchard plots (Scatchard, 1949), is typically in the region of 10^9 to 10^{11} litres/mole. The calculation and the definition of K_0 are of some importance, especially in the mixed populations of antibodies encountered in polyclonal antisera. The graphic representation shown in Fig. 1 is commonly obtained for a plot of r/c against r, where r is the ratio of bound antibody to total antibody and c the total free hapten concentration. The curve produced is a result of the interaction of, for instance, three subpopulations of antibody with high, medium and low affinity constants respectively. The average affinity of their populations is known as the avidity. K_0 is the reciprocal of the free hapten concentration when $r = 1$ or, alternatively, when half the sites of a divalent antibody are occupied. It is the construction of the rectangular y co-ordinate at this point. The equilibrium association constant encompasses both forward and reverse reactions of antibody with hapten, so although high affinity is desired, antibody with low dissociation or high 'avidity' is of prime importance (Peterfy *et al.*, 1983; Nimmo *et al.*, 1984). Affinity heterogenicity alone does not explain the typical sigmoidal ELISA titration curve, however, although the Law of Mass Action equation may be modified to include this effect (Lew, 1984). That maximal binding of antibody occurs in the linear portion of the curve has recently been demonstrated (Koertge, 1984) but for antibody detection systems at least, the sigmoidality at the upper end of the curve is more likely to be an effect of steric hindrance of the signal generating system rather than due to changes in antibody/conjugate binding (Koertge & Butler, 1985).

ENZYME-LABELLED CONJUGATES

Many developments and modifications have been made to ELISAs in order either to increase sensitivity or to decrease assay time, and although the antibody quality remains the most important limitation, many other factors can influence the performance of an ELISA. Considerations similar to those given to immunogen synthesis can also be applied profitably to the preparation of enzyme–hapten conjugates of defined characteristics, and also to immobilised haptens where these, rather than antibody, are used to coat microtitration plates. Additional considerations in conjugate preparation include the provision of spacer links and structurally dissimilar bridges linking hapten to enzyme or protein in order to reduce antibody recognition of the immunogen bridge and thus increase assay sensitivity (Exley & Abuknesha, 1978; Jackman, 1985). Selection of linking reagents should also consider their effects on the enzyme activity of the conjugates (Standefer, 1985). Greater attention is also being paid to the use of blocking agents, washing procedures and immobilisation techniques in order to lower non-specific binding (NSB), to increase the signal-to-noise ratio, and to decrease coefficients of variation from well to well and plate to plate.

ENHANCEMENT OF ASSAY SIGNAL

Providing the signal-to-noise ratio within the assay is sufficient, enhancement of the final detection system provides a useful means of speeding up chromogen formation. Fluorogenic substrates (see Ward *et al.*, p. 275, this volume) are available for the enzymes commonly used in

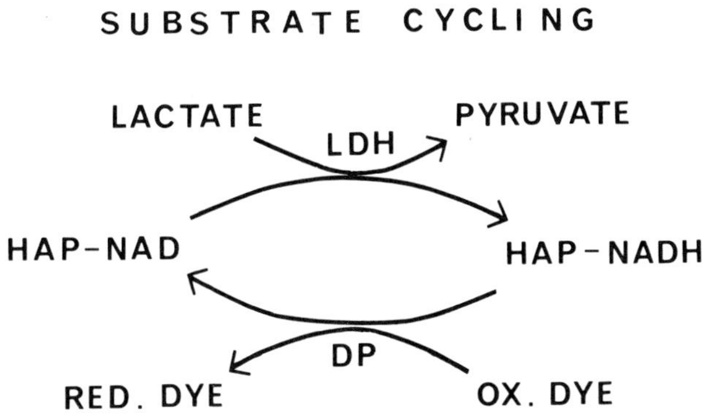

Fig. 2. An example of substrate cycling using the enzyme diaphorase (DP) to recycle oxidised hapten conjugated NAD (HAP–NAD) to feed the initial enzyme, lactate dehydrogenase (LDH) and produce the final signal.

ELISAs but are only practical in heterogeneous assay systems where background fluorescence from the sample can be removed. Direct substitution of fluorogenic for colorimetric substrates in an ELISA may increase both limits of detection and speed of assay unless the limit of detection of the assay is already restricted by the immunochemistry of the method. Similar considerations apply to the use of luminescent markers.

Substrate cycling offers an as yet unrealised potential for enhancement of signal. In systems such as that described in Fig. 2, the cycled substrate also takes part in the immunochemistry of the assay and may account for the cycling rate observed (Kohen *et al.*, 1978). Higher rates have been obtained, especially when using enzyme channelling systems (Ullman *et al.*, 1983).

Reports (Laurent, 1971) of increased enzyme activity in the presence of polymers, such as dextrans and polyethylene glycol, were tested at this laboratory for their ability to enhance the signal. Increases of up to 13% were obtained in an antibody–bound enzyme system where the immunoenzyme complex remained in solution. The effect was only apparent when rate-limiting concentrations of substrate were used. Under normal conditions of excess substrate, a small decrease in enzyme activity was noted. In addition, reaction rates were similar in the presence and absence of polymer when the enzyme was part of an immobilised complex.

True signal amplification, using a matrix of biotin–(strept)avidin to incorporate multiple enzyme molecules at a single immune reaction site, is shown in Fig. 3. The biotin–avidin system using commercially available reagents has been used to decrease colour development time in both a direct

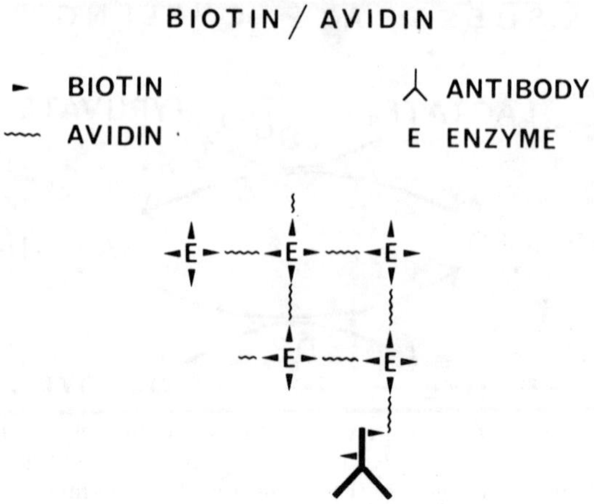

Fig. 3. Diagrammatic representation of the formation of a multiple enzyme matrix linked through avidin and biotin interaction at a single immunochemical locus.

competitive ELISA using immobilised antibody and biotinylated-hapten (chloramphenicol) and a sandwich-type competitive ELISA using immobilised antigen (aflatoxin) and biotinylated-antiimmunoglobulin (Jackman, unpublished data). Despite raised background, due to the biotinylated reagent, there was a significant increase in the signal-to-noise ratio. In spite of the extra step involved, the time taken for an ELISA was reduced from 3 h 50 min to 1 h 40 min.

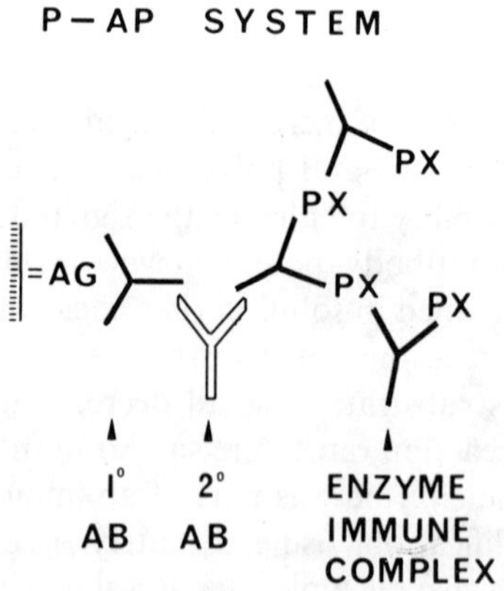

Fig. 4. Diagrammatic representation of the formation of a multiple enzyme matrix linked through anti-enzyme globulin and bridging antibody to a single immunochemical locus. PX, peroxidase.

A similar amplification procedure is provided by the soluble immuno-enzyme complexes such as the peroxidase–antiperoxidase system illustrated in Fig. 4. However, the need for excess bridging antibody and the additional steps involved have limited the majority of applications to immunohistochemistry and Western blotting procedures. This system has been used to measure distribution of antibodies among isotypes by simply changing the secondary (bridging) antibody and has the advantage of not requiring a series of specific antibody–enzyme conjugates (Butler *et al.*, 1983).

ELISA PROTOCOLS

There are now many variations on the simple principle. The competitive enzyme linked immunosorbent assay (CELIA), inhibition enzyme linked immunoassay (IELIA), immunoenzymometric assay (IEMA) and the enzyme-multiplied immunoassay technique (EMIT®) are now almost traditional methods and are well documented (Schall & Tenoso, 1980). Recently, a number of novel procedures has been described, offering interesting alternatives to the classical assay protocols.

The principle of the enzyme modulator mediated immunoassay (EMMIA) (Ngo, 1985) is shown in Fig. 5 and is an example of a homogeneous assay. Development of an EMMIA requires a suitable stable enzyme of high turnover number, whose activity can be easily quantified, and which can be markedly inhibited (or activated) by a modulator. Both the enzyme and modulator should be absent from the sample to be assayed. A covalent complex of the modulator and hapten is then prepared such that it retains

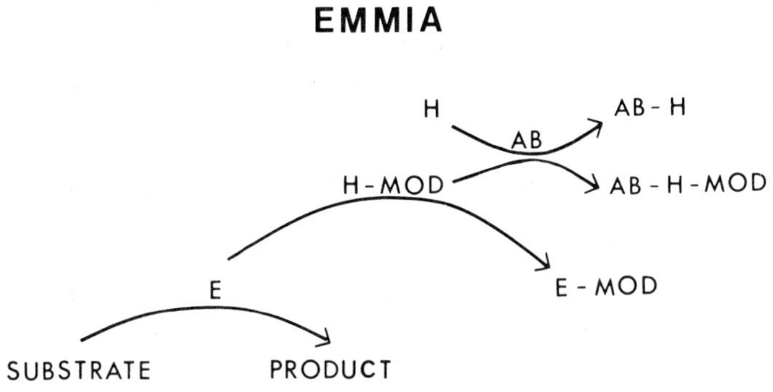

Fig. 5. Schematic of an enzyme modulator mediated immunoassay in which the hapten–modulator couple (H–MOD) competes with analyte (H) for antibody (AB). The enzyme (E) is inhibited by the free hapten–modulator only.

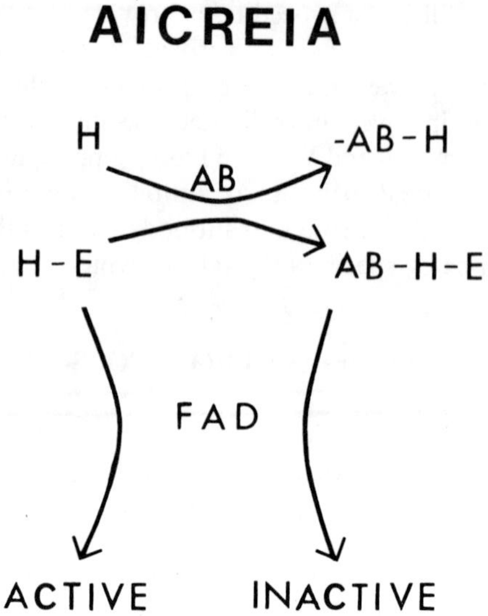

Fig. 6. Schematic of an antibody induced conformational restriction enzyme immunoassay in which the antibody-bound hapten–enzyme complex (AB–H–E) cannot undergo conformational change to the active holoenzyme under the influence of FAD.

both enzyme modulation and immunorecognition properties. In addition, capture of this complex by the antibody should interfere or suppress its modulator capacity. The modulator is normally an enzyme inhibitor, such as a phosphonate of acetylcholinesterase (Blecka *et al.*, 1983). This competes with free hapten in the sample for a limited amount of antibody. When bound to the antibody the hapten–modulator complex is unable to inhibit enzyme activity and the signal is inversely proportional to analyte concentration.

Another example of a non-separation protocol is the antibody induced conformational restriction enzyme immunoassay (AICREIA) (Fig. 6). The strict requirement is for an enzyme–hapten conjugate which, when attached to the antibody, will not combine with the enzyme modifier or prosthetic group. Ngo & Lenhoff (1983) have described such a system which incorporates a hapten–glucose oxidase apoenzyme complex requiring FAD for conversion or reconstitution into its catalytically active holoenzyme structure. Antibody attachment to the apoenzyme restricts the conformational mobility needed for FAD activation. Competition between free hapten in the sample and the hapten–apoenzyme conjugate for a

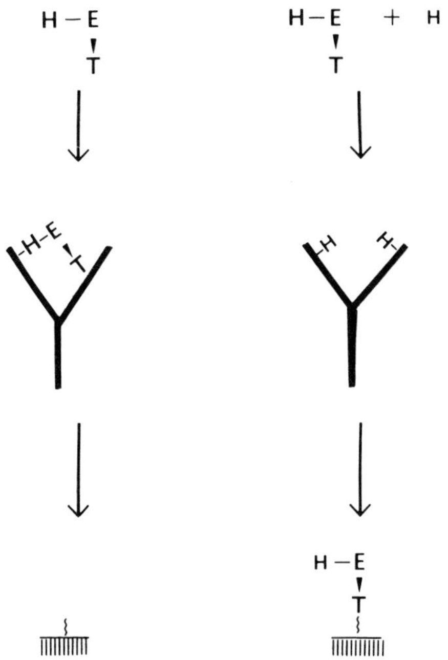

Fig. 7. Schematic of the antibody masking tag immunoassay in which the tag (T) on the hapten–enzyme–tag complex (H–E–T) is masked or sterically inhibited when bound to antibody.

limited amount of antibody results in the final signal being directly proportional to analyte concentration.

Two recently described heterogeneous EIAs differ from classical ELISAs in that the separation stage uses affinity-type gels for rapid sedimentation of one of the components of the assay system. One such protocol is the antibody masking tag immunoassay (AMETIA), the principle of which is shown in Fig. 7 (Ngo & Lenhoff, 1981). The enzyme–hapten complex also incorporates a tag such as biotin. When bound to antibody, the biotin is masked and therefore unable to attach to the tag receptor (avidin) immobilised on sepharose. In the absence of free hapten in the sample, almost all of the tagged-hapten–enzyme is bound to antibody. The presence of competing analyte allows the insolubilised avidin to bind with the tag. Separation of the phases is then undertaken and enzyme activity determined either in the supernatant, where it is inversely proportional to

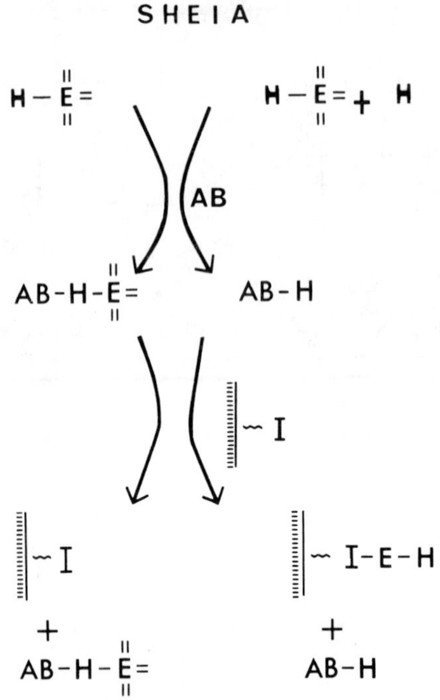

Fig. 8. Schematic of the steric hindrance enzyme immunoassay in which antibody binding of the hapten–enzyme complex (AB–H–E) restricts the uptake of enzyme by the immobilised inhibitor (I).

analyte concentration, or on the washed sepharose gel, in which case there is a direct relationship between sample hapten concentration and final signal.

Another new procedure is the steric hindrance enzyme immunoassay (SHEIA) (Castro & Monji, 1985). This also involves an affinity gel as the separation stage but differs from the preceding method in that a direct enzyme inhibitor is immobilised on the gel. A suitable system involves β-D-galactosamine linked to agarose through a 6-aminohexanoyl bridge. This is an inhibitor of the enzyme β-D-galactosidase. The sequence described in Fig. 8 requires the production of a β-D-galactosidase–hapten conjugate such that the binding of antibody to the enzyme–hapten complex sterically hinders the binding of this complex to the immobilised inhibitor. Following separation of the immobilised enzyme–hapten complex, the residual enzyme activity is measured in the supernatant and is inversely proportional to analyte concentration.

ELISA DEVELOPMENT STRATEGIES

All these procedures have practical applications and, as described earlier, remain dependent on antibody of high quality. Although the availability of so many options means that selection of the most appropriate protocol may be difficult, the practicality of the overall procedure must be the overriding criterion.

From this viewpoint the requirements for sample preparation must also be considered. This is often the most labour-intensive and costly stage of the analysis, especially when working with a wide range of complex sample matrices such as milk, meat and body fluids. It is therefore desirable to analyse body fluids and tissue homogenates directly. At the CVL, antibodies—either polyclonal or monoclonal—are selected not only for their affinity and specificity but also for their resistance to sample matrix effects.

REFERENCES

ANIDO, G. (1984) Seven ferritin kits compared with respect to 'Hook' effects. *Clinical Chemistry*, **30**, 500.

BLECKA, L. J., SHAFFOR, M. & DWORSCHACK, R. (1983) Inhibitor enzyme immunoassays for the quantitation of various haptens: a review. In: *Immunoenzymatic Techniques*, Avrameas, S., Druet, P., Masseyeff, R. & Feldman, G. (eds), Elsevier, Amsterdam, pp. 207–214.

BUTLER, J. E., CANTERO, L. A., SWANSON, P. & MCGIVERN, P. L. (1983) The amplified enzyme-linked immunosorbent assay (α-ELISA) and its applications. In: *Enzyme-Immunoassay*, Maggio, E. T. (ed.), CRC Press, pp. 197–212.

CASTRO, A. & MONJI, N. (1985) Steric hindrance enzyme immunoassay. In: *Enzyme Mediated Immunoassay*, Ngo, T. T. & Lenhoff, H. M. (eds), Plenum Press, pp. 291–298.

EXLEY, D. & ABUKNESHA, R. (1978) A highly sensitive and specific enzyme immunoassay for oestradiol-17-β. *FEBS Letters*, **91**, 162–165.

JACKMAN, R. (1985) Determination of aflatoxins by enzyme-linked immunosorbent assay with special reference to aflatoxin M_1 in milk. *Journal of the Science of Food and Agriculture*, **36**, 685–698.

JI, T. H. & JI, I. (1982) Macromolecular photoaffinity labelling with radioactive photoactivable heterobifunctional reagents. *Analytical Biochemistry*, **121**, 286–289.

JOEL, E. W., SCHONBERG, D. K., ILG, W. & KELLER, E. (1974) Problems of optimisation of double antibody RIA of HLH, HFSH and HGH: Hook phenomenon, false negative patient values and linearity of values from patient plasma dilutions. In: *RIA and Related Procedures in Medicine*, Volume 1. Proceedings of a symposium held in Istanbul, Turkey, September 10–14, 1973, International Atomic Energy Agency, Vienna; UNIPUB Inc., New York, pp. 45–58.

KIM, Y. T. & SISKIND, G. W. (1974) Studies on the control of antibody synthesis. VI. *Clinical and Experimental Immunology*, **17**, 329–338.

KOERTGE, T. E. (1984) A study of the quantitative capability of the enzyme linked immunosorbent assay with regard to the use of specific antibodies to study the transport of monomeric and polymeric antibodies. PhD Thesis, University of Iowa.

KOERTGE, T. E. & BUTLER, J. E. (1985) The relationship between the binding of primary antibody to solid phase antigen in microtitre plates and its detection by the ELISA. *Journal of Immunological Methods*, **83**, 283–300.

KOHEN, F., HOLLANDER, Z., YEAGER, F. M., CARRICO, R. J. & BOGUSLAKI, R. C. (1978) A homogeneous enzyme immunoassay for oestriol monitored by the enzyme cycling reactions. Proceedings of an International Symposium on Enzyme-labelled Immunoassays of Hormones and Drugs, Pal, S. (ed.). Ulm, FRG, July 1978, de Gruyter, Berlin, pp. 67–78.

LAURENT, T. C. (1971) Enzyme reactions in polymer media. *European Journal of Biochemistry*, **21**, 498–506.

LEW, A. M. (1984) The effect of epitope density and antibody affinity on the ELISA as analysed by monoclonal antibodies. *Journal of Immunological Methods*, **72**, 171–176.

MASUKO, Y., KISHIDA, K., SAITO, M., UNEMOTO, N. & HARA, T. (1982) Importance of the antigen-binding valency and the nature of the cross-linking bond in ricin A-chain conjugates with antibody. *Journal of Biochemistry*, **91**, 1583–1591.

MONJI, N., GOMEZ, N. O., KAWASHIMA, H., ALI, H. & CASTRO, A. (1980) Practical enzyme immunoassay for plasma cortisol using β-galactosidase as enzyme label. *Journal of Clinical Endocrinology & Metabolism*, **50**, 355–359.

NGO, T. T. (1985) Enzyme modulator as label in separation-free immunoassays: enzyme modulator mediated immunoassay (EMMIA). In: *Enzyme Mediated Immunoassays*, Ngo, T. T. & Lenhoff, H. M. (eds), Plenum Press, New York, pp. 57–72.

NGO, T. T. & LENHOFF, H. M. (1981) New approach to heterogeneous enzyme immunoassays using tagged enzyme–ligand conjugates. *Biochemical and Biophysical Research Communications*, **99**, 496–503.

NGO, T. T. & LENHOFF, H. M. (1983) Antibody induced conformational restriction as the basis for new separation-free enzyme immunoassay. *Biochemical and Biophysical Research Communications*, **114**, 1097–1103.

NIMMO, G. R., LEW, A. M., STANLEY, C. M. & STEWARD, M. W. (1984) Influence of antibody affinity on the performance of different antibody assays. *Journal of Immunological Methods*, **72**, 177–187.

PARSONS, G. H. (1981) Antibody coated plastic tubes in RIA. In: *Methods in Enzymology*, Volume 73, Langone, J. & Van Vunakis, H. (eds), Academic Press, New York, pp. 224–238.

PETERFY, F., KUNSELA, P. & MAKELA, O. (1983) Affinity requirements for antibody assays mapped by monoclonal antibodies. *Journal of Immunology*, **130**, 1809–1813.

SCATCHARD, G. (1949) The attractions of proteins for small molecules and ions. *Annals of the New York Academy of Science*, **51**, 660–667.

SCHALL, R. F. & TENOSO, H. J. (1980) Recent developments in heterogeneous immunoassays. In: *Immunoassays: Clinical Laboratory Techniques for the*

1980s, Nakamura, R. M., Dito, W. R. & Tucker, E. S. (eds), Alan R. Liss, New York, pp. 127–139.

STANDEFER, J. C. (1985) Separation required (heterogeneous) enzyme immunoassay for haptens and antigens. In: *Enzyme Mediated Immunoassays*, Ngo, T. T. & Lenhoff, H. M. (eds), Plenum Press, New York, pp. 203–222.

ULLMAN, E. F., GIBBONS, I., WENG, L., DINELLO, R., STISO, S. N. & LITMAN, D. J. (1983) Homogeneous immunoassays and immunometric assays employing enzyme channeling. In: *Diagnostic Immunology: Technology Assessment*, Nakamura, R. M. & Rippey, J. H. (eds), College of American Pathologists, Skokie, Illinois.

WELTMAN, J. K., JOHNSON, S. A., LANGEVIN, J. & RIESTER, E. F. (1983) 4-Succinimidyl (4-iodoacetyl) aminobenzoate: a new heterobifunctional crosslinker. *Biotechniques*, **1**, 148–152.

4

New Methods for Enzyme Labelling of Antigens and Antibodies and for Preparing Hapten Immunogens: EIA for Detection of Cephalexin Residues in Milk

T. KITAGAWA, K. UCHIHARA, W. OHTANI, Y. GOTOH, Y. KOHRI and T. KINOUE

Faculty of Pharmaceutical Sciences, Nagasaki University, Japan

INTRODUCTION

The general advantages of heterobifunctional cross-linkers, N-(*m*-maleimidobenzoyloxy)succinimide (MBS) and its analogues, over homobifunctional cross-linkers for the selective preparation of protein–protein conjugates are discussed. The application of the cross-linker in a new method and its improved method for enzyme labelling of insulin and other antigens are reviewed. Another application of the cross-linker in a new method and its modified procedures for preparing two hapten immunogens are also reviewed. Cephalexin (CEX) was labelled with β-D-galactosidase by using the improved enzyme labelling method. Both modified procedures of the new method for preparing hapten immunogens were applied for conjugating CEX with bovine serum albumin. Two anti-CEX antisera were produced in rabbits immunised with these conjugates. An EIA for CEX was developed using these antisera. The specificities of these two anti-CEX antisera were compared by EIA and the application of the EIA for measuring CEX in milk preparations is presented.

Recent progress in immunochemistry has required the preparation of protein–protein or protein–hapten conjugates for analytical and preparative techniques. Cross-linking reagents for preparing these conjugates have been studied extensively (Wold, 1972; Kennedy *et al.*, 1976). A general disadvantage of cross-linkers of the homobifunctional type is a lack of the controlled incorporation of protein and hapten molecules in the conjugate.

Protein I + X–R–X + Protein II

↓

(Protein I)$_x$–(R)$_y$–(Protein II)$_z$
(Protein I)$_x$–(R)$_y$–(Protein I)$_z$
(Protein II)$_x$–(R)$_y$–(Protein II)$_z$

X–R–X: Homobifunctional reagents

X = Cl, —N=C=O, —N=C=S
R = Alkylene or phenylene
x, y or z = 0, 1, 2, 3, 4

Fig. 1. Non-selective couplings for protein–protein conjugates using homobifunctional reagents.

Both groups of the cross-linkers react simultaneously, leading to a variety of complexes as shown in Fig. 1.

A series of heterobifunctional reagents, N-(*m*-maleimidobenzoyloxy)-succinimide (MBS) and its analogues, a maleimide succinimidyl ester type, was introduced by the authors for selective protein–protein conjugation (Kitagawa & Aikawa, 1976; Kitagawa *et al.*, 1978*a*; Kitagawa *et al.*, 1981; Kitagawa, 1986). These reagents prevented the formation of undesirable homopolymers (see Fig. 2).

The amine group of insulin was first acylated by the succinimidyl ester of MBS. This active ester had been used in peptide synthesis (Anderson *et al.*, 1964) under anhydrous conditions, but not in aqueous solution. In 1972, a procedure was developed to apply this active ester for acylation of viomycin in aqueous solution (Kitagawa *et al.*, 1972, 1976) and the established conditions were applied for MBS acylation of insulin.

The second step involved the addition of a free thiol group of

Protein I–NH_2 + X–R–Y ⟶ Protein I–NH–R–Y

↓ Protein II SH

Protein I–NH–R–S–Protein II

X = Succinimidyl ester
Y = Maleimide residue
R = Alkylene or phenylene

Fig. 2. Selective couplings for protein–protein conjugates using heterobifunctional reagents.

Table 1
EIAs for Antigens and Antibodies using the New Enzyme-labelling Method

Antigen/Antibody	*Reference*
Insulin	Kitagawa & Aikawa (1976)
Viomycin	Kitagawa *et al.* (1978*a*), Kitagawa (1986)
Human chorionic gonadotrophin	Kikutani *et al.* (1978)
Angiotensin I	Aikawa *et al.* (1979)
Heterobifunctional cross-linkers	Kitagawa *et al.* (1981)
Bradykinin	Ueno *et al.* (1981)
Neocarzinostatin (NCS)	Tanimori *et al.* (1981)
Rabbit IgG	Tanimori *et al.* (1983)
Specific IgG to NCS	Kitagawa *et al.* (1984)
Human IgG	Tanimori *et al.* (1985)

β-D-galactosidase (Kato *et al.*, 1975) to the double bond of maleimide of MBS-activated insulin. Both steps for conjugating insulin to β-D-galactosidase using MBS proceeded selectively and quickly under neutral aqueous conditions. This method has further improved the procedure by omitting the isolation of the intermediate, the MBS-activated antigen or antibody (Tanimori *et al.*, 1981, 1983; Kitagawa *et al.*, 1982*a*, *b*; Kitagawa, 1986), and these enzyme labelling methods have been applied to various EIAs for antigens and antibodies (Table 1).

NEW METHOD FOR THE PREPARATION OF HAPTEN IMMUNOGEN

During the course of developing an EIA for viomycin (VM), the preparation of VM-immunogen proved to be very difficult (Kitagawa *et al.*, 1978*a*). The synthetic route for VM-immunogen consisted of a five-step reaction sequence and essentially applied the mixed anhydride method of Erlanger (1980). Since no step was easy to perform, a new method was developed for preparing hapten immunogens using the heterobifunctional cross-linkers and linking the hapten molecule via thiol–ether bonds to carrier protein (Kitagawa *et al.*, 1978*b*,*c*). Two modifications were introduced to the method at the thiol-introducing step to simplify the original procedure (Fujiwara *et al.*, 1981*b*; Kitagawa *et al.*, 1982*a*). The free thiol reagent must be removed after the thiol-exchange reaction and sometimes this was not easy. By using these methods, a variety of EIAs for drugs was developed (Table 2).

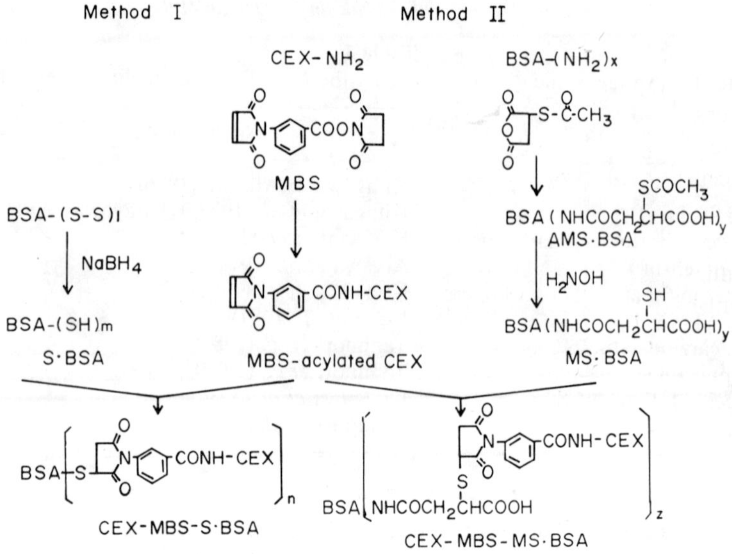

Fig. 3. Scheme for preparing two CEX immunogens, CEX–MBS–S.BSA and CEX–MBS–MS.BSA. Abbreviations: CEX, cephalexin; MBS, N-(*m*-maleimidobenzoyloxy)succinimide; BSA, bovine serum albumin.

Table 2
EIAs using the New Conjugation Method for Preparation of Hapten Immunogens

Antigen	*Reference*
Ampicillin	Kitagawa *et al.* (1978*c*)
Daunomycin and Adriamycin	Fujiwara *et al.* (1981*b*)
Pepleomycin	Fujiwara *et al.* (1981*c*)
Tobramycin	Suzuki *et al.* (1981)
Viomycin	Kitagawa *et al.* (1982*b*)
Mitomycin C	Fujiwara *et al.* (1982)
Blasticidin S	Kitagawa *et al.* (1982*a*)
Puromycin	Fujiwara *et al.* (1981*a*)
Bleomycin	Fujiwara *et al.* (1983*b*)
Kanamycin	Kitagawa *et al.* (1983)
Spermine and Spermidine	Fujiwara *et al.* (1983*a*)
Mitomycin C	Fujiwara *et al.* (1983*c*)
Mitomycin C analogue	Fujiwara *et al.* (1984)
Colistin	Kitagawa *et al.* (1985)
Aclacinomycin A	Sohda *et al.* (1985)
Chromomycin A_3	Fujiwara *et al.* (1985)
Mithramycin	Fujiwara *et al.* (1986)

Cephalexin (CEX), a semi-synthetic cephalosporin, is effective against a variety of Gram-positive and Gram-negative bacteria (Ryan *et al.*, 1969). Recent progress in EIA (Butler, 1978; Langone & Van Vunakis, 1981) has made possible the highly sensitive and specific assays for various drug concentrations. Cephalosporins possess an unstable β-lactam ring, and the ring cleavage is usually accompanied by successive degradative reactions of the cephalosporin molecule (Abraham & Loder, 1972). Consequently, an immunoassay has seldom been developed for any cephalosporin so far, owing to difficulty in preparing specific antisera.

Two selective modifications of proteins are required to develop an EIA for CEX. One is the preparation of CEX-immunogen and the other is enzyme-labelling. The method for preparation of hapten immunogen influences the specificity of the anti-hapten antiserum and the specificity to the enzyme-labelled hapten is affected by the labelling method (Van Weemen & Schuurs, 1975; Kitagawa *et al.*, 1983). A combination of two kinds of heterobifunctional reagents was applied for preparing hapten immunogens (Fig. 3) and for enzyme labelling (Fig. 4) in developing an EIA for CEX.

METHODS AND RESULTS

Preparation of the CEX-Immunogen

Both of the modified methods for preparing hapten immunogens (Kitagawa, 1986) were applied to the preparation of CEX-immunogen by using the heterobifunctional reagent (MBS) under mild conditions in a neutral aqueous solution.

Step 1: Acylation of CEX Hapten

The maleimide group was condensed with the amino group of CEX as shown in Fig. 3. A solution of 5·2 mg CEX in 1 ml 0·05 M phosphate buffer (pH 7·0) was incubated for 30 min at 30°C with 4·7 mg MBS in 0·5 ml tetrahydrofuran solution. The tetrahydrofuran was removed by flushing with nitrogen and excess MBS was then extracted from the reaction mixture with three 5-ml portions of methylene chloride–ether mixture (1:2 v/v). The aqueous layer was used for step 3.

Step 2: Activation of Carrier Protein

Free thiol groups were introduced into the BSA molecule using two methods as shown in Methods I and II of Fig. 3 and detailed below.

Method I: Reductive Cleavage of Disulphide Bonds of 17 Cystine Residues in BSA by Sodium Borohydride

A solution of 10 mg BSA in 2 ml of 6M urea–0·1M EDTA was reduced by 20 mg sodium borohydride at 25°C for 20 min. Excess reagent was decomposed by adding 0·4 ml acetone and the solution of reduced BSA (S.BSA) was used for step 3.

Method II: Conversion of BSA to Mercaptosuccinyl–BSA (MS.BSA) via S-Acetylmercaptosuccinyl–BSA (AMS.BSA)

BSA was converted to AMS.BSA by the use of S-acetylmercaptosuccinic anhydride according to the method of Klotz & Heiney (1962). (Note: AMS.BSA is now available commercially from Dojin Chemicals, Kumamoto, Kenguncho, Japan.) AMS.BSA (6·7 mg) was converted to MS.BSA by incubating it for 30 min at 30°C in 2 ml of 0·1M phosphate buffer containing 0·1M hydroxylamine. The mixture was diluted 1:10 with water and the MS.BSA formed was used immediately for step 3.

Step 3: Conjugation of MBS-acylated Cephalexin to S.BSA (CEX–MBS–S.BSA) or to MS.BSA (CEX–MBS–MS.BSA)

The solution of S.BSA (step 2-I) or of MS.BSA (step 2-II) (Fig. 3) was incubated for 2 h at 25°C with the aqueous layer of MBS-acylated CEX

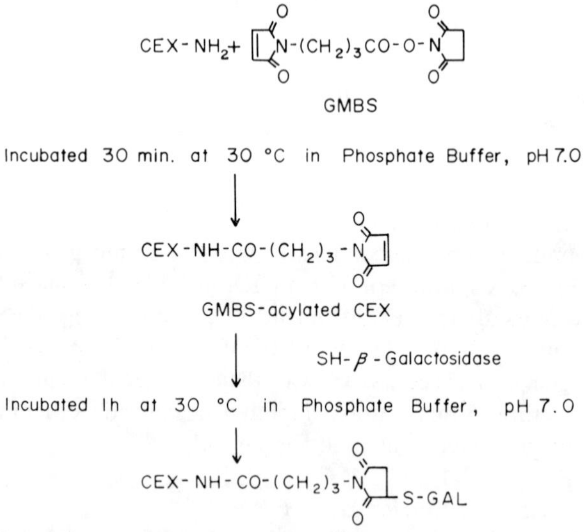

Fig. 4. Scheme for preparing the enzyme-labelled cephalexin, CEX–GMBS–GAL. Abbreviations: GMBS, N-(γ-maleimidobutyryloxy)succinimide; GAL, β-D-galactosidase.

(step 1). The reaction was terminated by the addition of 10 μl mercaptoethanol. All reaction steps were completed within 3 h and the mixtures were chromatographed on a Sephadex G-100 column (2·5 × 34 cm) using 3M urea as eluant.

Enzyme Labelling of CEX

Acylation of CEX with a heterobifunctional reagent, N-(γ-maleimidobutyryloxy)succinimide (GMBS), was performed at 25°C for 30 min in 0·05M sodium phosphate buffer (pH 7·0) at a molar ratio of 10:1 (Fig. 4). An aliquot of the GMBS-acylated CEX formed in the reaction mixture was immediately coupled with one-tenth of its molar amount of β-D-galactosidase (moles of GMBS-acylated CEX can be assumed to be 70% moles of GMBS used) (cf. Kitagawa *et al.*, 1981). No reduction in the enzyme activity was observed during the enzyme labelling process. After incubating for 2 h, the reaction mixture was chromatographed on a Sepharose CL 6B column to

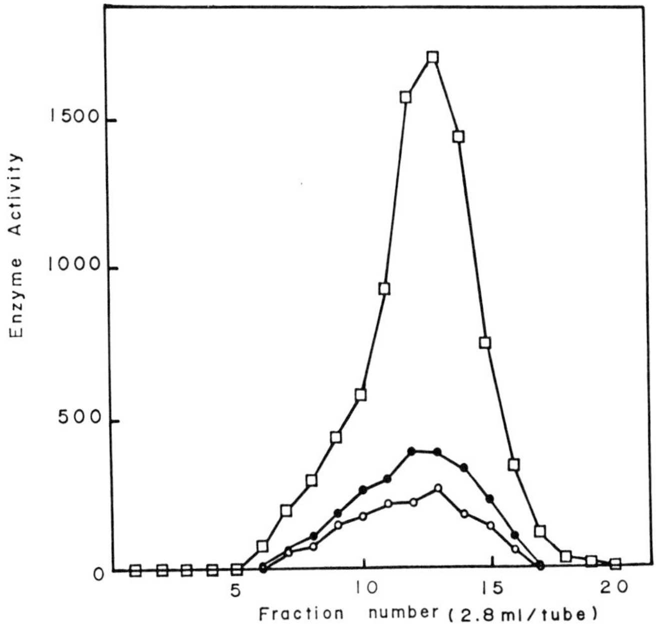

Fig. 5. Elution profiles of CEX–GAL from a Sepharose CL 6B column. Enzyme activity of the conjugate (□——□) measured with 5 μl of each fraction at 30°C for 5 min; immunoreactive enzyme activity (●——●) determined by EIA with use of 5 μl conjugate and a 1:1000 solution of anti-CEX–MBS–S.BSA antiserum in absence of CEX; immunoreactive enzyme activity (○——○) determined in competition with 100 ng of CEX in same manner.

remove any free CEX. The elution profiles determined by both enzyme and immunological activities are shown in Fig. 5. The maximum immunoreactivity of the conjugate was almost coincident with the enzyme activity in the presence and absence of 100 ng CEX. The fraction with the highest enzyme activity was used as a tracer for EIA of CEX.

Antibody Response

Each CEX-immunogen was injected into two rabbits. CEX antibody was produced in every rabbit immunised either with CEX–MBS–S.BSA or CEX–MBS–MS.BSA conjugate, and was detected by the reaction of the diluted antiserum with GAL-labelled CEX. The uptake of CEX–GAL conjugate by the precipitate gave a quantitative measure of the bound antibody. Typical binding curves for the sera from one of the two rabbits immunised with CEX–MBS–MS.BSA are shown in Fig. 6. The antibody titre, as determined with CEX–GAL, reached a maximum two weeks after the final injection. The titre of the final anti-CEX antiserum was excellent and a 10 000 000-fold dilution of the antiserum could bind CEX–GAL, with an enzyme activity value three times that of the blank determined in the same manner except that the antiserum was replaced by normal rabbit serum, as shown in Fig. 6.

Enzyme Immunoassay

After several sets of trials, the optimum condition for liquid phase EIA of CEX using the double antibody phase separation method was established: 50 micro-units of the enzyme label, and either a 1:300 000 dilution of anti-CEX–MBS–S.BSA or 1:30 000 of anti-CEX–MBS–MS.BSA were chosen as immunoreagents. Inhibition of the binding of CEX–GAL conjugate to these antisera by CEX is shown in Fig. 7. Addition of increasing quantities of CEX resulted in a progressive decrease in the amount of the enzyme-labelled conjugate precipitated.

Recovery and Precision of EIA

Recoveries of various doses of CEX ranging from 3 to 300 ng/tube were found to be between 89 and 118%. The coefficients of variation for within-assay and between-assay were less than 14·4% for doses of 10·0 to 300 ng and higher than 20% for samples of 3 ng.

Antibody Specificity

Cross-reactivities of four CEX analogues, two penicillins (the structures of which are shown in Fig. 8) and two unrelated antibiotics with both anti-CEX antisera were studied in the EIA for CEX; 50% cross-reaction values

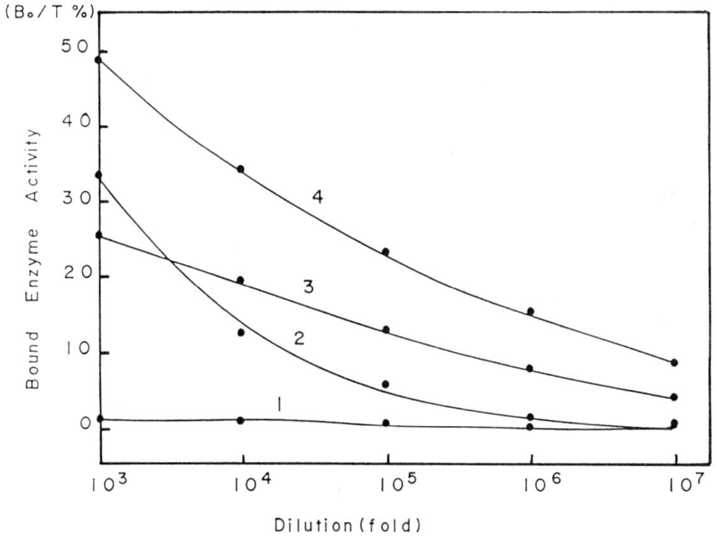

Fig. 6. Qualitative estimation of anti-CEX–MBS–MS.BSA antisera. Antiserum dilution curves 2, 3 and 4 are antisera collected 2, 4 and 6 weeks respectively after first injection. Normal rabbit serum sample (curve 1) obtained from rabbit bled before immunisation.

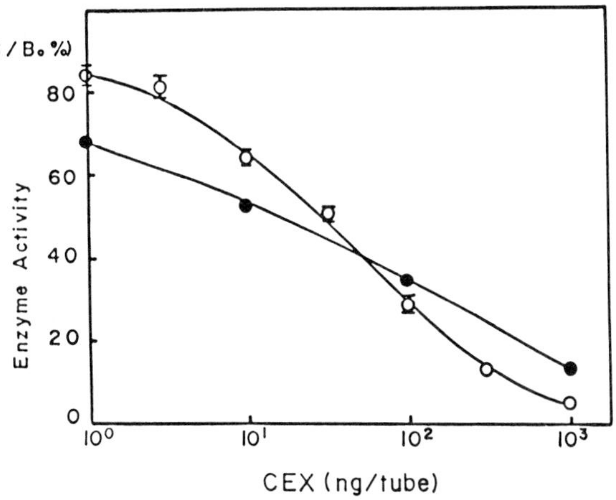

Fig. 7. Standard curves for EIA of CEX: ○——○, 1:30 000 dilution of anti-CEX–MBS–MS.BSA was used; ●——●, 1:300 000 dilution of anti-CEX–MBS–S.BSA was used. Curves show amount (%) of bound enzyme activity for various doses of CEX (B) (3–300 ng) with respect to that bound using CEX–GAL alone (B_0).

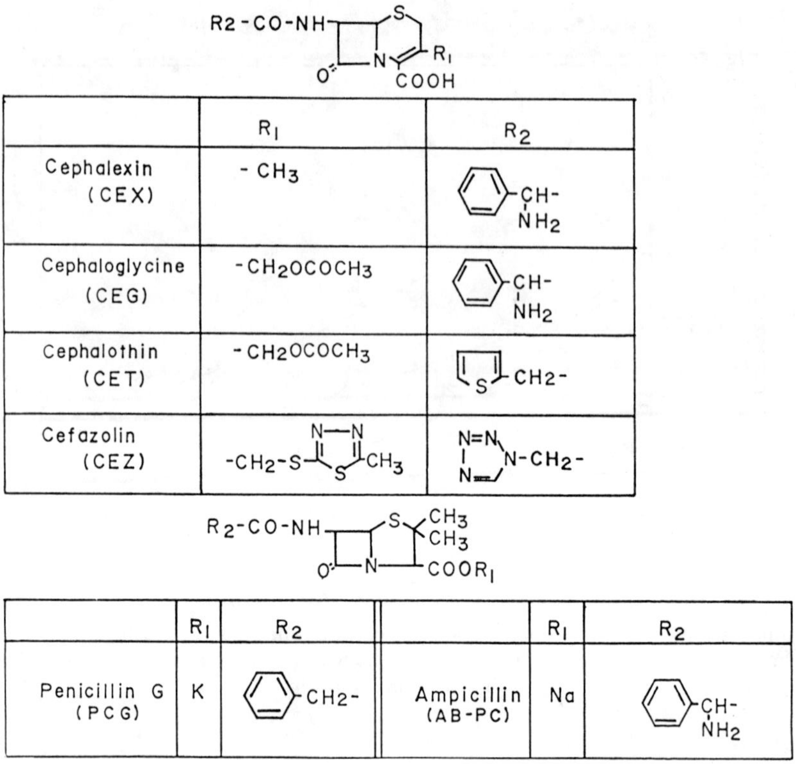

Fig. 8. Chemical structures of four cephalosporins and two penicillins.

Table 3

Cross-reaction Values of Four Cephalosporins, Two Penicillins and Two Other Antibiotics at B/B_0 50% Values determined by EIA for CEX, by using either Anti-CEX–MBS–S.BSA or Anti-CEX–MBS–MS.BSA

Sample	*Cross-reactivity* (%)	
	Anti-CEX–MBS–S.BSA	*Anti-CEX–MBS–MS.BSA*
Cephalexin	100	100
Cephalothin	0·32	126·7
Cephaloglycine	1·01	23·0
Cefazolin	0·001	0·1
Ampicillin	0·002	0·4
Penicillin G	0·018	0·4
Viomycin	<0·001	<0·001
Streptomycin	<0·001	<0·001

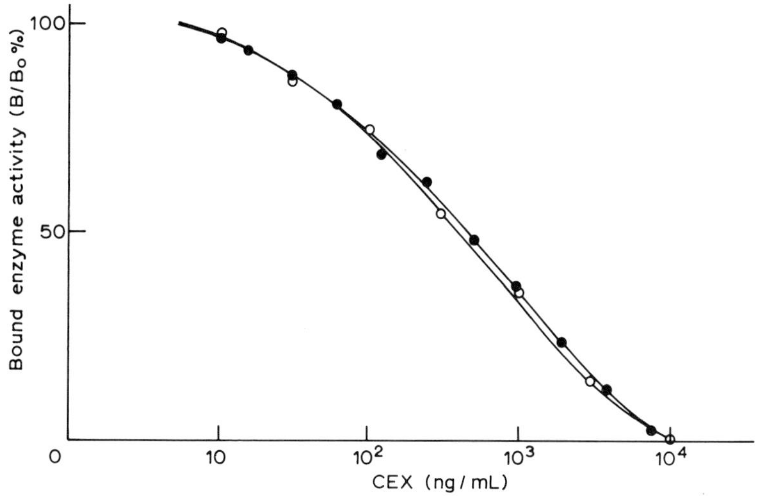

Fig. 9. Standard curves for EIAs of CEX with (○——○) and without (●——●) presence of 50 μl milk.

for the antibiotics are listed in Table 3. Anti-CEX–MBS–S.BSA is more specific for CEX than anti-CEX–MBS–MS.BSA.

Measurement of CEX in Milk

Dose–response curves for CEX were constructed with and without the addition of 50 μl CEX-free raw milk (Fig. 9). Both curves are essentially the same and 50 μl milk was found to have little matrix effect in this assay. Consequently, direct assay of milk samples by this assay is possible. Experiments were also performed to measure the change found in doses of CEX in a series of two-fold diluted solutions of some milk samples (Fig. 10). A sample of 0·12 μg/ml CEX in milk was easily detected and quantified by this dilution method. The present EIA is able to detect and quantify cephalexin easily in many milk samples without any pretreatment. The limit of detection of the assay was 0·12 μg/ml.

CONCLUSIONS

Today preparation of the two important immune reagents for developing competitive drug EIAs, namely an enzyme-labelled preparation of the

Editor's footnote: This method would be even simpler using an ELISA format.

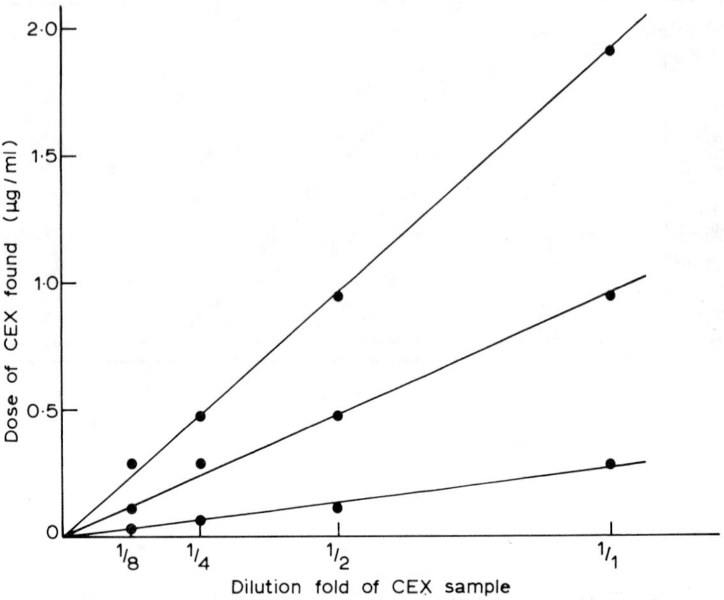

Fig. 10. Linear relationships between the detected CEX levels in three milk samples (2·0, 1·0 and 0·2 μg/ml) and their series of two-fold diluted solutions.

drug and an antiserum to the drug, has become much easier. Consequently, the EIA method will be a valuable tool for veterinary and food analysis, since the method is simple, able to handle many samples at the same time, without radio-isotope hazard, and does not require complicated pretreatment of the sample for separating the drug in question from foods prior to analysis.

REFERENCES

Abraham, E. P. & Loder, P. B. (1972) Degradation products of cephalosporin C. In: *Cephalosporins and Penicillins*, Flynn, E. H. (ed.), Academic Press, New York, pp. 15–19.

Aikawa, T., Suzuki, S., Murayama, M., Hashiba, K., Kitagawa, T. & Ishikawa, E. (1979) Enzyme immunoassay of angiotensin. I. *Endocrinology*, **105**, 1–6.

Anderson, G. W., Zimmerman, J. E. & Callahan, F. (1964) Esters of *N*-hydroxysuccinimide in peptide synthesis. *Journal of the American Chemical Society*, **86**, 1839–1842.

Butler, V. P. (1978) The immunological assay of drugs. *Pharmacological Reviews*, **29**, 103–184.

ERLANGER, B. F. (1980) The preparation of antigenic hapten-carrier conjugates: a survey. In: *Methods in Enzymology*, Volume 70, Van Vunakis, H. & Langone, J. L. (eds), Academic Press Inc., New York, pp. 85–104.

FUJIWARA, K., OGAWA, A., ASADA, H., SAIKUSA, H., NAKAMURA, H., ONO, S. & KITAGAWA, T. (1981*a*) Preparation of puromycin antibody and its use in enzyme immunoassay for the quantification using β-D-galactosidase as a label. *Journal of Biochemistry* (*Tokyo*), **92**, 1599–1605.

FUJIWARA, K., YASUNO, M. & KITAGAWA, T. (1981*b*) Novel preparation method of immunogen for hydrophobic hapten, enzyme immunoassay of daunomycin and adriamycin. *Journal of Immunological Methods*, **45**, 195–203.

FUJIWARA, K., YASUNO, M. & KITAGAWA, T. (1981*c*) Enzyme immunoassay for pepleomycin, a new bleomycin analog. *Cancer Research*, **41**, 4121–4126.

FUJIWARA, K., SAIKUSA, H., YASUNO, M. & KITAGAWA, T. (1982) Enzyme immunoassay for the quantification of mitomycin C using β-galactosidase as a label. *Cancer Research*, **42**, 1487–1491.

FUJIWARA, K., ASADA, H., KITAGAWA, T., YAMAMOTO, K., ITO, T., TSUCHIYA, R., SOHDA, M., NAKAMURA, N., HARA, K., TOMONAGA, Y., ICHIMARU, M. & TAKAHASHI, S. (1983*a*) Preparation of polyamine antibody and its use in enzyme immunoassay of spermine and spermidine with β-D-galactosidase as label. *Journal of Immunological Methods*, **61**, 217–226.

FUJIWARA, K., ISOBE, M., SAIKUSA, H., NAKAMURA, H., KITAGAWA, T. & TAKAHASHI, S. (1983*b*) Sensitive enzyme immunoassay for the quantification of bleomycin using β-D-galactosidase as a label. *Cancer Treatment Reports*, **67**, 363–369.

FUJIWARA, K., SAIKUSA, H., KITAGAWA, T., TAKAHASHI, S. & KONISHI, Y. (1983*c*) Specificity of antisera produced against mitomycin C. *Cancer Treatment Reports*, **67**, 1079–1084.

FUJIWARA, K., NAKAMURA, H., KITAGAWA, T., NAKAMURA, N., SAITO, A. & HARA, K. (1984) Development and application of a sensitive enzyme immunoassay for 7-*N*-(*p*-hydroxyphenyl)mitomycin C. *Cancer Research*, **44**, 4172–4176.

FUJIWARA, K., NAKAMURA, H. & KITAGAWA, T. (1985) Development of enzyme immunoassay for chromomycin A_3 and olivomycin using β-D-galactosidase as a label. *Cancer Research*, **45**, 5442–5446.

FUJIWARA, K., SAITA, T., NAKASHIMA, K. & KITAGAWA, T. (1986) Enzyme immunoassay for the quantification of mithramycin using β-D-galactosidase as a label. *Cancer Research*, **46**, 1084–1088.

KATO, K., HAMAGUCHI, Y., FUKUI, H. & ISHIKAWA, E. (1975) Enzyme-linked immunoassay. I. Novel method for synthesis of the insulin β-D-galactosidase conjugate and its applicability of insulin assay. *Journal of Biochemistry (Tokyo)*, **78**, 235–237.

KENNEDY, J. H., KRICKA, L. J. & WILDING, P. (1976) Protein–protein coupling reactions and the applications of protein conjugates. *Clinica Chimica Acta*, **70**, 1–31.

KIKUTANI, M., ISHIGURO, M., KITAGAWA, T., IMAMURA, S. & MIURA, S. (1978) Enzyme immunoassay of human chorionic gonadotrophin employing β-D-galactosidase as label. *Journal of Clinical Endocrinology and Metabolism*, **47**, 980–984.

KITAGAWA, T. (1986) Viomycin and ampicillin, In: *Methods of Enzymatic Analysis*, Volume 12, Bergmeyer, H. V. (ed.), VCH Publishers, Weinheim, pp. 200–215.

Kitagawa, T. & Aikawa, T. (1976) Enzyme coupled immunoassay of insulin using a novel coupling reagent. *Journal of Biochemistry (Tokyo)*, **79**, 233–236.

Kitagawa, T., Miura, T. & Taniyama, H. (1972) Characterization of viomycin and its acyl derivatives. *Chemical and Pharmaceutical Bulletin*, **20**, 2176–2184.

Kitagawa, T., Miura, T., Takaishi, C. & Taniyama, H. (1976) Studies on viomycin. IX. Amino acid derivatives of viomycin. *Chemical and Pharmaceutical Bulletin*, **24**, 1324–1330.

Kitagawa, T., Fujitake, T., Taniyama, H. & Aikawa, T. (1978*a*) Enzyme immunoassay of viomycin: New cross-linking reagent for enzyme labelling and a preparation method for antiserum to viomycin. *Journal of Biochemistry (Tokyo)*, **83**, 1493–1501.

Kitagawa, T., Kanamaru, T., Kato, H., Yano, S. & Asanuma, Y. (1978*b*) Novel enzyme immunoassay of three antibiotics: New methods for preparation of antisera to the antibiotics and for enzyme labelling using a combination of two hetero-bifunctional reagents. In: *Enzyme Labelled Immunoassay of Hormones and Drugs*, Pal, S. (ed.), Walter de Gruyter and Co., Berlin, pp. 59–66.

Kitagawa, T., Kanamaru, T., Wakamatsu, H., Kato, H., Yano, S. & Asanuma, Y. (1978*c*) A new method for preparation of an antiserum to penicillin and its application for novel enzyme immunoassay of penicillin. *Journal of Biochemistry (Tokyo)*, **84**, 491–494 (cf. 733, 735).

Kitagawa, T., Shimozono, T., Aikawa, T., Yoshida, T. & Nishimura, H. (1981) Preparation and characterization of hetero-bifunctional cross-linking reagents for protein modifications. *Chemical and Pharmaceutical Bulletin*, **29**, 1130–1135.

Kitagawa, T., Kawasaki, T. & Munechika, H. (1982*a*) Enzyme immunoassay of blasticidin S with a high sensitivity: A new convenient method for preparation of immunogenic (hapten–protein) conjugates. *Journal of Biochemistry (Tokyo)*, **92**, 585–590.

Kitagawa, T., Tanimori, H., Yoshida, K., Asada, H., Miura, T. & Fujiwara, K. (1982*b*) Studies on viomycin. XV. Comparative study on the specificities of two anti-viomycin antisera by enzyme immunoassay. *Chemical and Pharmaceutical Bulletin*, **30**, 2487–2491.

Kitagawa, T., Fujiwara, K., Tomonoh, S., Takahashi, K. & Koida, M. (1983) Enzyme immunoassays of kanamycin group antibiotics with high sensitivities using anti-kanamycin as a common antiserum: Reasoning and selection of a heterologous enzyme label. *Journal of Biochemistry (Tokyo)*, **94**, 1165–1172.

Kitagawa, T., Tanimori, H. & Yoshida, K. (1984) Enzyme immunoassay with high sensitivity and accuracy for specific antibody to neocarzinostatin. *Journal of Immunological Methods*, **72**, 297–303.

Kitagawa, T., Ohtani, W., Maeno, Y., Fujiwara, K. & Kimura, Y. (1985). Sensitive enzyme immunoassay of colistin and its application to detect residual colistin in rainbow trout tissue. *Journal of the Association of Official Analytical Chemists*, **68**, 661–664.

Klotz, I. M. & Heiney, R. E. (1962) Introduction of sulfhydryl groups into proteins using acetylmercaptosuccinic anhydride. *Archives of Biochemistry and Biophysics, Supplement*, **96**, 605–612.

LANGONE, J. J. & VAN VUNAKIS, H. (eds) (1981) Immunochemical techniques, part B. In: *Methods in Enzymology*, Volume 73, Academic Press, New York.

RYAN, C. W., SIMON, R. L. & VAN HEYNINGEN, E. M. (1969) Chemistry of cephalosporin antibiotics. XIII. Deacetoxy cephalosporins: Synthesis of cephalexin and some analogs. *Journal of Medicinal Chemistry*, **12**, 310–315.

SOHDA, M., SUJIWARA, K., SAIKUSA, H., KITAGAWA, T., NAKAMURA, N., HARA, K. & TONE, H. (1985) Sensitive enzyme immunoassay for the quantification of aclacinomycin A using β-D-galactosidase as a label. *Cancer Chemotherapy and Pharmacology*, **14**, 53–58.

SUZUKI, H., KATO, H., NAKANO, N., YANO, S. & KITAGAWA, T. (1981) Solid phase enzyme immunoassay of tobramycin. *The Journal of Antibiotics (Tokyo)*, **34**, 1195–1199.

TANIMORI, H., KITAGAWA, T., TSUNODA, T. & TSUCHIA, R. (1981) Enzyme immunoassay of neocarzinostatin using β-galactosidase as label. *Journal of Pharmacobio-Dynamics*, **4**, 812–819.

TANIMORI, H., ISHIKAWA, H. & KITAGAWA, T. (1983) A sandwich enzyme immunoassay of rabbit immunoglobulin G with an enzyme labeling method and a new solid support. *Journal of Immunological Methods*, **62**, 123–131.

TANIMORI, H., TAKAOKA, S., ISHII, N., KOJI, T., ISHIKAWA, F. & KITAGAWA, T. (1985) A new solid support for sandwich enzyme immunoassays of human immunoglobulin G. *Journal of Immunological Methods*, **83**, 327–336.

UENO, A., OH-ISHI, S., KITAGAWA, T. & KATORI, M. (1981) Enzyme immunoassay of bradykinin using β-D-galactosidase as a labeling enzyme. *Biochemical Pharmacology*, **30**, 1659–1664.

VAN WEEMEN, B. K. & SCHUURS, A. H. W. M. (1975) The influence of heterologous combinations of antiserum and enzyme labelled oestrogen on the characteristics of oestrogen enzyme immunoassay. *Immunochemistry*, **12**, 667–670.

WOLD, F. (1972) Bifunctional reagents. In: *Methods in Enzymology*, Volume 25, Hirs, C. H. W. & Reimasheff, A. N. (eds), Academic Press, New York, pp. 623–651.

5

The Use of Enzymes in Ultrasensitive Immunoassays

B. J. GOULD

Department of Biochemistry, University of Surrey, Guildford, UK

COMPETITIVE VERSUS TWO-SITE IMMUNOMETRIC (NON-COMPETITIVE) ASSAYS

Before reviewing this area of the application of enzymes, it is necessary to consider the two different types of ELISA technique (Fig. 1). The competitive ELISA for antigen uses a limited amount of antibody whereas the two-site immunometric (or capture, sandwich or non-competitive) ELISA uses an excess of solid-phase antibody. As a consequence, with the competitive ELISA the signal decreases with increasing antigen concentration whilst the opposite is true for the two-site immunometric assay. Although the competitive assay produces its greatest signal for low concentrations of antigen, the two-site immunometric assays have the theoretical and practical advantage of giving lower detection limits as demonstrated by Jackson & Ekins (1986). This point is discussed below.

Two-site immunometric assays also offer the advantage of greater specificity, since the two separate binding sites for the antigen which are recognised by the antibodies used are of different epitope specificity. This also allows simpler one-step assays to be performed, especially if monoclonal antibodies are employed; in this case the antigen and labelled monoclonal antibody can be added at the same time. One-step assays have the benefit of being quicker, but an important washing step is eliminated, which allows the possibility of greater matrix effects.

Since these assays require the binding of the antigen by two distinct antibodies, they are not usually applicable to the determination of haptens; nevertheless, a way round this problem has been found so that immunometric hapten assays, with the possibility of increased sensitivity,

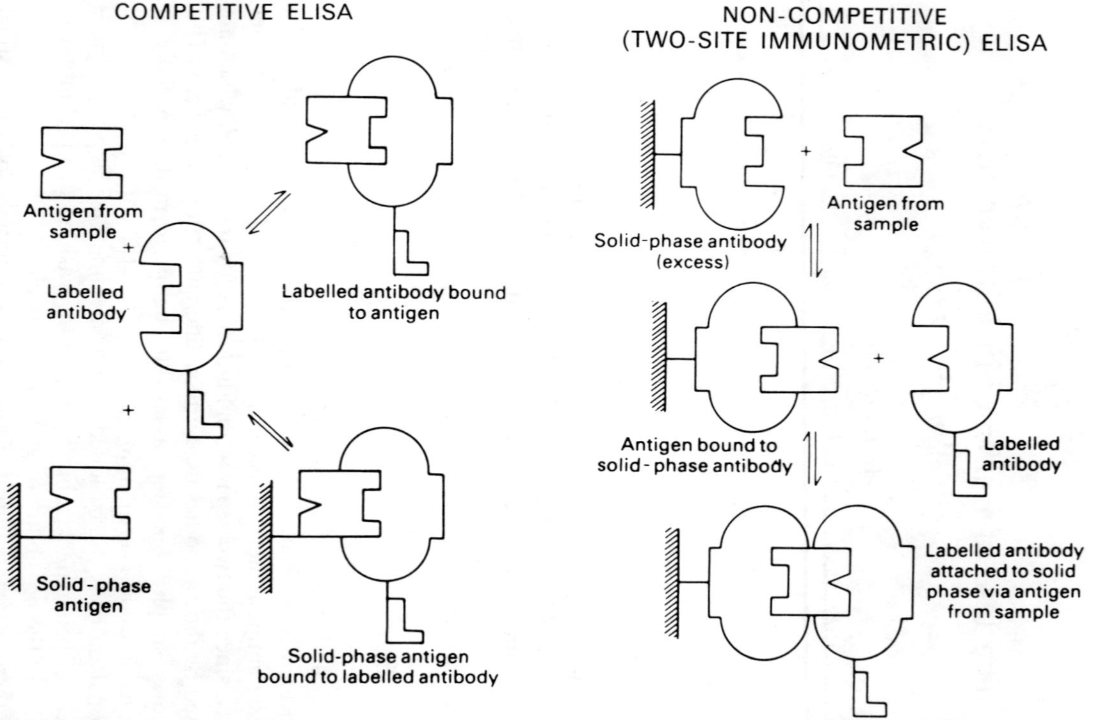

Fig. 1. Diagrammatic representation of competitive ELISA and two-site immunometric ELISA. Extensive washing is carried out between each stage of the immunometric assays and prior to the addition of substrate to measure enzyme activity for both types of immunoassay. (After Blake & Gould, 1984.)

may now be developed (Freytag *et al.*, 1984) and these will be discussed later.

Two other advantages of immunometric assays are that the affinity of the capture antibody is less important than in the competitive assay, since excess antibody is used. Secondly, the accuracy of pipetting of the capture antibody is less critical since it is no longer a limiting factor.

As a consequence of these advantages, the immunometric assays are characterised by being more rapid, more reliable and more rugged than competitive assays, with the added advantages of improved sensitivity and specificity.

SENSITIVITY OF TWO-SITE IMMUNOMETRIC ASSAYS

The greater potential sensitivity of these non-competitive over competitive assays is not immediately apparent, but this advantage has now been established (Ekins, 1985). Figure 2 shows the plots of log sensitivity versus log affinity constant, K_{Ab}, for the two types of immunoassay; in both cases it is assumed that measurements are performed on the bound fraction. The 'potential' straight lines are based on the assumption of a 1% experimental error (minimal pipetting errors, counting errors) for the competitive assay and a 1% or 0·01% fractional non-specific binding in the case of the non-competitive assays. More extensive mathematical treatment is given in Ekins (1985) and Jackson & Ekins (1986). The ^{125}I-label curves represent the predicted sensitivities assuming one ^{125}I/molecule of antibody or antigen and 'reasonable' values for counter efficiency and counting time. The sensitivity gap, i.e. the difference between the 'potential' line and the ^{125}I-curve, increases as K_{Ab} increases. For a K_{Ab} of $10^{12}\,M^{-1}$, which is a relatively high affinity constant, the sensitivity gap is small for the competitive assay, implying that alternative labels can do little to improve the sensitivity of these assays.

Comparison of the competitive and two-site immunometric assays reveals two important features:

(i) even with ^{125}I-labels the two-site immunometric assays are more sensitive by a factor of 10–100;
(ii) there is a larger sensitivity gap with two-site immunometric assays and this is increased as the non-specific binding decreases.

The size of the sensitivity gap can be reduced by the use of high turnover labels. In the case of ^{125}I-labels, there is a compromise between half-life and

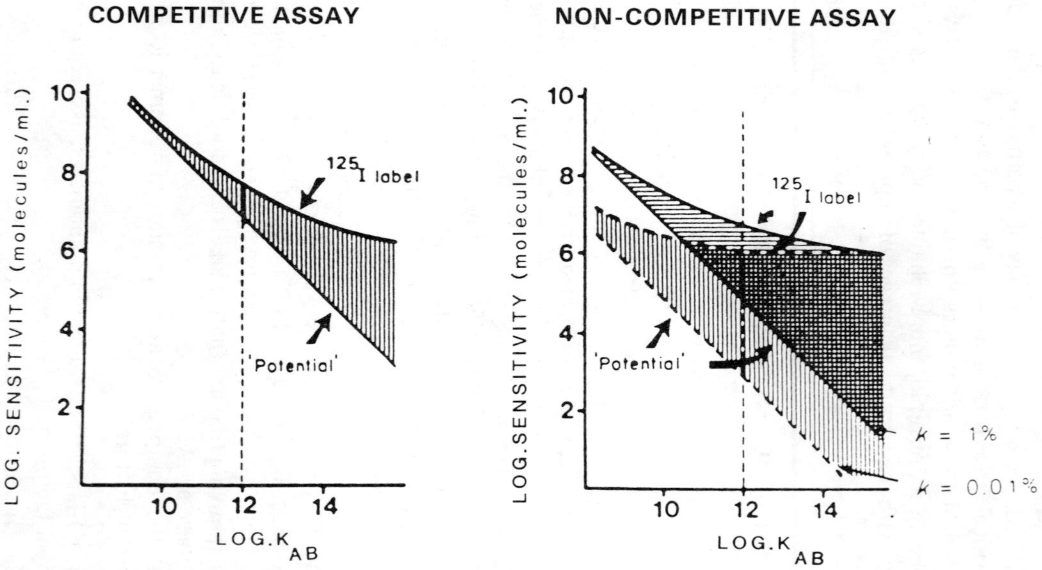

Fig. 2. Sensitivity against antibody equilibrium constant (K_{Ab}) for competitive and immunometric assays for the bound fraction. The 'potential' lines represent the maximal sensitivity assuming 1% experimental errors for competitive assays and 1% and 0·01% of fractional non-specific binding for the immunometric assays. The ^{125}I-label curves represent the predicted sensitivities with one atom of ^{125}I per molecule and 'reasonable' values for counter efficiency, counting time, pipetting, etc. (After Dakubu *et al.*, 1984 and Elkins, 1985.) Reprinted from *Practical Immunoassay—the State of the Art* edited by W. R. Butt, p. 82, by courtesy of Marcel Dekker, Inc.

shelf-life. However, enzymes can be stable for a year or more and all those commonly used in immunoassay have turnover rates in excess of 10^5. Every molecule of enzyme can contribute to the signal, whereas only a small fraction of ^{125}I (about 1 in 10^5 molecules) is detected per minute. The sensitivity of ELISA can also be improved by increasing the surface area of the solid phase, so that more capture antibody is available. Increases in the enzyme assay time also enhance the signal, although the response may deviate from linearity. Probably the most important characteristic of a sensitive assay is a very low non-specific binding, which may be achieved by using affinity purified or monoclonal antibodies. Using serum from the same species providing the indicator antibody as a blocking reagent may also produce the same effect, thus preventing non-specific binding of enzyme-labelled antibody to the unoccupied sites (Shields & Turner, 1986). Other ways of overcoming unwanted interactions in immunoassays involving food are discussed by Windemann (see Chapter 11).

PRACTICAL APPROACHES TO INCREASED IMMUNOASSAY SENSITIVITY USING ENZYMES

There are various approaches for producing more sensitive enzyme immunometric assays. These are based on (a) increasing the molar ratio of enzyme to antigen, (b) amplifying the signal produced or (c) using a more sensitive detection method.

Figure 3 shows how this can be achieved using (strept)avidin. Streptavidin is produced by *Streptomyces avidinii*, whereas avidin is isolated from egg-white. Both have four very high affinity sites (10^{15} M^{-1}) for biotin, but avidin has a higher isoelectric point (pH 10, cf. pH 6 for streptavidin) and is a glycoprotein; both properties, however, can lead to unwanted non-specific binding (Buckland, 1986). Figure 3(a) shows one molecule of enzyme per molecule of antigen (Guesdon *et al.*, 1979); this can be increased to three by using all the available binding sites of streptavidin (Fig. 3(b)) or to much higher ratios if a three-dimensional network of streptavidin and biotinylated enzyme is produced before addition of the complex to the biotinylated antibody (Fig. 3(c)). The main drawbacks of this system are the cost and possibility of steric hindrance, but the procedure is simple to apply.

A similar enhancement can be produced by using enzymes entrapped in a liposome. This system has only been used in homogeneous EIA (Litchfield *et al.*, 1984) but could be used in an immunometric assay, as indicated in

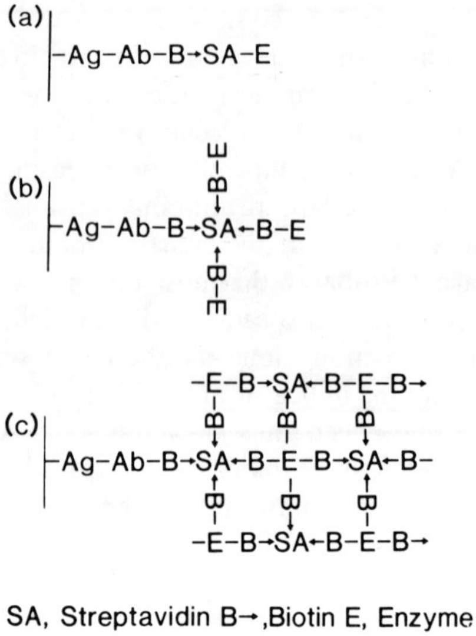

Fig. 3. Systems showing how (strept)avidin and biotin can be used to increase the ratio of enzyme to antigen in immunometric assays. Ratio of enzyme to antigen is (a) 1:1, (b) 3:1 and (c) very large.

Fig. 4. The liposomal membrane incorporates specific antibodies to the antigen. After washing to remove excess liposomes, the enzymes are released, by addition of a cytolytic agent, and assayed. Again there may be problems of steric hindrance, but for very sensitive assays this may be reduced by using a less dense antigen coat on the solid phase.

A simple way of enhancing the signal is to use fluorimetric rather than

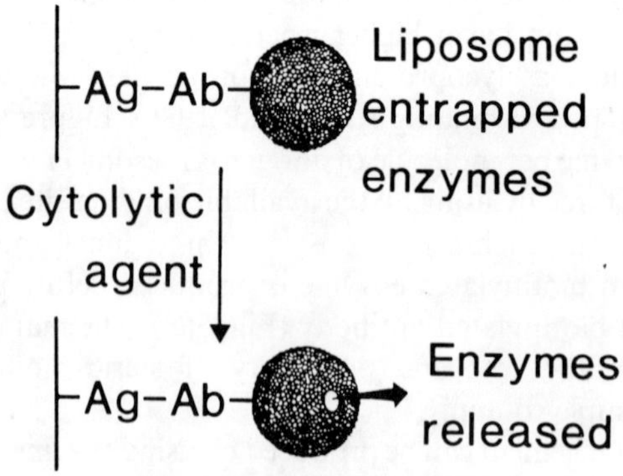

Fig. 4. Possible use of liposome entrapped enzymes to increase ratio of enzyme to antigen in immunometric assays.

Table 1
Enzymes and Substrates used for Fluorimetric and Spectrophotometric Immunometric Assays

Enzymes	*Substrates*	*Product and measurement*
β-D-Galactosidase	*o*-nitrophenyl-β-D-galactopyranoside	*o*-nitrophenol (A)
	chlorophenyl red-β-D-galactopyranoside	chlorophenol red (A)
	4-methylumbelliferyl-β-D-galactopyranoside	4-methylumbelliferone (Fl)
Glucose-6-phosphate dehydrogenase	(glucose-6-phosphate) + $NAD(P)^+$	NAD(P)H (A) NAD(P)H (Fl)
Alkaline phosphatase (calf intestine)	*p*-nitrophenylphosphate	*p*-nitrophenol (A)
	4-methylumbelliferyl phosphate	4-methylumbelliferone (Fl)

A = Absorbance; Fl = Fluorescence.
Further details of fluorimetric assays are available for β-galactosidase (Labrousse *et al.*, 1982), glucose-6-phosphate dehydrogenase (Shah *et al.*, 1984) and alkaline phosphatase (Yolken & Stopa, 1979).

spectrophotometric methods. Table 1 shows three enzymes with which this approach has been used. The coloured or fluorescent products are shown. Even different coloured products may give enhanced signals; e.g. chlorophenol red has a molar absorbance coefficient which is 10 times greater than that of *o*-nitrophenol. The main disadvantages of fluorescent detection are the equipment, which tends to be more expensive, and the greater chance of background fluorescence from biological materials. This is normally removed by the extensive washing used in ELISA procedures. Several of the advantages and disadvantages of the use of fluorescence in ELISA are illustrated in the assay of quinidine presented (see Ward *et al.*, p. 275, this volume).

The increase in sensitivity that can be achieved by fluorimetry is indicated in Fig. 5, taken from the work of Shalev *et al.* (1980). They also studied the effect of increasing the surface area for antigen binding and

	Increase in sensitivity
(a) Fluorimetric detection versus colorimetric detection of alkaline phosphatase	× 16 to 39
(b) Four-fold increase in antigen binding surface area	× 100
(c) Prolonged enzyme assay incubation up to 30 h at 10°C	× 10 to 50
(d) (a) + (b) + (c) combined	10^8

Fig. 5. High-sensitivity ELISA. Effect of altering different factors to increase the sensitivity of an ELISA.

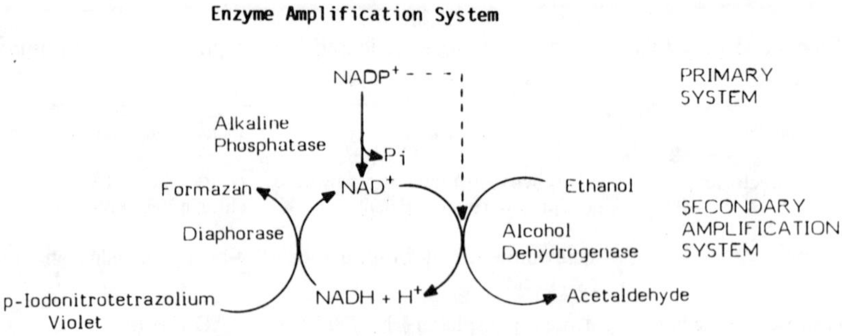

Fig. 6. Enzyme amplification system.

obtained a dramatic and not easily explained increase in binding. Prolonging the enzyme assay incubation time also increased sensitivity, providing that background is not also increased. When these three approaches were used together, they achieved a 'high-sensitivity ELISA' (HS-ELISA), where the combined effect was greater than expected from the sum of their individual improvements.

A different approach is to produce amplification by enzymic cycling. This approach has been patented (Self, 1981) and the system described (Fig. 6) is commercially available as a kit. This method employs alkaline phosphatase as the primary enzyme system to convert $NADP^+$ to NAD^+. This is then used in a secondary amplification system involving alcohol dehydrogenase and excess ethanol. The NADH generated is then utilised by diaphorase to regenerate NAD^+ with simultaneous formation of a formazan dye. The dye accumulates, since each molecule of NAD^+ formed in the primary system is recycled many times, whilst the level of NAD^+ is not depleted. Typically, a 100-fold increase in absorbance can be obtained for the same amount of enzyme activity in the primary system. The primary and secondary systems may proceed simultaneously or sequentially (Self, 1985). This method has been shown to facilitate detecting 0·01 attomole of alkaline phosphatase and 0·4 attomole of thyroid stimulating hormone (Johannsson *et al.*, 1986). A slight problem with the system is that $NADP^+$ can also act as a substrate for alcohol dehydrogenase. This reaction must be minimised to avoid obtaining a high background. The system has the advantage of a colorimetric endpoint and has been used to develop more sensitive immunoassays of *Clostridium botulinum* toxins (Modi *et al.*, 1986).

In another amplification system, use was made of the blood-coagulation cascade (Blake *et al.*, 1984). Although originally used in a homogeneous enzyme immunoassay, it could be adapted to an immunometric assay, as

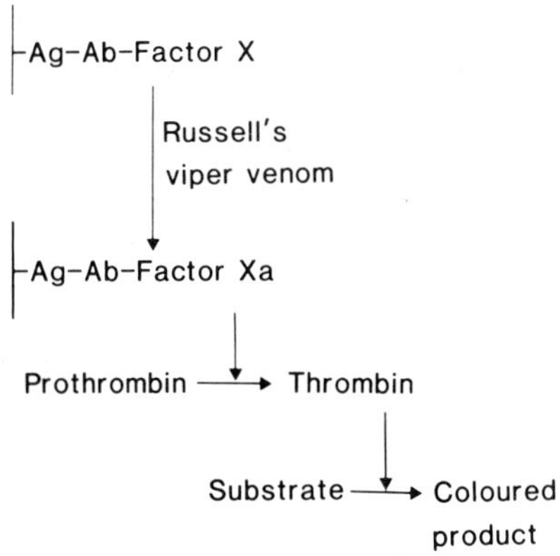

Fig. 7. Possible use of blood-coagulation cascade enzymes in immunometric assay.

shown in Fig. 7. Factor X is activated by a proteinase to factor Xa in an amount equivalent to the antigen concentration. Factor Xa drives two enzymically catalysed amplification steps which result in the formation of a coloured product. A potential problem with this type of assay is that depletion of one of the substrates is more likely to occur than with enzymic cycling.

Other methods for endpoint detection include radioactivity counting as used in 'ultrasensitive enzymatic radioimmunoassay' (USERIA) (Harris *et al.*, 1979). Tritium allows the development of sensitive assays and avoids the use of the potentially more hazardous ^{125}I. This system is illustrated in Fig. 8; immobilised alkaline phosphatase was used as the enzyme label and the substrate was tritiated adenosine monophosphate. The tritiated product,

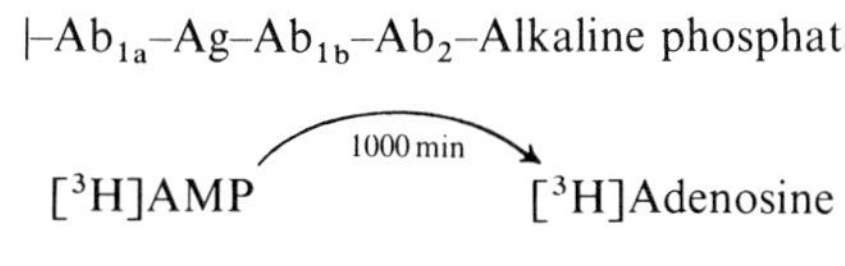

Separate [^{3}H]AMP and [^{3}H]Adenosine on DEAE Sephadex.
Count [^{3}H]Adenosine.
USERIA for cholera toxin 1000 × more sensitive than RIA and 100 × more sensitive than ELISA.
Detection limit 10^{-16} g *or* 600 molecules of cholera toxin.

Fig. 8. Ultrasensitive enzymatic radioimmunoassay (USERIA). Outline of combined enzyme and radioimmunoassay to give a very sensitive assay for cholera toxin.

adenosine, was separated from the substrate by ion-exchange chromatography and counted. When this assay was applied to the measurement of cholera toxin, using prolonged incubation, it became 100–1000 times more sensitive than the previously used RIA or ELISA. It was estimated that as few as 600 molecules of toxin could be detected by this method (Harris *et al.*, 1979).

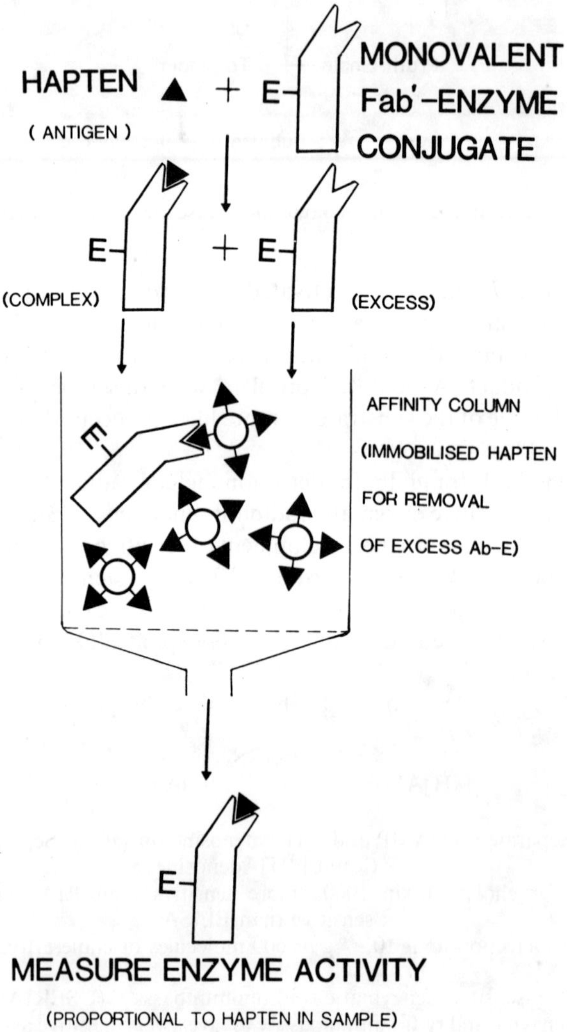

Fig. 9. Immunometric assay of haptens.

Another sensitive method of endpoint detection is to use enzymes as labels in conjunction with chemiluminescent substrates. Horseradish peroxidase catalyses the oxidation of luminol and, if this reaction takes place in the presence of an enhancer such as luciferin, photons are produced and measured in a luminometer (Whitehead *et al.*, 1983). If qualitative assays alone are satisfactory, the photon production system can be measured using high-speed photographic film (Thorpe *et al.*, 1984).

IMMUNOMETRIC ASSAYS FOR HAPTENS

A novel immunometric technique, termed 'affinity column mediated immunometric assay' (ACMIA), combines the advantages of an immunometric assay with a requirement for only a single antigenic site (Freytag *et al.*, 1984). It can therefore be used for haptens as well as for high molecular weight antigens (see Fig. 9). The technique uses $F_{(ab')_2}$ fragments, produced from IgG with pepsin, which are separated into two parts, giving monovalent-$F_{(ab')}$. This is then conjugated to enzyme. Excess enzyme-labelled $F_{(ab')}$ is incubated with a sample containing hapten and the mixture passed through an affinity column containing immobilised hapten in large excess. The column retains unreacted antibody but permits the enzyme-labelled antibody–hapten complex to pass through and be collected. Its enzyme activity is directly proportional to the original amount of hapten in the sample. Freytag *et al.* describe an assay for digoxin using this method, which enabled 10 pmol of this hapten to be measured in less than 7 min. This type of assay could be combined with the enhancement enzyme assays described above to produce very sensitive assays for haptens. A disadvantage of this method is the possibility of interfering materials in the specimen passing straight through the column with the enzyme-labelled antibody–antigen complex.

ROLE OF ULTRASENSITIVE IMMUNOASSAYS FOR VETERINARY AND FOOD ANALYSIS

This article has emphasised some ways of producing more sensitive EIA using enzymes. These are likely to be of practical value in immunoassays for toxins and residues, where low concentrations may be significant. They may also be useful if any analyte is greatly diluted during extraction or if non-specific (matrix) effects have to be diluted out to decrease background. The techniques discussed above may also be used to shorten assay time when this greater sensitivity is not necessary. This will be relevant for assays where the result is required urgently. These methods can also allow miniaturisation or aid the production of more convenient assay formats, thus enabling reagent costs to be reduced.

REFERENCES

Blake, C. & Gould, B. J. (1984) Use of enzymes in immunoassay techniques: a review. *Analyst*, **109**, 533–545.

Blake, D. A., Skarstedt, M. T., Shultz, J. L. & Wilson, D. P. (1984) Zymogen activation: a new system for homogeneous ligand-binding assay. *Clinical Chemistry*, **30**, 1452–1456.

Buckland, R. M. (1986) Strong signals from streptavidin–biotin. *Nature*, **320**, 557–558.

Dakubu, S., Ekins, R., Jackson, T. & Marshall, N. J. (1984) High sensitivity, pulsed-light time resolved fluoroimmunoassay. In: *Practical Immonoassay—the State of the Art*, Butt, W. R. (ed.), Marcel Dekker, Inc., New York, pp. 71–101.

Ekins, R. P. (1985) Current concepts and future developments. In: *Alternative Immunoassays*, Collins, W. P. (ed.), J. Wiley, Chichester, pp. 219–237.

Freytag, J. W., Dickinson, J. C. & Tseng, S. Y. (1984) A highly sensitive affinity-column-mediated immunometric assay, as exemplified by digoxin. *Clinical Chemistry*, **30**, 417–420.

Guesdon, J.-L., Ternynck, T. & Avremeas, S. (1979) The use of avidin–biotin interactions in immunoenzymatic techniques. *Journal of Histochemistry and Cytochemistry*, **27**, 1131–1139.

Harris, C. C., Yolken, R. H., Krokan, H. & Hsu, I. C. (1979) Ultrasensitive enzymatic radioimmunoassay: application to detection of cholera toxin and rotovirus. *Proceedings of the National Academy of Sciences, USA*, **76**, 5336–5339.

Jackson, T. M. & Ekins, R. P. (1986) Theoretical limitations on immunoassay sensitivity. *Journal of Immunological Methods*, **87**, 13–20.

Johannsson, A., Ellis, D. H., Bates, D. L., Plumb, A. M. & Stanley, C. J. (1986) Enzyme amplification for immunoassays. Detection limit of one hundredth of an attomole. *Journal of Immunological Methods*, **87**, 7–11.

Labrousse, H., Guesdon, J.-L., Ragimbeau, J. & Avremeas, S. (1982). Miniaturization of β-galactosidase immunoassays using chromogenic and fluorogenic substrates. *Journal of Immunological Methods*, **48**, 133–147.

Litchfield, W. J., Freytag, J. W. & Adamich, M. (1984) Highly sensitive immunoassays based on use of liposomes without complement. *Clinical Chemistry*, **30**, 1441–1445.

Modi, N. K., Shone, C. C., Hambleton, P. & Melling, J. (1986) Monoclonal antibody-based amplified enzyme-linked immunosorbent assays for *Clostridium botulinum* toxin types A and B. In: *Proceedings of 2nd World Congress Foodborne Infections and Intoxications*, Institute of Veterinary Medicine, Robert von Ostertag-Institute, Berlin (West), **2**, 1184–1188.

SELF, C. H. European Patent Application No. 0027036. Date of filing 2.10.80; date of publication of application 15.4.81. Assay method using enzymes as labelling substances.

SELF, C. H. (1985) Enzyme amplification—a general method applied to provide an immunoassisted assay for placental alkaline phosphatase. *Journal of Immunological Methods*, **76**, 389–393.

SHAH, H., SARANKO, A.-M., HÄRKÖNEN, M. & ADLERCREUTZ, H. (1984) Direct solid-phase fluoroimmunoassay of 5β-pregnane-3α,20α-diol-3α-glucuronide in urine. *Clinical Chemistry*, **30**, 185–187.

SHALEV, A., GREENBERG, A. H. & MCALPINE, P. J. (1980) Detection of attograms of antigen by a high sensitivity enzyme-linked immunosorbent assay (HS-ELISA) using a fluorogenic substrate. *Journal of Immunological Methods*, **38**, 125–139.

SHIELDS, J. G. & TURNER, M. W. (1986) The importance of antibody quality in sandwich ELISA systems. *Journal of Immunological Methods*, **87**, 29–33.

THORPE, G. H. G., WHITEHEAD, T. P., PENN, R. & KRICKA, L. J. (1984) Photographic monitoring of enhanced luminescent immunoassays. *Clinical Chemistry*, **30**, 806–807.

WHITEHEAD, T. P., THORPE, G. H. G., CARTER, T. J. N., GRONCUTT, C. & KRICKA, L. J. (1983) Enhanced luminescence procedure for sensitive determination of peroxidase-labelled conjugates in immunoassay. *Nature*, **305**, 158–159.

YOLKEN, R. H. & STOPA, P. J. (1979) Enzyme-linked fluorescence assay: ultrasensitive solid-phase assay for detection of human rotavirus. *Journal of Clinical Microbiology*, **10**, 317–321.

SESSION II

Veterinary Applications

6

The Need for Immunoassays in Disease Surveillance and Meat Hygiene within the State Veterinary Service

W. A. WATSON

Central Veterinary Laboratory, New Haw, Weybridge, Surrey, UK

INTRODUCTION

The State Veterinary Service in Great Britain has a staff of about 1350 and comprises the Field Service, the Veterinary Investigation Service and the Central Veterinary Laboratories (CVL). The former operates on a regional and divisional basis with primary responsibility for implementing the statutory controls for notifiable diseases, for import/export of animals and animal products, and for meat hygiene. It also has responsibility for animal welfare, the operation of the pig and poultry health schemes, and certain specific voluntary health schemes such as those for enzootic bovine leucosis and Maedi visna.

The Veterinary Investigation Service, with its national network of 19 laboratories, works closely with the CVL and Field Headquarters at Tolworth. Diagnostic and consultancy support is provided to the livestock industry through private veterinary surgeons in practice. It also provides laboratory facilities for some of the statutory work and there is a close involvement with the Public Health Laboratory Service in the diagnosis and control of zoonoses.

The Central Veterinary Laboratory at Weybridge is principally involved with the diagnosis of certain scheduled diseases, research into diseases of farm livestock, the provision of a diagnostic and consultancy support centre, and the import/export testing of animals and animal products. In addition, it is an international reference centre for brucellosis, Newcastle disease, avian influenza and many standardised diagnostic materials. The scope for the use of immunoassays is therefore considerable, especially in the areas of animal disease diagnosis and surveillance, and with implications for the zoonoses and for meat hygiene.

INFECTIOUS DISEASES

Although detailed data on the losses due to specific diseases are limited, the cost of disease to the livestock sectors of the agricultural industry in losses due to mortality are estimated to be approximately £400m out of a total annual output of £6000m. A major part of this is due to disease or accident, although the proportion preventable by the use of veterinary measures already available or measures which could be developed through R&D efforts is probably between £250m and £325m per annum. Further losses due to morbidity are difficult to calculate, but in cattle alone they are likely to approach the equivalent of 10% of a total output of £4310m. In addition, there are many 'knock-on' economic effects for the industry which are particularly important in the case of epidemic diseases.

All too often there is a failure by those responsible for funding animal disease research to appreciate the dynamic nature of animal disease and a tendency to adopt the attitude that once the resources have been set aside for a research programme and the work done, the problem is solved for good. It must be recognised that existing agents are constantly changing and new disease problems emerging, necessitating flexibility in the commitment of R&D funding and continuous progress in the development of improved methods for the identification of pathogens, disease diagnosis, monitoring, surveillance and control, many of which can and do involve immunoassays.

Over the years the State Veterinary Service has had major success in eradication of the most important epidemic diseases of livestock, such as sheep pox, rinderpest, rabies, bovine tuberculosis and most recently Aujeszky's disease. ELISA (Banks, 1983) and ELISA disc (Banks, 1985) techniques have been central to the eradication programme for Aujeszky's disease (Cartwright *et al.*, 1984), with many hundreds of thousands of sera examined. Nevertheless, extreme vigilance is required to prevent reintroduction of this and other diseases.

The vulnerability of our livestock industry (and the necessity for rapid immunoassays) has been clearly illustrated by the reintroduction of sheep scab in 1973 after 20 years of freedom, the introduction of foot and mouth disease to the Isle of Wight in 1981 (fortunately confined to a single outbreak), the occurrence of paramyxovirus 1 (PMV 1) as a pigeon variant in domestic poultry in 1983, and the reintroduction of classical swine fever in April 1986.

Other diseases not previously recognised in the UK but introduced in the

1970s, and which are diagnosed by immonoassay, include *Mycoplasma bovis* (see Thorns *et al.*, Chapter 7), swine vesicular disease (SVD) (Hamblin & Crowther, 1982), a more virulent strain of infectious bovine rhinotracheitis (Hebert *et al.*, 1985), enzootic bovine leucosis (Dawson, 1984; Perrin *et al.*, 1984) and Maedi visna (Houwers & Gielkens, 1979). Of these, only SVD has been eradicated.

The problems of rapid, specific and cost-effective diagnosis of a number of these diseases have been overcome by the use of immunoassays. For instance, collaboration between the Animal Virus Research Institute and the CVL has resulted in the development and evaluation of an ELISA for the detection of foot and mouth disease (McCullough *et al.*, 1985).

The avian PMV of the Newcastle disease type have required the use of a panel of monoclonal antibodies in an indirect immunoperoxidase test in order to differentiate between antigenically distinct groups and to define the episode of disease caused by PMV1 (Alexander, 1985).

Existing notifiable diseases are not easy to eradicate and the programmes for bovine tuberculosis and brucellosis have been long and expensive, firstly with the voluntary establishment of accredited herds, followed by compulsory eradication. A specific IgG and IgM ELISA is of particular value in detecting brucella antibody in pregnant cattle before a response to traditional tests such as Rose Bengal, serum agglutination, or complement fixation develops (Rylatt *et al.*, 1985). An important part of the warble fly eradication programme is the detection of antibodies to *Hypoderma* species in cattle by ELISA (Sinclair *et al.*, 1983). The wildlife reservoir of bovine tuberculosis in badgers in the South West remains a difficult problem with spill-over of infection to cattle. For diagnosis of the disease in cattle an ELISA is now in use which is capable of resolving non-specific reactors to the tuberculin test. Considerable improvements are also being made in the diagnosis and control of bovine *Leptospira* infections due to the development and use of immunofluorescent analysis (Stevens *et al.*, 1985) and a specific ELISA.

The production of monoclonal antibodies to the K88 and K99 fimbrial adhesins produced by some strains of *E. coli* has led to the development of slide agglutination tests widely used for routine identification of enteropathogenic *E. coli* (Morris *et al.*, 1985; Thorns *et al.*, 1987). The detection of toxic products of pathogenic bacteria rather than the infectious agent itself has resulted in the use of an ELISA for *Clostridium perfringens* epsilon toxin (see Thorns *et al.*, Chapter 7).

It is self-evident that as progress is made towards the eradication of any disease the low incidence of infection makes detection more difficult and costly. There is, therefore, a need for more sensitive, specific and cheaper tests (Harkness, 1985), especially if these can be automated.

In the field of virological identification and diagnosis many traditional techniques have been, or are being, replaced by immunoassays. ELISA is now used instead of tissue culture to confirm infection and to complement electron microscopy (Reynolds *et al.*, 1984) for the diagnosis of rotavirus (Coulson & Holmes, 1984) and coronavirus (Crouch *et al.*, 1984). An ELISA screening procedure is being developed to replace the EEC approved agar gel immunodiffusion test (Bau *et al.*, 1984) for the detection of enzootic bovine leucosis in bulk milk samples.

Parasitological uses of ELISA currently include an *Eimeria* specific assay (Sinclair *et al.*, 1983) to study coccidial infection and the transfer of maternal antibody in lambs (Nolan *et al.*, 1987). The monitoring of sarcocystic infection which is increasingly being associated with reproductive failure in sheep is also being carried out with the aid of ELISAs.

At the present time the most important endemic infectious disease problems are as follows: in cattle, respiratory and enteric disease and salmonellosis, especially *Salmonella typhimurium* and mastitis; in pigs, respiratory and enteric disease, especially swine dysentery; in sheep, enteric and respiratory disease, particularly pasteurellosis and ovine abortion, especially due to chlamydiosis and toxoplasmosis; in poultry, respiratory disease, particularly infectious bronchitis and turkey rhinotracheitis.

Suitable immunoassays are required for the diagnosis and monitoring of many of these disease problems and will be an essential part of future programmes of disease surveillance.

MEAT HYGIENE

In comparison with many developed countries, Britain has been slow to introduce improvements in the slaughter, inspection and processing of farm livestock. However, certain events have brought changes in the last few years:

1. Entry into the EEC with common requirements for intracommunity trade and the introduction of community legislation covering trade from Third World countries for red meat and poultry meat, and specific standards for export-approved slaughterhouses.
2. Improved markets, particularly in Europe, and others which are now opening up in the Middle East, North American and Far East.

3. Consumer pressures, first developing in continental Europe and now more evident here in respect of a wide range of environmental issues and more particularly residue-free food.
4. Concentration of the market in the hands of a small number of large marketing companies wishing to supply products of a standard quality to meet consumer demands and with a long shelf-life.
5. Public interest in the welfare of livestock during transport, handling and slaughter.

The export market in red meat and poultry meat is now valued at £779m and that for meat products at £308m. The slaughter, processing and marketing of livestock has undergone rapid changes. Although meat inspection responsibilities still rest with local authorities, there is increased central involvement by the Veterinary Service working through local veterinary inspectors and official veterinary surgeons.

Both the Food Science Division and the State Veterinary Service of the Ministry of Agriculture, Fisheries and Food are involved in the National Scheme for Residues in Meat, testing for antimicrobials and growth promoter residues, many of which are screened by immunoassays (see Calverley *et al.*, Chapter 8). Some importing countries have introduced very specific certification requirements such as testing for trichinosis, but particularly for antimicrobials and growth promoters.

In order to meet the increased requirements of both the EEC and the National Surveillance Scheme for residues in meat in a climate of decreased human, laboratory and financial resources, cheaper screening procedures with high throughput have been developed such as RIAs for zeranol (Dixon & Mallinson, 1986), diethylstilboestrol (Bates *et al.*, 1985; see Calverley *et al.*, Chapter 8), and trenbolone and ELISAs for chloramphenicol and aflatoxin (Jackman, 1985). Similar immunoassays are under development for other antimicrobial substances such as sulphonamides, penicillins, tetracyclins, streptomycin and cephalosporins.

DIAGNOSTIC TESTS AND SURVEILLANCE

Diagnostic tests must be simple to use with the minimum of training, rapid, easy to read and interpret, and have good reproducibility. They must also be developed to replace the use of experimental animals in laboratory diagnosis and in quality control procedures in the pharmaceutical industry. Some problems still remain to be resolved in their use for disease surveillance as developing techniques have not kept pace with the present needs.

In addition, disease problems in farm livestock are increasingly being recognised as multi-factorial and complex, and outbreaks can seldom be attributed to individual pathogens. Not only do the host, pathogen, nutritional and environmental aspects interact but also a wide variety of infectious agents, particularly those associated with respiratory and enteric syndromes. Because of this, a word of caution must be aimed at enthusiasts for penside tests. It is often difficult enough to develop a suitable test for a specific agent, but much more difficult to interpret the significance of the results obtained, not only in the context of the animal tested but particularly the population at risk. Without adequate attention to interpretation and correct diagnosis on a herd basis, many results will be misinterpreted and much harm will be done.

IMMUNOASSAYS—FUTURE REQUIREMENTS AND POTENTIAL DEVELOPMENTS

More reliable diagnostic techniques are required for tuberculosis in cattle and if possible in the badger using either serum samples or improved, more specific tuberculins.

A more sensitive and specific test is needed for *Mycobacterium johnei* infection in cattle and sheep to replace the complement fixation test.

Immunoassays are required to assist in the identification and differentiation of mycoplasmas, ureaplasmas, acholeplasmas and spiroplasmas.

Better methods are needed for the differentiation of *Chlamydia psittaci* isolates from animals and birds, and to establish the importance of these infections, particularly in sheep, poultry and cattle. In addition, their epidemiological patterns and sources of infection to humans require study as well as improvement in the available vaccines.

More specific *Leptospira* immunoassays are required to facilitate the differentiation between subgroups and the epidemiological study of this zoonosis. Improved diagnostic methods for swine dysentery to establish herds free from infection need to be developed.

Immunoassays could also be used to improve the diagnosis of mastitis and for epidemiological studies of the disease.

Suitable techniques could assist in the diagnosis of sheep scab in infected flocks and improve epidemiological information and control.

There is an urgent need for immunoassays for antibiotic residue detection, especially to meet export certification requirements and to assess risk to both animal and public health.

CONCLUSIONS

The importance of immunoassays has been clearly recognised by the Veterinary Service for many aspects of its work. Some such tests have been developed and evaluated at the Central Veterinary Laboratory, and are at a stage where they could be taken up by commercial laboratories. Conversely, other commercially developed immunoassays could be used by the Veterinary Service, providing they are not too expensive. Closer collaboration with immunoassay kit manufacturers is desirable for the development and use of immunoassays in the future.

REFERENCES

ALEXANDER, D. J. (1985) Advances in the diagnosis of Newcastle disease. In: *Veterinary Viral Diseases: Their Significance in Southeast Asia and the Western Pacific*, Della Porta, A. J. (ed.), Academic Press, New York, pp. 317–325.

BANKS, M. (1983) Rapid ELISA for Aujeszky's disease eradication. *Veterinary Record*, **113**, 94–95.

BANKS, M. (1985) Detection of antibodies to Aujeszky's disease virus in whole blood by ELISA disc. *Journal of Virological Methods*, **12**, 41–45.

BATES, M. L., WARWICK, M. J., SHEARER, G., HARWOOD, D. J., HERRIMAN, I. D., HEITZMAN, R. J. & WATSON, D. H. (1985) Distribution of diethylstilboestrol in pigs. *Journal of the Science of Food and Agriculture*, **36**, 31–36.

BAU, T., WIEGAND, D. & MANZ, D. (1984) Comparative serological investigations with blood and milk samples for diagnosis of enzootic leucosis in cattle using AGIDT and ELISA. *Tierärztliche Wochenschrift*, **91**, 313–317.

CARTWRIGHT, S. F., BANKS, M. & FLOWERS, M. (1984) Laboratory involvement in the Aujeszky's disease eradication programme in England and Wales. *8th International Pig Veterinary Society Proceedings*, Ghent, Belgium, August 27–31, 1984, International Pig Veterinary Society, Ghent, p. 42.

COULSON, B. S. & HOLMES, I. H. (1984) An improved ELISA for the detection of rotavirus in faeces of neonates. *Journal of Virological Methods*, **8**, 165–179.

CROUCH, C. F., RAYBOULD, T. J. G. & ACRES, S. D. (1984) Monoclonal antibody capture ELISA for detection of bovine enteric coronavirus. *Journal of Clinical Microbiology*, **19**, 388–393.

DAWSON, M. (1984) Development and assessment of an avidin–biotin ELISA for bovine leucosis virus antibodies in milk. In: *5th International Symposium on Bovine Leucosis*, Straub, O. C. (ed.), Edinburgh, September 13–14, 1983, Commission of the European Communities, Luxembourg, p. 147.

DIXON, S. N. & MALLINSON, C. B. (1986) RIA of the anabolic agent zeranol. III: Zeranol concentrations in the faeces of steers implanted with zeranol (Ralgro). *Journal of Veterinary Pharmacology and Therapeutics*, **9**, 88–93.

HAMBLIN, C. & CROWTHER, J. R. (1982) A rapid ELISA for the serological confirmation of swine vesicular disease. *British Veterinary Journal*, **138**, 247–252.

HARKNESS, J. W. (1985) Classical swine fever and its diagnosis: a current view. *Veterinary Record*, **116**, 288–293.

HEBERT, C. N., EDWARDS, S., BUSHNELL, S., JONES, P. C. & PERRY, C. T. (1985) Establishment of a statistical base for the use of ELISA in diagnostic serology for infectious bovine rhinotracheitis. *Journal of Biological Standardisation*, **13**, 243–253.

HOUWERS, D. J. & GIELKENS, A. L. J. (1979) An ELISA for the detection of maedi visna antibody. *Veterinary Record*, **65**, 680–684.

JACKMAN, R. (1985) Determinations of aflatoxins by ELISA with special reference to aflatoxin M_1 in raw milk. *Journal of the Science of Food and Agriculture*, **36**, 685–698.

McCULLOUGH, K. C., CROWTHER, J. R. & BUTCHER, R. N. (1985) A liquid phase ELISA and its use in the identification of epitopes on foot and mouth disease virus antigens. *Journal of Virological Methods*, **11**, 329–338.

MORRIS, J. A., THORNS, C. J., BOARER, C. D. H. & WILSON, R. A. (1985) Evaluation of a monoclonal antibody to the K99 fimbrial adhesin produced by *Escherichia coli* enterotoxigenic for calves, lambs and piglets. *Research in Veterinary Science*, **39**, 75–79.

NOLAN, A., GOLDRING, O. L., CATCHPOLE, J., GREGORY, M. W. & JOINER, P. (1987) Demonstration of antibodies to *Eimeria* species in lambs by an ELISA. *Research in Veterinary Science*, **42**, 119–123.

PERRIN, B., PERRIN, M. & FEDIDA, M. (1984) The detection of enzootic bovine leucosis. The ELISA test. *Bulletin d'Information des Laboratoires des Services Veterinaires*, **15/16**, 37–41.

REYNOLDS, D. J., CHASEY, D., SCOTT, A. C. & BRIDGES, J. C. (1984) Evaluation of ELISA and electron microscopy for the detection of coronavirus and rotavirus in bovine faeces. *Veterinary Record*, **114**, 397–401.

RYLATT, D. B., WYATT, D. M. & BUNDESEN, P. G. (1985) A competitive enzyme immunoassay for the detection of bovine antibodies to *Brucella abortus* using monoclonal antibodies. *Veterinary Immunology and Immunopathology*, **8**, 261–271.

SINCLAIR, I. J., TARRY, D. W. & WASSALL, D. A. (1983) Persistance of antibody in calves after an infection with *Hypoderma bovis*. *Research in Veterinary Science*, **37**, 383–384.

STEVENS, A. E., HEADLAM, S. A., PRITCHARD, D. G., THORNS, C. J. & MORRIS, J. A. (1985) Monoclonal antibodies for diagnosis of infection with *Leptospira interrogans* serovar *hardjo* by immunofluorescence. *Veterinary Record*, **116**, 593–594.

THORNS, C. J., BOARER, C. D. H. & MORRIS, J. A. (1987) Production and evaluation of monoclonal antibodies directed against the K88 fimbrial adhesin produced by *Escherichia coli* enterotoxigenic for piglets. *Research in Veterinary Science*, **43**, 233–238.

7

Monoclonal Antibodies in the Diagnosis of Infectious Diseases

C. J. THORNS, A. NOLAN, C. D. H. BOARER and P. L. ROEDER

Central Veterinary Laboratory, New Haw, Weybridge, Surrey, UK

INTRODUCTION

In the eleven years since Kohler & Milstein (1975) first developed the technology to produce monoclonal antibodies (MAbs) by means of *in vitro* hybridoma systems, their impact in many areas of human and veterinary medical research has been considerable; yet the advances made in the research laboratory have been slow to find application in the immunodiagnosis of infectious diseases, although progress has been most evident in the diagnosis of human infections (Nowinski *et al.*, 1983; Macario & Conway de Macario, 1984; Brooks & York, 1985; Pereira, 1985) and animal viral diseases (Forman, 1985).

MONOCLONAL AND POLYCLONAL ANTIBODIES IN IMMUNOASSAY

The arguments for using MAbs in immunoassays have been extensively reviewed (Macario & Conway de Macario, 1984; Allen, 1985). The production and adequate characterisation of MAbs is laborious, labour-intensive and thus expensive, at least in the short term. The benefits to be gained from specificity, homogeneity and indefinite availability must be balanced against the constraints of economics; currently most commercially available MAbs are more expensive than polyclonal reagents. Enthusiasm for MAb technology must not be allowed to encourage the replacement of all polyclonal reagents with MAbs, since both have their uses. The broader spectrum reactivity of polyclonal reagents may even be preferable in some circumstances, for example as capture antibodies in antigen detection assays, whereas MAbs are used to probe for individual epitopes. The property of exquisite specificity offered by MAbs, whilst essential for the precise definition of an infectious agent, may itself be a disadvantage in primary diagnosis, unless the epitope recognised is common to all antigenic variants of the agent, as illustrated for classical swine fever virus by van Zaane (1984). The specificity of an assay may be tailored by selection of the MAb and the search to find an appropriate MAb may be a long one. It is essential that candidate MAbs are evaluated in assays to detect reactivity relevant to the formulation of the assay being developed, as this can markedly alter the apparent epitope detection (McCullough *et al.*, 1985).

Brooks & York (1985) emphasised the importance of the predictive value of an assay in disease diagnosis. For a new immunodiagnostic assay, developed with a 95% sensitivity and specificity, the predictive value of a positive test is highly dependent on the prevalence of the disease (Galen & Gambino, 1975). If the prevalence of the disease is low, the predictive value is low and the individual cost of a positive diagnosis is prohibitively high. However, if subpopulations can be defined such that the prevalence of the disease approaches 50%, the predictive value of a positive test rises to 95%, which then becomes cost-effective. Thus, in the case of a disease of low incidence where positive results are obtained infrequently, even a considerable expected improvement in assay efficiency may not justify the cost of producing MAb reagents. Future economic constraints must affect the type of and rate at which new diagnostic assays (many of which will use MAbs) are applied in the veterinary field.

DETECTION OF AN INFECTIOUS AGENT OR ITS PRODUCTS

The most rapid method available for the primary diagnosis of infection is the detection and identification of antigens either directly in tissues and body fluids or after isolation in culture. Antigens can be identified directly by immunofluorescence, immunoperoxidase and electron microscopy (using colloidal gold labelled antibodies) or indirectly using such techniques as ELISA and agglutination of the agent or antibody-coated particles. MAbs have been used successfully in all these assays.

Several characteristics are desirable when selecting MAbs for this use:

(a) high affinity for antigen—this enables detection of low antigen concentrations and can displace host antibody in biopsy material;

(b) direction towards repeating epitopes allows detection of low concentrations of antigen;
(c) direction towards epitopes not seen by the host avoids antigen 'masking' by host antibody;
(d) IgM antibodies have a greater avidity than those of the IgG class—this may increase assay sensitivity (Wands *et al.*, 1981);
(e) direction towards non-carbohydrate determinants of viral glycosylated polypeptides as carbohydrate determinants can be influenced by the host cell in which the virus replicates (Klenk & Rott, 1980).

Mycobacteria

The traditional ways of detecting and identifying mycobacteria rely on biological, cultural and biochemical techniques. Although a combination of these can detect low numbers of organisms, the procedures are slow and expensive. Studies using MAbs indicate that many *Mycobacterium bovis* antigens contain epitopes common to other micro-organisms and even host tissue (Thorns & Morris, 1985, 1986). Table 1 illustrates some of these cross-reactions.

For this reason, the production of specific antisera has proved problematical and their use in detecting and serotyping mycobacteria has been largely unsuccessful. In our laboratory MAbs have been produced to *M. bovis*-specific epitopes (Morris *et al.*, 1985*a*) and these are currently being evaluated for use in assays designed to detect *M. bovis* antigen directly in tissues and body fluids or after culture *in vitro* (Fig. 1). MAbs have been used successfully to detect *M. avium* in the body fluids of AIDS patients (Kolk, A. H., 1985, pers. comm.).

Table 1
Common Antigens of Mycobacteria defined by Monoclonal Antibodies raised against *Mycobacterium bovis*

	Groups of common antigens				
	a	*b*	*c*	*d*	*e*
Mycobacteria and related genera	+	+	+	+	+
Other bacteria	−	+	+	+	−
Parasites	−	−	−	+	−
Fungi	−	−	−	+	−
Host tissue	−	−	+	+	+

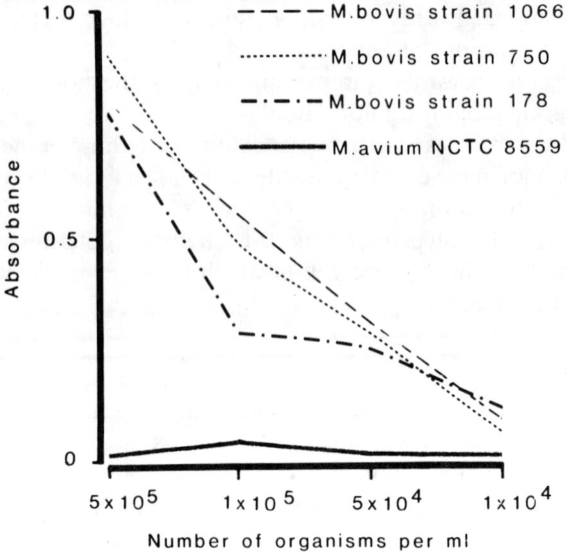

Fig. 1. Sensitivity of a MAb-based ELISA in detecting heat-killed mycobacteria grown in Middlebrook's 7H11 liquid medium.

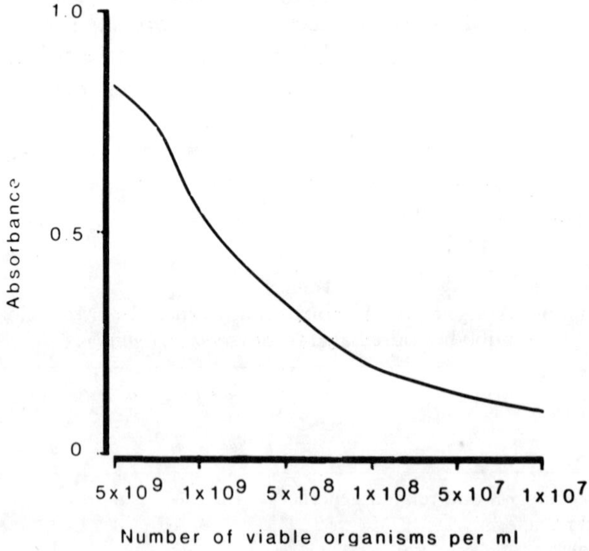

Fig. 2. Detection of K88 fimbrial adhesin in faeces of a piglet infected with enterotoxigenic *Escherichia coli* K88 was captured by polyclonal monospecific K88 antiserum and detected with enzyme-labelled K88 MAb.

E. coli

MAbs directed against the K88 and K99 fimbrial adhesins produced by certain enteropathogenic strains of *Escherichia coli* (Morris *et al.*, 1985*b*; Thorns *et al.*, 1987) have replaced polyclonal antisera in the slide agglutination test for routine identification in many laboratories. These same MAbs can be used in immunoperoxidase staining of gut tissue for the direct diagnosis of colibacillosis in piglets.

Mills & Tietze (1984) have used an antigen capture ELISA to detect K99 positive *E. coli* isolates using a MAb against a repeating epitope on the adhesin. The nature of the epitope recognised enables the same MAb to be used for capture and detection with a sensitivity as low as $3{\cdot}5 \times 10^5$ bacteria per millilitre. Similar techniques have been applied in our laboratory to the detection of K88 and K99 antigens in faeces. The results indicate a good correlation with conventional isolation and adhesin identification (Fig. 2). An assay for K99 detection in faeces based on the same principle is commercially available (Coli-Tect ™99, Molecular Genetics Inc., USA) and is formulated for field use.

Bacterial Toxins

In addition to the antigens comprising the agents themselves, it is also feasible to detect their toxic products. One assay for the heat labile toxin produced by enteropathogenic strains of *E. coli* relies on capturing toxin with GM1 ganglioside and detecting its binding with a MAb (Svennerholm, A. M., pers. comm.). A sandwich assay with signal amplification detects *Clostridium botulinum* Type A toxin with high sensitivity (Shone *et al.*, 1985), and in our laboratory we have produced a monoclonal antibody which neutralises the biological activity of *C. perfringens* epsilon toxin in the mouse protection test and is capable of detecting the toxin when used in ELISA (Fig. 3).

Leptospira

MAbs have recently been applied to the diagnosis of *Leptospira interrogans* serovar *hardjo* infection by immunofluorescent analysis of clinical specimens (Stevens *et al.*, 1985).

Viruses

From the foregoing it is clear that the combined use of MAb and enzyme immunoassay methods is increasingly finding application in the detection of antigens, frequently directly in clinical samples (Yolken, 1985), maximal sensitivity being achieved by assays which capture antigen on to the solid phase (Moudallal *et al.*, 1984). Rapid and sensitive MAb capture ELISAs,

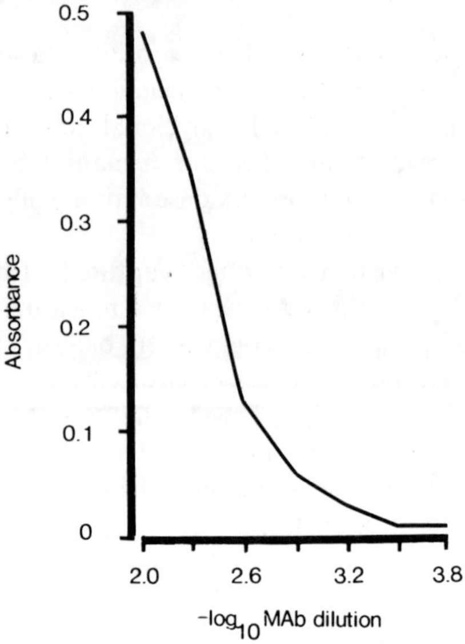

Fig. 3. Reactivity of neutralising MAb against *C. perfringens* epsilon toxin in antigen capture ELISA.

suitable for testing large numbers of faeces samples, have been developed for bovine coronavirus (Crouch *et al.*, 1984) and canine parvovirus (Mildbrand *et al.*, 1984). The latter assay employs two MAbs directed against different epitopes of the specific haemagglutinin. This enables the simultaneous addition of test sample and enzyme-conjugated MAb and allows completion of the test within 30 min. Clinical studies revealed 95% correlation between ELISA and haemagglutination detection. A similar assay described for the detection of infectious bovine rhinotracheitis (IBR) virus in nasal swabbings was, however, less sensitive than conventional virus isolation techniques (Collins *et al.*, 1985).

MONOCLONAL ANTIBODY TYPING PANELS

One recent development of significance is the international collaboration which is providing panels of monoclonal antibodies for 'finger-printing' closely related viruses. Typing by this method is a powerful tool which reveals subtle differences between isolates and, although embryonic at present, is providing data of profound epidemiological significance in several important areas of animal disease.

Until recently it seemed that rabies viruses were all very similar but the use of a large panel of monoclonal antibodies directed against nucleocapsid antigens in immunofluorescent assays not only differentiates between classical rabies and rabies-related viruses, such as Mokola, Duvenhage and Lagos bat viruses, but even defines types within closely related classical rabies viruses (King, A. & Crick, J., pers. comm.; Wiktor *et al.*, 1980). This approach is being used to investigate the epidemiology of bat rabies which is currently causing concern in Europe and to explore the likely efficacy of available vaccines.

The control of foot and mouth disease in many countries relies heavily on the use of vaccines but the virus exists as seven types with more than 60 subtypes being recognised. Cross-protection is variable and for a serviceable degree of protection to be obtained the vaccine virus strains must be matched accurately to field strains. This is extremely laborious and slow using reciprocal neutralisation assays as currently practised. A novel approach to strain differentiation, necessary both for vaccine matching and epidemiological studies, uses panels of monoclonal antibodies in an indirect sandwich ELISA. This has been applied so far to the O and A virus types with promising results (Crowther, J. R., 1986, pers. comm.).

The upsurge in incidents of classical swine fever in Europe has given new incentive to refining diagnostic methodology. Several European laboratories are including in their approach the production of monoclonal antibodies to both classical swine fever virus and the related bovine viral diarrhoea virus which is capable of infecting pigs and complicating diagnostic procedures (Harkness, J. W., 1986, pers. comm.). The typing panel approach may again help to clarify a complex disease epidemiology and improve the precision of diagnostic methods.

The avian paramyxoviruses (PMV) were one of the first groups of agents to yield to this approach. What had seemed by conventional serological techniques to be an antigenically homologous Newcastle disease virus group was differentiated into eight distinct antigenic groupings of PMVs, each with shared biological and epidemiological properties, by the use of nine monoclonal antibodies in an indirect immunoperoxidase test (Russell & Alexander, 1983). Subsequently the use of this test proved to be valuable in defining the episode of this disease in pigeons in Britain caused by PMV1 (Alexander, 1985).

Terpstra *et al.* (1985) have produced a panel of 13 MAbs to serovars of *Leptospira interrogans* which allows the classification of almost all serovars of the Sejroe group. The epidemiological significance of subgroup classification of rotavirus isolates can now be investigated using MAbs directed against the subgroup-specific proteins (Greenberg *et al.*, 1983).

ANTIBODY DETECTION

With the advent of MAbs it has become possible to dissect, with relative ease, the individual components of the polyclonal antibody response by allowing antibodies in the test sample to compete with a MAb for the single epitope against which it is directed. Certain general considerations apply when using MAbs in blocking/competition assays and these include the following:

(a) The degree of competition will be affected by the relative affinity of the antibody response. It is not practicable to determine this for each test sample but MAb of very high or low affinity should be avoided as these may give spuriously low or high antibody estimations respectively.
(b) Specificity for an immunodominant epitope as seen by the infected animal is essential.
(c) For most applications the MAb selected should compete with antibodies produced by the animal throughout the course of infection. This is not always possible but a deficit in this respect can be compensated for by using a panel of MAbs to detect antibodies produced at different stages of infection.

The central problem in developing a serodiagnostic test for bovine tuberculosis in cattle and badgers is that of differentiating the antibody response to *M. bovis*-specific epitopes from that induced by highly conserved microbial epitopes. Healthy animals and those infected with agents other than *M. bovis* may possess antibodies which react with antigen preparations currently employed in serological assays for bovine tuberculosis (Morris & Thorns, 1985). Using MAbs an *M. bovis*-specific antibody response has been detected in naturally and experimentally infected calves, but no single MAb was able to detect all infected animals. It may be necessary, therefore, to use a battery of specific MAb probes to increase the sensitivity of the assay (Thorns, unpublished data), as in the approach to the diagnosis of leprosy and human tuberculosis (Ivanyi *et al.*, 1983; Sina *et al.*, 1983). A MAb-based competition ELISA for detecting bovine antibody to *Brucella abortus* has been shown to be more selective and sensitive than conventional complement fixation or agglutination procedures (Rylatt *et al.*, 1985).

As with foot and mouth disease virus the detection of infection with bluetongue virus is complicated by the existence of multiple serotypes. Group-specific gel precipitation tests are relatively insensitive and type-

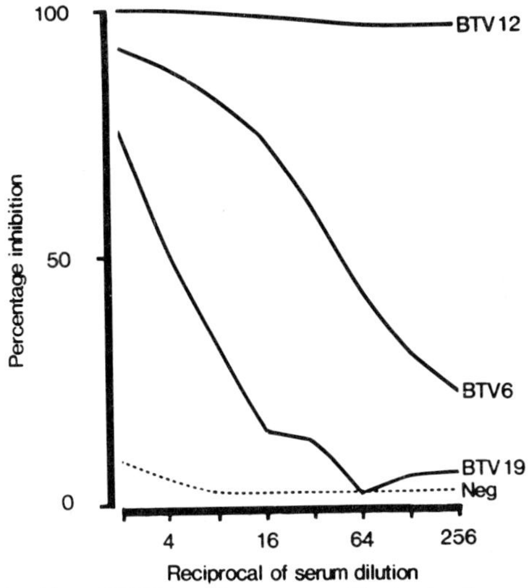

Fig. 4. MAb blocking ELISA. Three sera illustrate the range of reactions obtained with hyperimmune guinea pig sera raised against all 22 types of bluetongue virus. A negative serum control is included. Data by courtesy of J. Anderson.

specific neutralisation assays are extremely laborious and expensive to perform. Anderson (1984) has overcome these problems by developing and validating a blocking ELISA which uses a MAb directed against a group-specific antigen. It is interesting to note that only one of the 24 candidate MAbs which showed group reactivity was suitable for use in the assay. The others tested, although able to react to high levels in an indirect ELISA, were not substantially inhibited even by high concentrations of positive sera. The ELISA has proved sensitive and specific for the detection of group-specific ovine, bovine and guinea pig antibodies. Antibody to all 22 serotypes of BTV resulted in high levels of inhibition of the MAb reactivity with bluetongue virus antigen whereas antisera to epizootic haemorrhagic disease viruses (an arbovirus closely related to bluetongue virus) gave little or no inhibition even at low serum dilutions (Fig. 4). It should now be possible to standardise bluetongue virus serodiagnosis between laboratories.

In contrast, the use of MAbs specific for the haemagglutinins of two different isolates of avian PMV1 in haemagglutination inhibition assays clearly differentiates between infections with the closely related pigeon and classical isolates of PMV1 (Collins, M. & Alexander, D. J., 1986, pers. comm.).

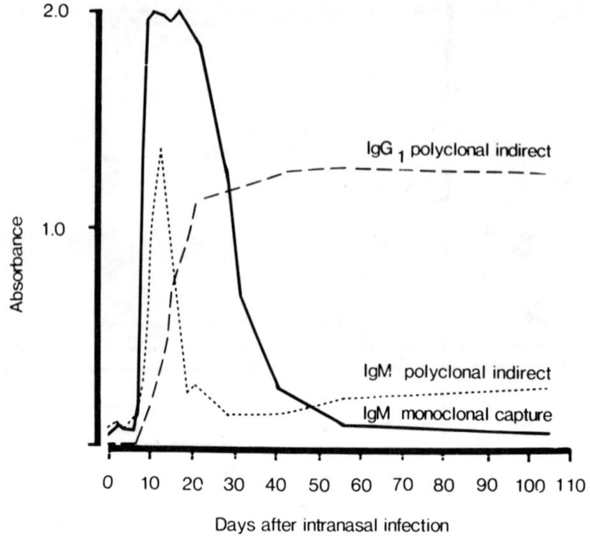

Fig. 5. Primary serological response of a calf to IBR virus infection as measured by ELISA. Data by courtesy of S. Edwards.

As in antigen detection, the use of two MAbs directed against different epitopes of the same antigen can increase the speed of performance of an assay by reducing the number of steps required in an ELISA. Houwers & Wensvoort (1986) have used this principle to design antibody assays to detect infection with classical swine fever virus in pigs and Maedi visna virus in sheep. Their novel 'complex trapping blocking' ELISA uses plates coated with one MAb followed by the simultaneous addition of antigen and test serum diluted appropriately. After a short incubation the second MAb (conjugated) is added for a further incubation. After washing, the addition of substrate reveals the presence of antibody in the test sample by the inhibition of binding of the labelled MAb.

Also contributing to the refinement of serodiagnostic assays is the use of MAbs produced against immunoglobulins to provide immunoglobulin class-specific tests. Class-specific MAbs made in our laboratory to bovine immunoglobulins are being evaluated in several applications. An antibovine IgG is being used in an ELISA designed to detect antibodies to *Brucella abortus* in milk and serum samples. Preliminary results indicate that the MAb shows a higher specificity and sensitivity than the commercially-available polyclonal antiglobulins used previously (MacMillan, A., 1986, pers. comm.). Similarly, another MAb specific for

IgM is being evaluated as a capture antibody for the detection of primary antibody responses to IBR virus infection. Again results indicate a greater sensitivity than that obtained with polyclonal reagents (Edwards, S., 1986, pers. comm.; Fig. 5).

SECONDARY APPLICATIONS

Besides being used directly in diagnostic assays, MAbs provide useful tools for the purification of individual antigens by immunoaffinity chromatography (Young, 1985). Such preparations may be used to improve the performance of immunoassays for a number of infectious diseases. However, the supply of antigens purified in this way will always be limited and the cloning and expression of microbial genes in an appropriate host is seen as a major breakthrough in the production of purified proteins. The identification and purification of expression products from cloned DNA can be achieved using MAbs. In our laboratory, *M. bovis* proteins produced by recombinant DNA technology at Surrey University and immunoaffinity purified are being evaluated as potential skin test reagents for the diagnosis of bovine tuberculosis in cattle.

Being of uniform specificity, MAbs can be used relatively easily to prepare anti-idiotype antibodies, some of which should theoretically behave structurally as an 'internal image' of the original antigen (Thanavala *et al.*, 1985) with potential for use as surrogate antigens in immunodiagnostic tests. The production of monoclonal surrogate antigens in this way is an attractive proposition since it would make available a virtually unlimited supply of a standardised reagent (Potocnjak *et al.*, 1982; Mitchell *et al.*, 1983). This approach is being applied in our laboratory to the diagnosis of bovine tuberculosis in an attempt to provide novel reagents for use in skin tests and other diagnostic assays.

CONCLUSION

Clearly some MAbs are already making a significant impact on the diagnosis of infectious animal disease and this will surely increase as more MAbs become available.

It is to be hoped that the general lack of research funding and the incentives to commercialise will not inhibit the intra- and international cooperation which has allowed the exchange of MAb reagents essential for the assembly of panels of antibodies for agent typing. As the antigenic components of numerous infectious agents become progressively defined and electrophoretic and immunoblotting techniques enable the precise characterisation of MAb reactivity, it should become commonplace to design immunoassays of appropriate specificity with relative ease.

ACKNOWLEDGEMENTS

We would like to record our grateful thanks to numerous colleagues who have given permission for us to refer to work in progress.

REFERENCES

ALEXANDER, D. J. (1985) Advances in the diagnosis of Newcastle Disease. In: *Veterinary Viral Diseases: Their Significance in South-east Asia and the Western Pacific*, Della-Porta, A. J. (ed.), Academic Press, New York, pp. 317–325.

ALLEN, J. (1985) Immunodiagnostics in clinical microbiology. In: *Rapid Detection and Identification of Infectious Agents*, Kingsbury, D. T. & Falkow, S. (eds), Academic Press, New York, pp. 279–292.

ANDERSON, J. (1984) Use of monoclonal antibody in a blocking ELISA to detect group specific antibodies to bluetongue virus. *Journal of Immunological Methods*, **74**, 139–149.

BROOKS, G. F. & YORK, M. K. (1985) Technological advances in the clinical microbiology laboratory: sensitivity, specificity and cost effectiveness. In: *Rapid Detection and Identification of Infectious Agents*, Kingsbury, D. T. & Falkow, S. (eds), Academic Press, New York, pp. 3–17.

COLLINS, J. K., BUTCHER, A. C., TERAMOTO, Y. A. & WINSTON, S. (1985) Rapid detection of bovine herpesvirus type 1 antigens in nasal swab specimens with an antigen capture enzyme-linked immunosorbent assay. *Journal of Clinical Microbiology*, **21**, 375–380.

CROUCH, C. F., RAYBOULD, T. J. G. & ACRES, S. D. (1984) Monoclonal antibody capture enzyme-linked immunosorbent assay for detection of bovine enteric coronavirus. *Journal of Clinical Microbiology*, **19**, 388–393.

FORMAN, A. J. (1985) Diagnosis of virus diseases of veterinary importance. In: *Veterinary Viral Diseases: Their Significance in South-east Asia and the Western Pacific*, Della-Porta, A. J. (ed.), Academic Press, New York, pp. 49–52.

GALEN, R. S. & GAMBINO, S. R. (1975) In: *Beyond Normality: The Predictive Value and Efficiency of Medical Diagnosis*, Wiley, New York.

GREENBERG, H., MCAULIFFE, V., VALDESUSO, J., WYATT, R., FLORES, J., KALICA, A., HOSHINO, Y. & SINGH, N. (1983) Serological analysis of the subgroup protein of rotavirus, using monoclonal antibodies. *Infection and Immunity*, **39**, 91–99.

HOUWERS, D. J. & WENSVOORT, G. (1986) Application of monoclonal antibodies in ELISAs: complex trapping blocking (CTB), novel one-step assays for the detection of antibodies to Maedi-visna and classical swine fever virus. *4th International Symposium of Veterinary Laboratory Diagnosticians*, (Abstracts), June 1–6, 1986, Amsterdam, The Netherlands, Borst, G. H. A. *et al.* (eds), The Royal Netherlands Veterinary Association, Amsterdam, pp. 50–52.

IVANYI, J., KRAMBOVITS, E. & KEEN, M. (1983) Evaluation of monoclonal antibody (TB72) based serological test for tuberculosis. *Clinical and Experimental Immunology*, **54**, 337–345.

KLENK, H. D. & ROTT, R. (1980) Co-translational and post-translational processing of viral glycoproteins. *Current Topics in Microbiology and Immunology*, **90**, 19–48.

KOHLER, G. & MILSTEIN, C. (1975) Continuous cultures of fused cells secreting antibody of pre-defined specificity. *Nature (London)*, **256**, 495–497.

MACARIO, A. J. L. & CONWAY DE MACARIO, E. (1984) Antibacterial monoclonal antibodies and the dawn of a new era in the control of infection. *Survey and Synthesis of Pathology Research (Basel)*, **3**, 119–130.

MCCULLOUGH, K. C., CROWTHER, J. R. & BUTCHER, R. N. (1985) Alteration in antibody reactivity with foot-and-mouth disease virus (FMDV) 146 S antigen before and after binding to a solid phase or complexing with specific antibody. *Journal of Immunological Methods*, **82**, 91–100.

MILDBRAND, M. M., TERAMOTO, Y. A., COLLINS, J. K., MATHYS, A. & WINSTON, S. (1984) Rapid detection of canine parvovirus in faeces using monoclonal antibodies and enzyme-linked immunosorbent assay. *American Journal of Veterinary Research*, **45**, 2281–2284.

MILLS, K. W. & TIETZE, K. L. (1984) Monoclonal antibody enzyme-linked immunosorbent assay for identification of K99-positive *Escherichia coli* isolates from calves. *Journal of Clinical Microbiology*, **19**, 498–501.

MITCHELL, G. F., GARCIA, E. G. & CRUISE, K. M. (1983) Competitive radioimmunoassays using hybridoma and anti-idiotype antibodies in identification of antibody responses to, and antigens of, *Schistosoma japonicum*. *Australian Journal of Experimental Biology and Medical Sciences*, **61**, 27–36.

MORRIS, J. A. & THORNS, C. J. (1985) Evidence for the reaction of bovine autoantibodies with *Mycobacterium bovis*. *The Veterinary Record*, **117**, 169.

MORRIS, J. A., THORNS, C. J. & WOOLLEY, J. (1985*a*) The identification of antigenic determinants on *Mycobacterium bovis* using monoclonal antibodies. *Journal of General Microbiology*, **131**, 1825–1831.

MORRIS, J. A., THORNS, C. J., BOARER, C. & WILSON, R. A. (1985*b*) Evaluation of a monoclonal antibody to the K99 fimbrial adhesin produced by *Escherichia coli* enterotoxigenic for calves, lambs and piglets. *Research in Veterinary Science*, **39**, 75–79.

MOUDALLAL, Z. AL., ALTSCHUH, D., BRIAND, J. P. & VAN REGENMORTEL, M. H. V. (1984) Comparative sensitivity of different ELISA procedures for detecting monoclonal antibodies. *Journal of Immunological Methods*, **68**, 35–43.

NOWINSKI, R. C., TAM, M. R., GOLDSTEIN, L. C., STONG, L., KUO, C.-C., COREY, L., STAMM, W. E., HANDSFIELD, H. H., KNAPP, J. S. & HOLMES, K. K. (1983) Monoclonal antibodies for diagnosis of infectious diseases in humans. *Science*, **219**, 637–644.

PEREIRA, L. (1985) Serodiagnosis of herpes simplex virus and cytomegalovirus infection with monoclonal antibodies. In: *Rapid Detection and Identification of Infectious Agents*, Kingsbury, D. T. & Falkow, S. (eds), Academic Press, New York, pp. 49–69.

POTOCNJAK, P., ZAVALA, F., NUSSENZWEIG, R. & NUSSENZWEIG, V. (1982) Inhibition of idiotype–anti-idiotype interaction for detection of a parasite antigen: a new immunoassay. *Science*, **215**, 1637–1639.

RUSSELL, P. H. & ALEXANDER, D. J. (1983) Antigenic variation of Newcastle disease virus strains detected by monoclonal antibodies. *Archives of Virology*, **75**, 243–253.

RYLATT, D. B., WYATT, D. M. & BUNDESEN, P. G. (1985) A competitive enzyme immunoassay for the detection of bovine antibodies to *Brucella abortus* using monoclonal antibodies. *Veterinary Immunology and Immunopathology*, **8**, 261–271.

SHONE, C., WILTON-SMITH, P., APPLETON, N., HAMBLETON, P., MODI, N., GATLEY, S. & MELLING, J. (1985) Monoclonal antibody-based immunoassay for type A *Clostridium botulinum* toxin is comparable to the mouse bioassay. *Applied and Environmental Microbiology*, **50**, 63–67.

SINA, S., SENGUPTA, U., RAMU, G. & IVANYI, J. (1983) A serological test for leprosy based on competitive inhibition of monoclonal antibody binding to the MY2a determinant of *Mycobacterium leprae*. *Transactions of the Royal Society of Tropical Medicine and Hygiene*, **77**, 869–871.

STEVENS, A. E., HEADLAM, S. A., PRITCHARD, D. G., THORNS, C. J. & MORRIS, J. A. (1985) Monoclonal antibodies for diagnosis of infection with *Leptospira interrogans* serovar *hardjo* by immunofluorescence. *The Veterinary Record*, **116**, 593–594.

TERPSTRA, W. J., KORVER, H., LEEUWEN, J. V., KLATSER, P. R. & KOLK, H. H. J. (1985) The classification of Sejroe group serovars of *Leptospira interrogans* with monoclonal antibodies. *Zentralblatt für Bakteriologie, Mikrobiologie und Hygiene. Series A, Medical Microbiology, Infectious Diseases, Virology, Parasitology*, **259**, 498–506.

THANAVALA, Y. M., BOND, A., TEDDER, R., HAY, F. C. & ROITT, I. M. (1985) Monoclonal 'internal image' anti-idiotypic antibodies of hepatitis B surface antigen. *Immunology*, **55**, 197–204.

THORNS, C. J. & MORRIS, J. A. (1985) Common epitopes between mycobacterial and certain host tissue antigens. *Clinical and Experimental Immunology*, **61**, 323–328.

THORNS, C. J. & MORRIS, J. A. (1986) Shared epitopes between mycobacteria and other microorganisms. *Research in Veterinary Science*, **47**, 275–276.

THORNS, C. J., BOARER, C. D. H. & MORRIS, J. A. (1987) Production and evaluation of monoclonal antibodies directed against the K88 fimbrial adhesin produced by *Escherichia coli* enterotoxigenic for piglets. *Research in Veterinary Science*, **43**, 233–238.

WANDS, J. R., CARLSON, R. I., SCHOEMAKER, H., ISSELBACHER, K. J. & ZURAWSKI, V. R. Jr (1981) Immunodiagnosis of hepatitis B with high affinity IgM monoclonal antibodies. *Proceedings of the National Academy of Science, USA*, **78**, 1214–1218.

WIKTOR, T. J., FLAMAND, A. & KOPROWSKI, H. (1980) Use of monoclonal antibodies in diagnosis of rabies virus infection and differentiation of rabies and rabies-related viruses. *Journal of Virological Methods*, **1**, 33–46.

YOLKEN, R. H. (1985) Enzymatic assays for the diagnosis of infectious diseases. In: *Rapid Detection and Identification of Infectious Agents*, Kingsbury, D. T. & Falkow, S. (eds), Academic Press, New York, pp. 19–32.

YOUNG, D. B. (1985) Cloning and expression of mycobacterial genes in *E. coli*. *Immunology Today*, **6**, 296–297.

ZAANE, D. VAN (1984) Use of monoclonal antibodies in virus diagnosis. In: *Recent Advances in Virus Diagnosis*, McNulty, M. S. & McFerran, J. B. (eds), Martinus Nijhoff, Dordrecht, pp. 145–156.

8

Solid-phase Sample Preparation Techniques for Immunoassays

R. A. CALVERLEY
Analytichem International, Cambridge, UK

R. JACKMAN and J. J. PEMBROKE-HATTERSLEY
Central Veterinary Laboratory, New Haw, Weybridge, Surrey, UK

INTRODUCTION

The need for sample preparation procedures prior to immunoassays can arise for a number of reasons. In many samples that are of food or veterinary origin, the first step of an assay is to homogenise the sample with a solvent that will solubilise the isolates of interest and provide the means of separating these compounds from the bulk of the matrix material.

For many applications the solvents that are appropriate for this initial extraction procedure are selected solely on their ability to solubilise the isolates and many of these solvents are not compatible with the immunoassay procedures that follow. In these cases it may only be necessary to exchange the solvent for one that is compatible with the immunoassay and this may simply involve an evaporation and reconstitution procedure. In some applications however, the specificity of the assay may not be sufficient and the extract must be submitted to a purification procedure in order to enhance specificity. For example, this purification step is often used to separate a drug from pharmacologically inactive metabolites which cross-react in the immunoassay (Pankey *et al.*, 1986). Although sensitivity is not always a problem with immunoassay procedures, on those occasions where it is a concentration step is desirable.

A traditional approach to these sample preparation problems has been to employ liquid–liquid extraction procedures. Because of the large volumes of solvent used, this approach invariably necessitates a time-consuming evaporation and reconstitution step at the end of the procedure.

Unfortunately this approach often lacks selectivity and can lead to emulsion formation, and the efficiency of the procedure can be operator-dependent. Liquid–liquid extraction also tends to be rather slow and tedious, and can be the rate-determining step in an assay procedure.

An alternative approach to solving the problems of solvent exchange, sample purification and concentration is to utilise a solid-phase sample preparation technique, which makes use of the properties of a wide range of commercially available extraction columns (Bond-Elut™, Analytichem International Inc., USA) containing bonded silica sorbents to selectively extract, purify and concentrate isolates from both aqueous and non-aqueous solutions.

BONDED SILICA SORBENTS

Silica gel is now the material of choice for the preparation of bonded-phase sorbents. It has the advantages of being available as a highly porous, high surface-area material (approximately 500 m^2/g for the Bond-Elut sorbents) and this property facilitates relatively large sample loadings on to the extraction columns.

Bonded silica sorbents are prepared by reaction of the surface hydroxyl groups (silanols) with halo- or alkoxysilyl derivatives, resulting in the covalent bonding of a wide range of functional groups (Fig. 1). The high surface coverage that can be achieved during the bonding process means that the adsorptive characteristics of the bonded silica sorbent are largely a function of the characteristics of the phase covalently bonded to the silica surface.

Bonded silica sorbents exhibit unusual physical stability. They do not shrink or swell in contact with aqueous or organic solvents. The bonded silica particles are rigid and will tolerate a high velocity flow of samples and solvents when these materials are packed into small extraction columns (Fig. 2). When samples and solvents are passed through the extraction columns rapidly, the bonded silica sorbents are stable over a wide pH range.

When using bonded silica extraction columns for sample preparation, there are a number of options available as far as the general approach to separating the isolates from the interferences is concerned. Without any consideration of the properties of the isolate or the choice of bonded silica sorbent extraction column, these options are illustrated in Fig. 3. Methods 1–3 offer a major advantage over method 4 because they involve retention of the compound of interest and, unlike method 4, can combine both

Sorbent structures

C_{18}	Octadecyl	$-Si-C_{18}H_{37}$
C_8	Octyl	$-Si-C_8H_{17}$
C_2	Ethyl	$-Si-C_2H_5$
CH	Cyclohexyl	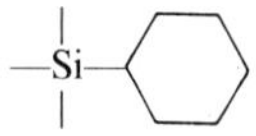
PH	Phenyl	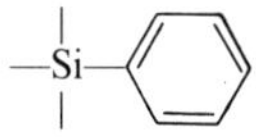

Polar

CN	Cyanopropyl	$-Si-CH_2CH_2CH_2CN$
2OH	Diol	$-Si-CH_2CH_2CH_2OCH_2CH(OH)-CH_2(OH)$
SI	Silica	$-Si-OH$
NH_2	Aminopropyl	$-Si-CH_2CH_2CH_2NH_2$
PSA	N-propylethylenediamine	$-Si-CH_2CH_2CH_2NHCH_2CH_2NH_2$

Ion exchange

SCX	Benzenesulphonylpropyl	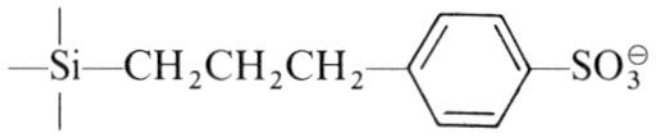
PRS	Sulphonylpropyl	$-Si-CH_2CH_2CH_2-SO_3^{\ominus}$
CBA	Carboxymethyl	$-Si-CH_2COO^{\ominus}$
DEA	Diethylaminopropyl	$-Si-CH_2CH_2CH_2\overset{\oplus}{N}H(CH_2CH_3)_2$
SAX	Trimethylaminopropyl	$-Si-CH_2CH_2CH_2\overset{\oplus}{N}(CH_3)_3$

Fig. 1. Functional groups available on bonded silica sorbents.

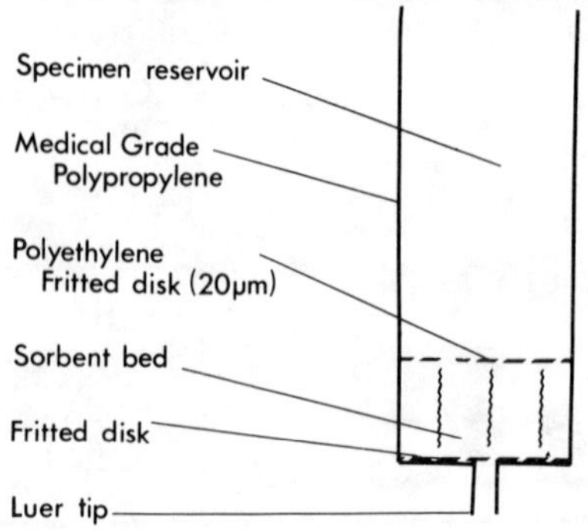

Fig. 2. Bonded-phase extraction column.

purification and concentration steps, assuming that the sample volume is larger than the final isolate elution volume. However, if concentration of the isolate is not a requirement, method 4 provides the fastest approach.

The extraction columns are available packed with various amounts of sorbent (typically between 100 and 1000 mg). Optimisation of column capacity will ensure high isolate recovery and also facilitate elution of the isolates in the minimum volume of solvent. This will ensure that the

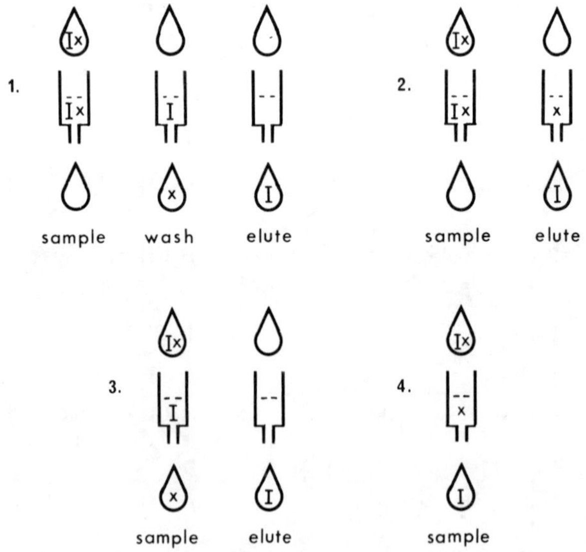

Fig. 3. Options for the separation of isolate (I) from interfering material (X).

concentration of the isolate in the elution solvent is as high as possible without recourse to a time-wasting evaporation step.

Multiple samples can be processed simultaneously using a commercially available vacuum-operated sample processing station (Vac-Elut™, Analytichem International Inc., USA). This device provides a controllable vacuum which can pull the sample solution, interference and isolate elution solvents through the extraction columns at a controlled and reproducible flow rate, an important consideration when developing robust sample preparation procedures. Alternatively, single samples can be processed by attaching the Bond-Elut extraction column to a Luer tipped syringe fitted with an adaptor. Positive pressure is then used to load the sample and subsequently elute the interferences and isolates.

Sorbent/Isolate Interactions

The selectivity of extraction procedures achievable using bonded silica sorbents is largely due to the wide range of sorbents available. The solvated bonded phases offer an array of chemical environments which can be selected for specificities suitable for the isolate. This is possible because the immobilisation of the solvated bonded phase precludes the necessity for immiscibility, which is a requirement in liquid–liquid extraction. The selection of appropriate interference and isolate elution solvents is another means of achieving selectivity. The range of Bond-Elut phases is illustrated in Fig. 1. The sorbents can be conveniently divided into three classes according to the nature of the interactions between the isolates and the sorbents, i.e. non-polar, polar and ion exchange.

Non-polar Interactions

Non-polar interactions are those based on the dispersion forces (van der Waal's forces) that occur between the carbonaceous component of the isolate and the sorbent functional group (Fig. 4). The principal non-polar phases are those with the C_{18}, C_8, C_2, cyclohexyl and phenyl groups. However, since most sorbent functional groups are bonded to the silica substrate through a carbon chain, all of the bonded silica sorbents illustrated in Fig. 1 are capable of exhibiting non-polar interactions. The strongest non-polar interactions are normally attained using the C_{18} phase. For many isolates the affinity for the C_{18} phase will be too strong and the isolates are only removed by using a large volume of a relatively strong eluting solvent.

The use of a sorbent with a shorter chain, e.g. C_2, CN or diol phase, will often provide sufficient retention of the isolate by the sorbent to give good extraction efficiency yet facilitate elution of the isolate by a small volume of a weaker solvent, e.g. a methanol/water mixture. The result of optimising choice of phase using this selection criterion is often a more pure and concentrated sample.

Non-polar interactions between sorbent and isolate are strongest when the sample matrix and interference eluting solvents are polar in nature. Aqueous-based samples will maximise retention of the isolates by the sorbents and this is one reason why the extraction of isolates from biological fluids such as whole blood, plasma, urine and bile using non-polar sorbents is such a successful technique.

Elution of isolates from non-polar sorbents is normally achieved using solvents or solvent mixtures with sufficient non-polar characteristics to disrupt the isolate/sorbent interaction. For many weakly retained compounds even an aqueous-based solvent containing a small percentage of methanol or acetonitrile will have enough non-polar characteristics to disrupt the non-polar interactions. In some circumstances the elution of non-polar isolates is only possible when a relatively non-polar solvent such as chloroform or even hexane is used. The choice of solvent will normally be governed by the solubility of the isolates in these solvents.

Many compounds containing ionisable functional groups can be retained by non-polar interactions. Control of retention and elution will often be dramatically influenced by changes in the pH of the sample and

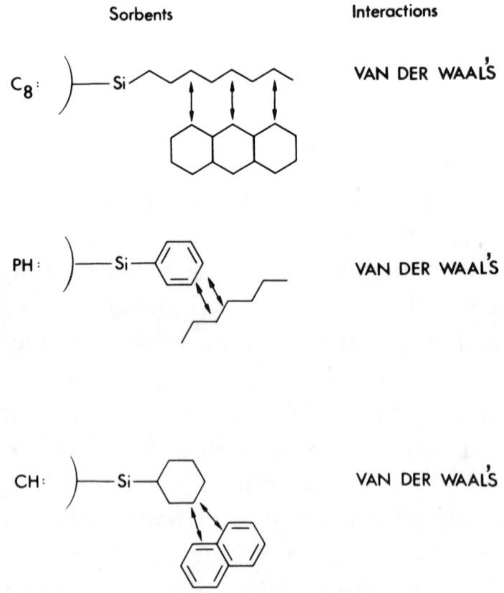

Fig. 4. Non-polar interactions between sorbent phase and isolate.

eluting solvent. This applies equally to isolates and interferences and is another means of achieving selective extraction and elution procedures.

Almost all isolates have the potential for non-polar interactions. The exceptions include inorganic ions, extremely polar molecules with high water solubility such as carbohydrates, and very small molecules. In these cases the probability of dispersive interactions providing adequate retention on a bonded silica extraction column is minimal.

Polar Interactions

Polar interactions are exhibited by a number of different sorbents and functional groups on isolates. Retention of polar compounds by polar-phase columns can be achieved using hydrogen bonding, dipole–dipole, induced dipole–dipole and π–π interactions (Fig. 5). As well as the polar phases, cyanopropyl, diol, aminopropyl (NH_2) and N-propyl-ethylene-diamine (PSA), silica also capable of strong polar interactions.

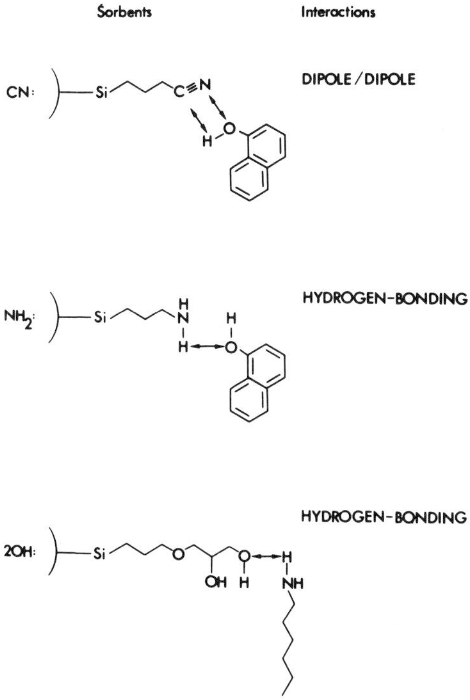

Fig. 5. Polar interactions between sorbent phase and isolate.

However, in many applications the tendency for silica to adsorb moisture from the atmosphere and the resulting unpredictable retention characteristics can make unbonded silica a poor choice of sorbent. The substitution of a polar-bonded sorbent such as diol will often make an extraction procedure more robust.

Hydrogen bonding interactions are the polar interactions most widely used in this mode of extraction. Hydroxyl and amine groups are the most common hydrogen bond donors and these typically interact with other groups containing oxygen, nitrogen and sulphur atoms. The aminopropyl sorbent is an ideal phase to retain isolates containing hydroxyl groups. Conversely, the diol phase is particularly effective at retaining isolates containing an amino group.

Retention of isolates on polar-phase extraction columns is facilitated by a non-polar environment. The exclusion of water from the sample is generally necessary unless the isolate is extremely polar, as is the case for sugars. A typical approach to exploit these polar interactions is to homogenise the sample in a relatively non-polar solvent such as hexane, chloroform, ether, ethylacetate or acetonitrile. The solvent of choice should facilitate efficient solubilisation of the isolate. After filtering and drying the solvent, the sample can be loaded on to an appropriate polar-phase column. Elution of isolates is achieved using a polar solvent. This can either be a non-polar solvent to which is added a polar solvent or an aqueous-based solvent such as a methanol/water mixture.

The possibility of being able to homogenise a food sample with a non-polar solvent that is required to isolate a component from a complex matrix and end up with the isolate dissolved in an aqueous-based solvent that is compatible with an ELISA is an approach that has yet to be widely exploited. This approach is fast and simple, and negates the need for time-consuming solvent evaporation and reconstitution steps.

Polar interactions are often capable of producing a more selective sample preparation procedure compared with the non-polar interactions. This is due in part to the fact that fewer molecules capable of polar interactions are likely to be present in a sample compared with the number of molecules that will be capable of non-polar interactions.

Ionic Interactions

The third class of interactions available using bonded silica sorbents is ionic. These interactions occur when one of the ion-exchange phases in Fig. 1 (including the NH_2 and PSA phases in the polar phase group) carries a charge (either positive or negative) and attracts an isolate molecule of

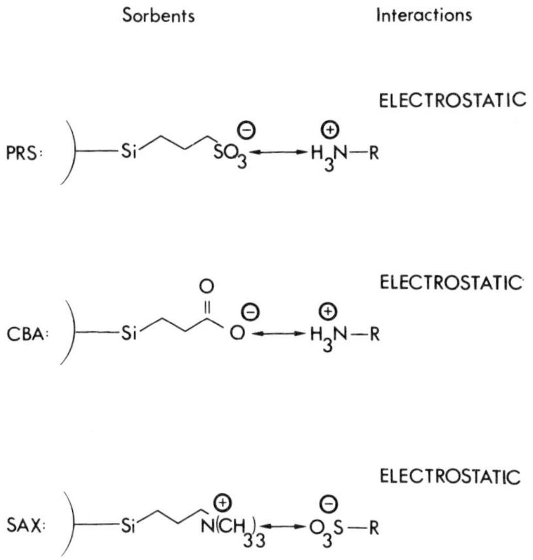

Fig. 6. Ionic interactions between sorbent phase and isolate.

opposite charge (Fig. 6). An ideal environment for these interactions to be effective would be one of low ionic concentration. Isolate retention by ion-exchange phases generally occurs from an aqueous sample. However, ionic interactions are also capable of extracting isolates from organic solvents. The control of retention and elution of isolates on these ion-exchange sorbents can normally be achieved by controlling the pH of the sample, interference and isolate elution solvents.

For effective retention of an isolate molecule by an ion-exchange sorbent, the sample/solvent pH must be adjusted to facilitate a charge on both the sorbent and the isolate. It is also important that the sample does not contain a high concentration of strongly competing ionic species of the same charge as the isolate. The use of pH as a means of controlling elution of the interferences and isolates can be achieved by eliminating the charge on either the sorbent or the isolate. Another means of elution is to use a high ionic-strength buffer.

Like polar interactions, and for the same reasons, the ionic extraction mechanism is often capable of a more selective extraction when compared with the selectivity attainable using non-polar interactions.

Many isolate molecules are capable of retention by more than one type of interaction. The choice of interaction most likely to result in a selective and robust sample preparation procedure will normally be determined by careful consideration of the isolate properties (Harris, 1985) and the properties and major components of the matrix (Van Horne, 1985).

A review of the properties of bonded silica sorbents and guidance on their selection for use in sample preparation has recently been published (Blevins *et al.*, 1985).

APPLICATIONS

As part of a National Surveillance Scheme for residues in animal tissues undertaken at the Central Veterinary Laboratory, Weybridge, solid-phase extraction procedures on Bond-Elut columns have been used to prepare samples for immunoassay. The numbers of samples involved and constraints on staffing levels and capital investment have precluded traditional chromatographic techniques for initial screening purposes although these have been retained, coupled with mass spectrometry, for confirmatory testing. The immunoassay reagents and methods available at present for residues, such as chloramphenicol, zeranol, hexoestrol and diethylstilboestrol (DES), require some sample clean-up and/or concentration prior to assay.

CHLORAMPHENICOL

The immunoassay applied is the E-Z Screen Card Test as supplied by Environmental Diagnostics, Irvine, California. This consists of absorbent material backed by a plastic card similar to a credit card and covered in soft plastic in which are two small cutouts. The two cutouts in the top cover contain an area of immobilised anti-chloramphenicol antibody. The sample, positive or negative control, is applied to the cutout and after complete penetration of the solution a quantity of enzyme-labelled chloramphenicol conjugate is added, followed by the substrate. A blue coloration due to conjugate binding to the immobilised antibody constitutes a negative result. Saturation of the antibody with sample or standard chloramphenicol prevents conjugate binding and no colour results. The limit of detection is 10 ng/ml chloramphenicol, and although this may be decreased to 1–2 ng/ml by applying larger amounts of sample, the same procedure cannot be carried out with samples of tissue homogenate due to false positive results. Since the maximum allowable limit for chloramphenicol in meat is 10 ng/g, a sample preparation stage was

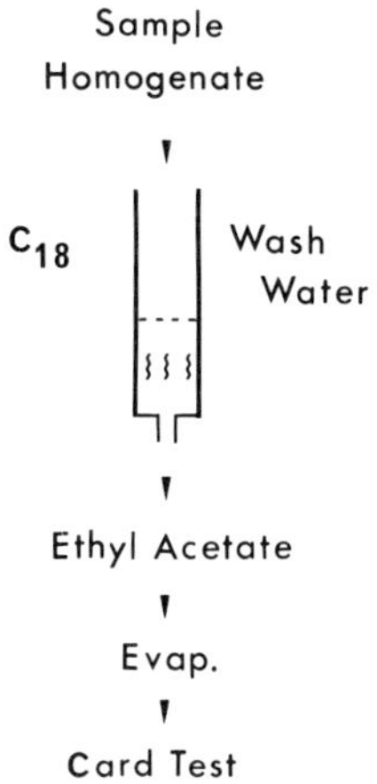

Fig. 7. Scheme for extraction, clean-up and isolation of chloramphenicol from a 10% aqueous meat homogenate.

necessary, both to gain sensitivity and to eliminate false positives. This was carried out according to the scheme in Fig. 7, with a 10% aqueous meat homogenate being placed directly on to a C_{18} column. Following a water wash, the chloramphenicol was selectively eluted from the column with ethylacetate and evaporated to dryness. Reconstitution to an equivalent tissue concentration of 1 g muscle/ml in phosphate buffered saline allows a reliable assay sensitivity of 10 ng/g for each drop of sample applied. This may be reduced to <2 ng/g with increased sample application.

AFLATOXIN M_1

The second application of solid-phase extraction has been to both increase the sensitivity of the analysis of aflatoxin M_1 in milk and to provide a convenient transport and storage medium for the milk sample. The immunoassay is a competitive ELISA (Jackman, 1985) with a limit of detection of 10 pg/ml. The solid-phase extraction method utilises a C_{18} Bond-Elut column previously washed with methanol, 15% chloroform in acetonitrile and water. A milk sample of up to 20 ml is applied and the column washed with water.

At this stage the aflatoxin is stabilised on the column and can be stored or transported in this condition for at least 13 days (Table 1). This procedure alleviates the problems associated with the analysis of milk as samples

Table 1
Stability of Aflatoxin M_1 (AFM_1) on C_{18} Bond-Elut Columns During Storage

Days	0	1	4	6	10	13
AFM_1 (pg)	108	96	92	118	86	92

rapidly spoil and lose homogeneity, making accurate sampling a difficult procedure. Acetonitrile is used to elute the aflatoxin from the column and, after evaporation of the solvent, is re-dissolved in phosphate buffered saline containing 0·1% gelatin for immunoassay. In this way the limit of detection may be lowered to 0·5 pg/ml. Extraction efficiencies for spiked milk samples in the range 1–200 pg/ml of milk were 87·6–108·1%. Individual columns could be re-used a number of times depending on the amount of milk processed.

GROWTH PROMOTERS

The sensitivity and specificity of RIAs for both zeranol and stilbenes in bile are substantially improved if the initial ether extracts of the bile hydrolysate are subjected to clean-up on a Bond-Elut C_{18} column (Table 2). The ether extract is evaporated to dryness, re-dissolved in methanol/water (1/10) and applied to the C_{18} column. Zeranol is eluted with methanol/water (9/1) and stilbenes with methanol/water (8/1). Analyses were carried out using standard RIA procedures, developed in-house using a commercial monoclonal antibody for zeranol (Dixon, 1980) and polyclonal antisera for DES and hexoestrol. In cases where the total anabolic content of meat samples are required, necessitating the hydrolysis of conjugated DES with glucuronidase, or where bile is unavailable and liver or other tissue must be used, even C_{18} columns proved to be inadequate for preparing samples suitable for RIA. In addition, traditional solvent/solvent partition methods and the use of silica, alumina, florisil and charcoal as clean-up agents also gave very poor recoveries. The procedure outlined in Fig. 8 incorporates two different solid-phase columns in tandem and eliminates the considerable sample matrix effects in the RIA which occur when conjugate-releasing agents are used on tissue samples. Recoveries of spiked samples and standards are compared with unextracted standards in Fig. 9, where the matrix effect of a single ether extraction is evident. In order to present pictorially the degree of clean-up of bile in this procedure, HPLC

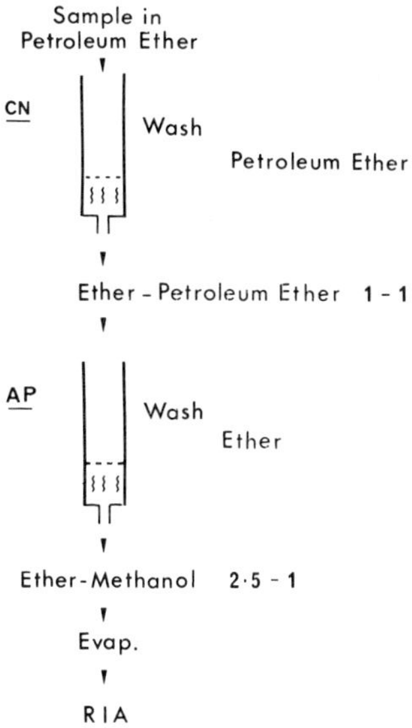

Fig. 8. Scheme for extraction, clean-up and isolation of DES from ether extracts of tissue.

Table 2
Effect of Solid-phase Extraction on the RIA of Anabolics in Bile

Sample	*Ether extract*		C_{18} *Bond-Elut*	
	pg	*% rec.*	*pg*	*% rec.*
Zeranol				
Bile A	195		351	
+50 pg	236	82	415	129
+100 pg	257	62	452	102
Bile B	55		114	
+100 pg	140	85	206	92
+200 pg	224	85	309	97
Bile C	130		198	
+50 pg	177	94	254	111
+100 pg	204	74	282	84
Diethylstilboestrol				
Bile D	38		51	
+50 pg	69	63	107	113
+100 pg	100	63	159	107
+200 pg	114	38	216	83

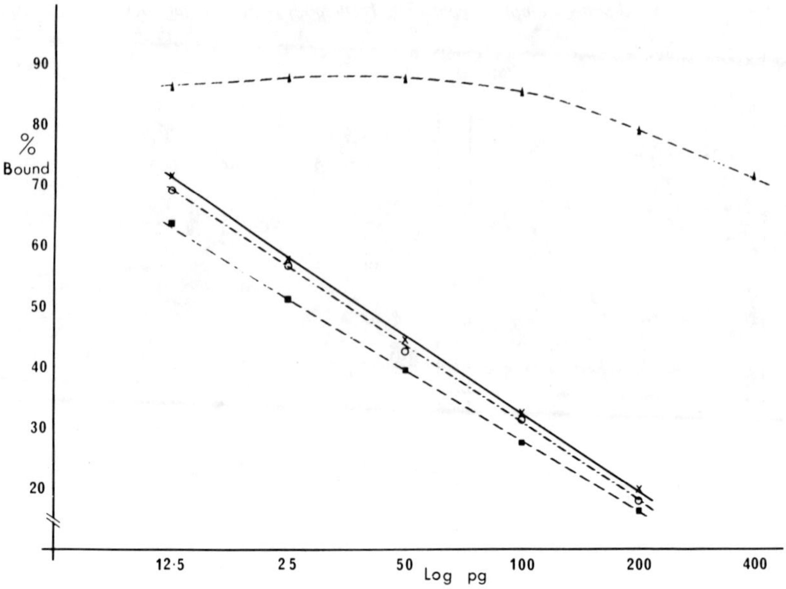

Fig. 9. Comparison of RIA standard curves for DES in spiked tissue extracts before and after clean-up by solid-phase extraction: ▲---▲, ether extract of spiked tissue; ×---×, direct standard assay; ○---○, solid-phase extraction of standard solutions; ■---■, solid-phase extraction of standards in spiked tissue.

Extraction of bile. 1. Diethyl ether

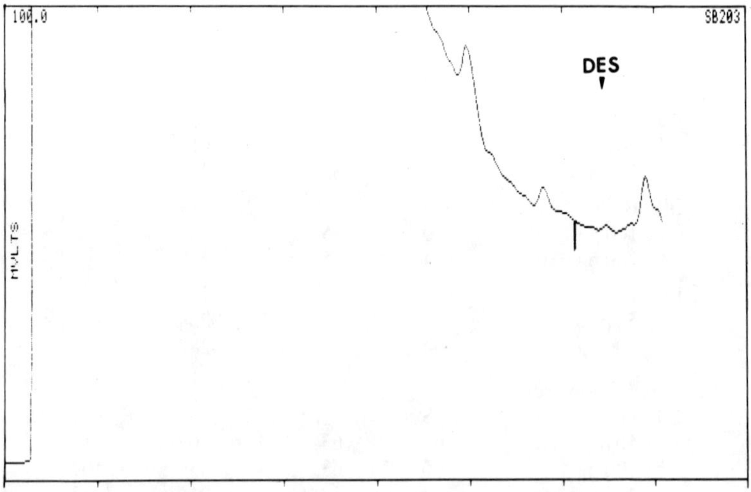

Fig. 10. HPLC of an ether extract of bile.

Extraction of bile. 2. Aminopropyl column

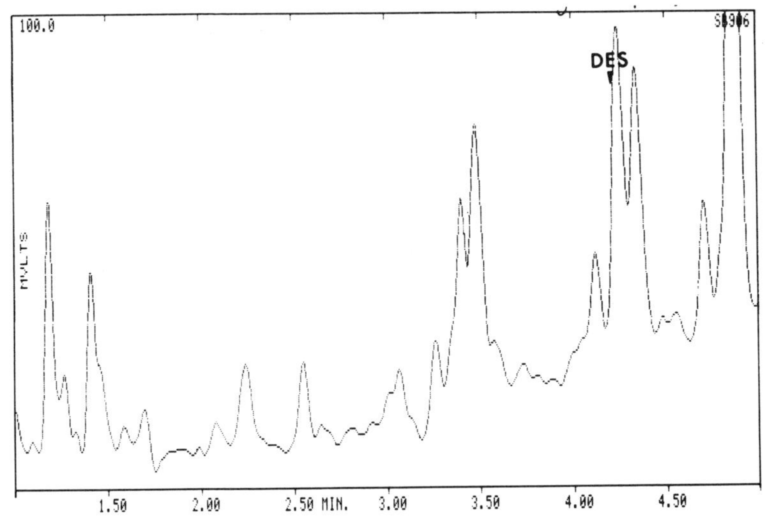

Fig. 11. HPLC of a single solid-phase column clean-up of an ether extract of bile.

Extraction of bile. 3. Cyanopropyl + Aminopropyl columns

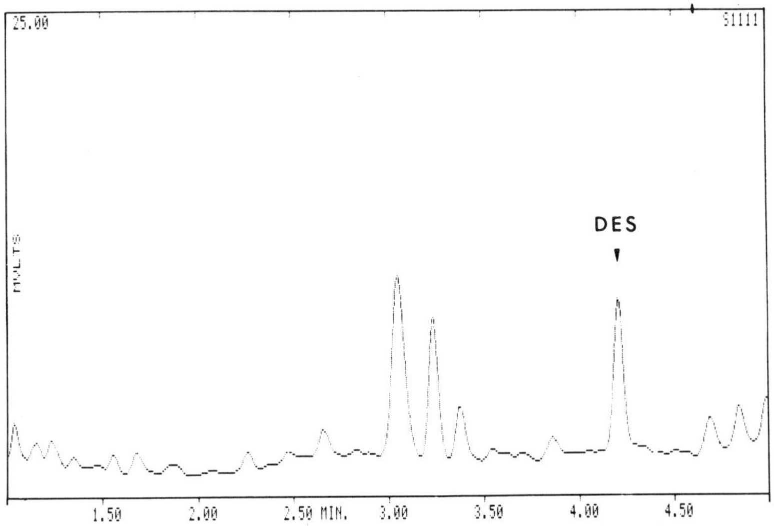

Fig. 12. HPLC of a tandem solid-phase clean-up procedure of an ether extract of bile.

separations of untreated ether extract, single-column clean-up (aminopropyl) and tandem (cyanopropyl + aminopropyl) eluates are shown in Figs 10–12. Using solid-phase clean-up less than 1% false positives have been obtained during the initial screen. Commercial or custom-built vacuum manifolds designed to facilitate the sample addition, washing and elution steps also enable large numbers of columns to be handled in a single batch. At present, however, there is no suitable automated equipment available, especially with regard to tandem column operation, with which to speed up further the preparation of samples for immunoassay.

CONCLUSION

Some benefits of using solid-phase extraction procedures in sample clean-up operations prior to immunoassay have been demonstrated. More widespread applications of these methods can be expected as their advantages become more generally appreciated.

REFERENCES

BLEVINS, D. D., BURKE, M. F., GOOD, T. J., HARRIS, P. A., VAN HORNE, K. C. & YAGO, L. S. (1985) *Sorbent Extraction Technology*, Van Horne, K. C. (ed.) Analytichem International Inc., Harbor City, USA.

DIXON, S. N. (1980) Radioimmunoassay of the anabolic agent zeranol. 1. Preparation and properties of a specific antibody to zeranol. *Journal of Veterinary Pharmacology and Therapeutics*, **3**, 177–181.

HARRIS, P. A. (1985) Rationale of method development. In: *Proceedings of the Second Annual International Symposium on Sample Preparation and Isolation using Bonded Silicas*, January 14–15, 1985, Philadelphia, USA, Analytichem International Inc., Harbor City, USA. pp. 3–9.

JACKMAN, R. (1985) Determination of aflatoxins by ELISA with special reference to aflatoxin M_1 in milk. *Journal of the Science of Food and Agriculture*, **36**, 685–698.

PANKEY, S., COLLINS, C., JAKLITSCH, A., HU, M., PIRIO, M. & SINGH, P. (1986) Quantitative homogeneous enzyme immunoassays for amitriptyline, imipramine and desipramine. *Clinical Chemistry*, **32**, 768–772.

VAN HORNE, K. C. (1985) Method development—sample matrix considerations. In: *Proceedings of the Second Annual International Symposium on Sample Preparation and Isolation using Bonded Silicas*, January 14–15, 1985, Philadelphia, USA, Analytichem International Inc., Harbor City, USA, pp. 45–56.

9

Graphical Presentation of ELISA-based Flock Profiling Data: Applications for Veterinary Diagnostics, Research and Quality Control

E. T. MALLINSON, D. B. SNYDER,
W. W. MARQUARDT and S. L. GORHAM

Maryland Cooperative Extension Service and Virginia–Maryland Regional College of Veterinary Medicine, College Park, Maryland, USA

INTRODUCTION

Diagnosticians now find that uncomplicated diseases with clearly defined aetiologies are encountered less frequently whilst complex problems with obscure aetiologies have become more common. This scenario, and the advent of ELISA technology promising one analytical method for most diseases, has led workers in Maryland to utilise ELISA-based sequential mass testing to improve the diagnosis and definition of today's production problems (Marquardt *et al.*, 1982; Snyder *et al.*, 1984; Snyder *et al.*, 1985). The immunological 'macroscope' that has evolved is generally termed flock profiling or population diagnostics.

ELISA-based flock profiling, as practised in Maryland and other states, is either qualitative or quantitative. The intended purpose of qualitative profiling is diagnostic. Besides being time-consuming and complex, it often requires dedicated organisation and analysis of data before useful conclusions can be obtained.

Ideally it is also the forerunner of quantitative profiling. Quantitative profiling, hopefully utilising knowledge and insights already gained from qualitative profiling, is direct, simple and less time-consuming.

The complexities and dynamics of today's disease problems in food animal production resemble a musical chord. Flock profiling enables

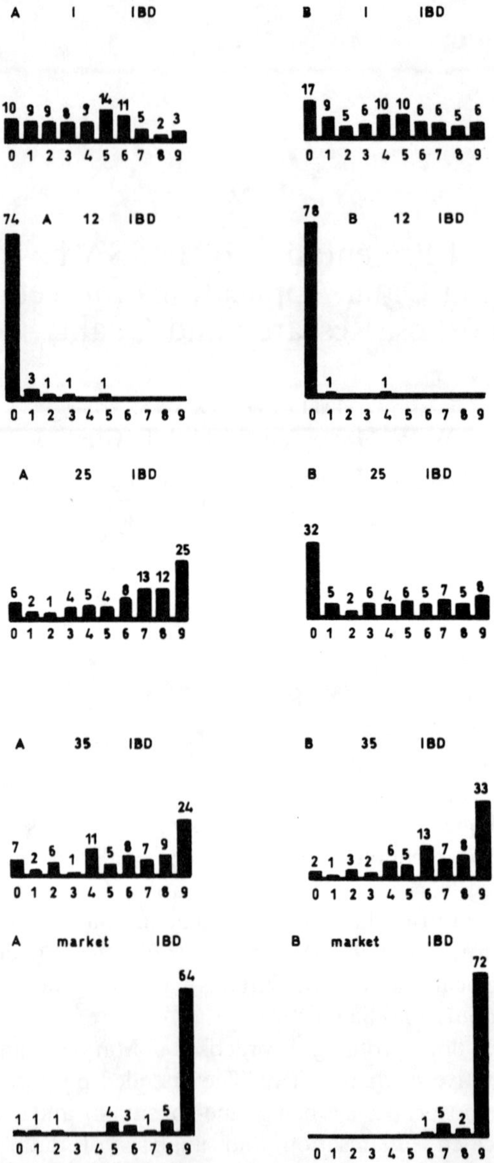

Fig. 1. Temporal Graphic distribution of IBD titres in broiler flock groups A (high grow-out mortality) and B (low grow-out mortality). Numbers on the abscissa repesent the relative titre group levels obtained by ELISA. Reciprocal endpoint titres of 0–50 are group 0, 51–150; group 1, 151–300; group 2, etc., with a titre of >19 201 comprising group 9. Numbers above each bar represent the number of samples reacting at each level at days 1, 12, 25 and 35 of age and at market time. From *Avian Diseases*, **30**, 139–148 (1986).

veterinarians and scientists to discern many of the notes and harmonics in the chord—to 'hear' what is in and out of tune with good performance.

A flock profiling system begins with the very basic medical principle of diagnostic serology, the paired serum sample. It starts to take shape as a flock profile when immunodiagnostic data are acquired and analysed over three or more sequential samplings. It evolves further with the inclusion of tests for more than one infectious agent. This step, although providing a better opportunity to detect other infections, makes interpretation difficult and adds complexity when different test systems are used simultaneously.

These problems are in part circumvented by the test flexibility and data display that ELISA technology and computer graphics provide (Mallinson *et al.*, 1985). Figures 1–3 provide examples of the diagnostic and disease surveillance power of an ELISA-based computer-assisted flock profiling system. Figure 4 illustrates the relatively low between-assay variation obtained with the Maryland prototype ELISA as compared to many other immunological methods.

Figure 1 compares the antibody titres of broiler flock group A (high grow-out mortality) with flock group B (low grow-out mortality). Both groups obviously experienced early field outbreaks of infectious bursal disease (IBD). However, the 'mirror-image' pattern differences between these two groups were detectable only at 25 days of age. Close-interval profiling, in this instance, revealed significant differences between flocks that may easily have been missed by conventional data analysis.

During the past year our ELISA system was used in the analysis of 16 000 immunodiagnostic and 100 000 management data points. These were collected to uncover disease management factors responsible for excessive broiler grow-out mortality and increased condemnations due to airsacculitis in an 80 million bird broiler population under the management of nine integrated poultry companies. This stimulated further evolution of our total flock profiling menu, which now includes pathology, virology, management and performance data (Figs 2 and 3).

Beyond using bar graphs of titre patterns at different ages, plots of mean titre ranges are now employed in comparisons with various additional performance parameters. Although the delineation of promising correlations can be very time-consuming, database graphics are now significantly alleviating this situation, by providing rapid access to the enormous numbers of comparisons that must be made. Furthermore, comparisons and correlations obtained are available in a clear, readily interpreted graphic format.

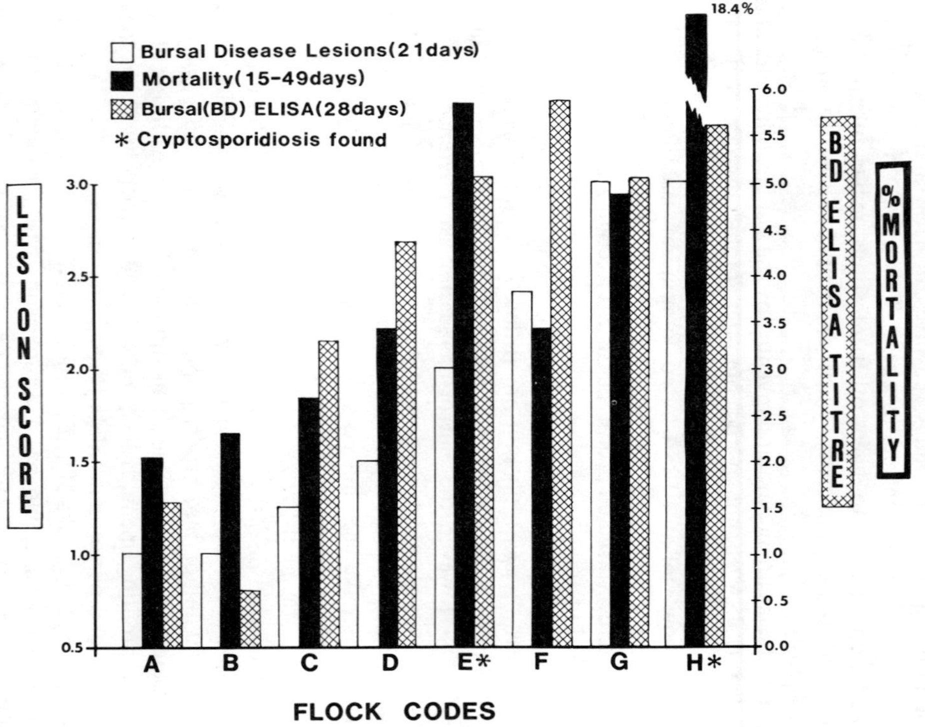

Fig. 2. Correlations between bursal disease serology, histopathology, other diseases and grow-out mortality. (Comparison between eight flocks of broiler chickens.)

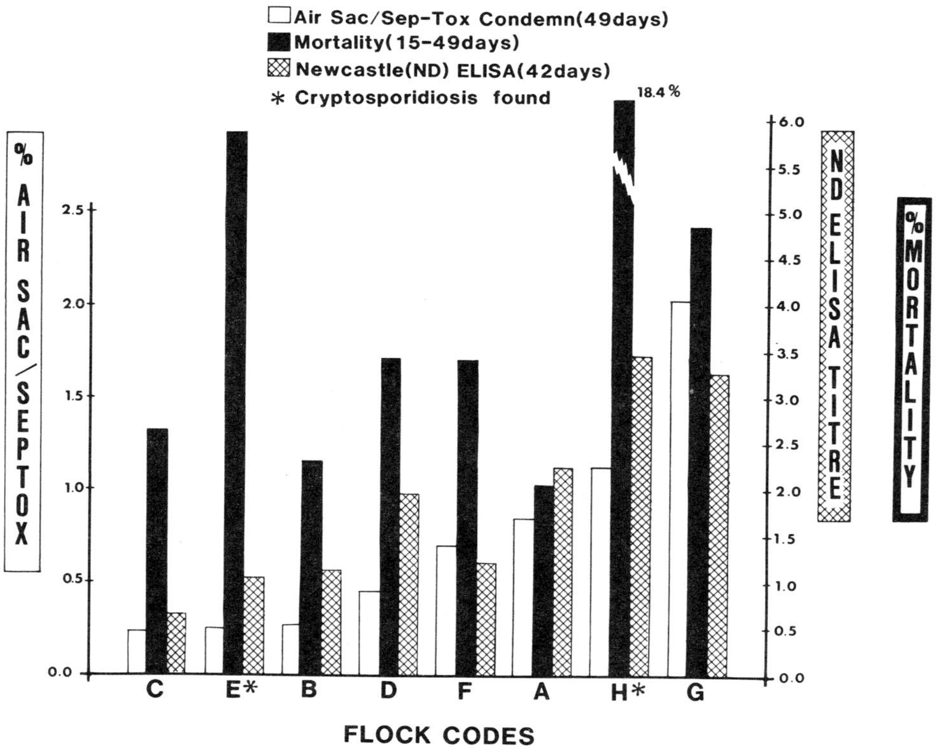

Fig. 3. Correlation between Newcastle disease serology and airsacculitis/septicaemia–toxaemia condemnations at market time. (Comparison between eight flocks of broiler chickens.)

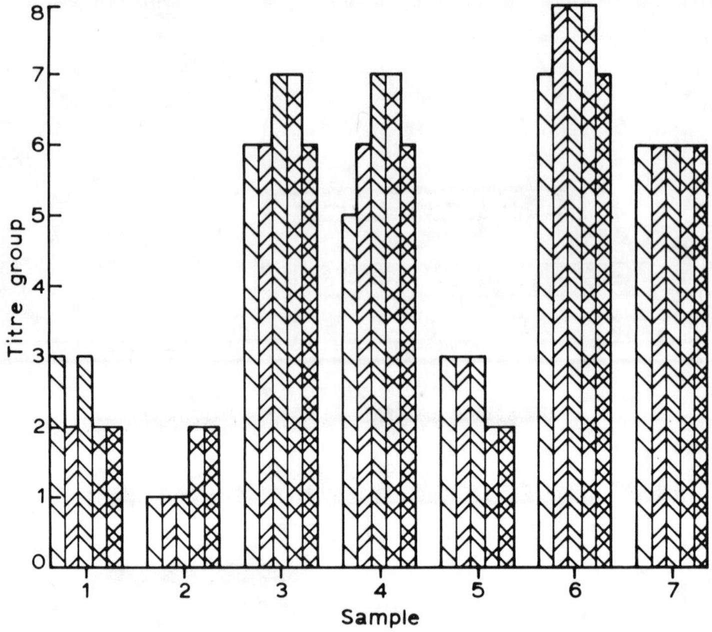

Fig. 4. A random selection of Newcastle disease (NDV) ELISA titre group values for the same sera tested on six different days. Refer to Fig. 1 for titres represented by titre group levels 0–9. (Adapted from Table III, Snyder *et al.*, 1984.)

Veterinarians using a full qualitative profiling menu should, nonetheless, be prepared to invest considerable time with either pen and paper or at a computer console, and perhaps with both, to obtain all the insights that ELISA profiling and good data organisation can provide. Investigative epidemiology, with the mass of data now available for analysis, advanced computers notwithstanding, generally remains somewhat tedious and time-consuming, but worth the effort.

ELISA-based profiling has proved useful to veterinarians in many professional environments. For those in academia, it provides a better view of the true field situation. It erases misconceptions about field conditions and points out unexpected needs and opportunities for additional research. It sharpens research directions and priorities. By virtue of the availability of a broad array of sequential data on factors that influence the outcome of field trials and studies, it brings a heretofore unattainable measure of internal control to these and similar investigations.

For those in industry, profiling offers unique opportunities to understand the dynamics of disease and their inter-relationships to management, performance and profitability. It detects deficiencies in disease control and prevention that would ordinarily have been missed by conventional diagnostic programmes. It establishes a more logical basis for vaccination programmes and immunological standards.

For those in regulatory veterinary medicine, ELISA profiling provides a cheaper means of multiple disease surveillance. As part of a government-sponsored general diagnostic service, it provides an opportunity to obtain a global view on diseases which, although initially of only marginal interest to producers, might be of much greater interest to government with its different set of priorities.

When using ELISA technology, samples may also be collected on filter paper strips (Lana *et al.*, 1983), dried and sent in a simple mailing envelope to a distant central laboratory for analysis. This strategy minimises the problems variously associated with use by relatively untrained personnel in remote areas, or where bio-security precautions must be especially tight, or where refrigeration or laboratory services may not exist. ELISA can also be used for detecting antibodies in egg yolk. Collection and testing of eggs instead of blood is another example of ELISA compatibility with sample collection techniques.

ELISA STANDARDISATION

1. Premature standardisation of the assay protocols at this time may impede improvement of this developing technology. Correlations between virus neutralisation (VN) and haemagglutination inhibition (HI) titres appear to be age-dependent, reflecting relative levels of IgG and IgM. These and other issues may need to be settled before ELISA methodology and interpretations are standardised.
2. There is enthusiasm for the development of international standard ELISA reference sera. The US Department of Agriculture (USDA) appears to be interested in collaborating with the International Association for Biological Standardization or similar groups. The National Veterinary Services Laboratory in Iowa, South-Eastern Poultry Research Laboratory in Georgia and Plum Island Animal Disease Laboratory in New York may be able to provide assistance.
3. Many lay users of ELISA kits experience problems with ELISA titre standardisation and comparable values between different test kits. The use or reporting of these results as 'ELISA Equivalent' VN or HI values

in the short term may or may not alleviate the confusion experienced by some lay poultry managers in the interpretation of these tests.*

CONCLUSIONS

Flock profiling represents an excellent marriage between computers and biotechnology. The foundations should now be laid for handling the exhaustive epidemiological analysis of the enormous quantities of data that can now be generated. High priority must be given to combining experienced veterinary intuition with sound biometrics to produce good technology and good medicine.

ELISA-based flock profiling is most productive when veterinary epidemiologists, immunologists and statisticians combine to ask the most penetrating questions and work co-operatively to seek the best answers.

ACKNOWLEDGEMENTS

The authors wish to thank Larry Crouse and Terry Bowen for Figs 2 and 3, and Anna Mathers and Peggy Sandridge for typing assistance.

* Whilst the Editors appreciate the reasons why lay poultry managers who have used VN and HI values for many years might prefer to have ELISA titres expressed as VN or HI equivalents, so as to be able to interpret them in the light of their previous experience with the older methods, such a conversion of ELISA data should not be attempted.

Immunoassay procedures involve different aspects of the antigen–antibody reaction from those involved in VN or HI techniques, both of which are precipitation methods. In HI, for example, the ability of the antibody to inhibit the aggregation of red blood cells is measured. Some antibodies are able to do this, whilst others are not. Therefore HI measures that proportion of the total antibody population which is capable of doing this, whereas immunoassay measures the total number present. After all, an antibody is secreted *in vivo* to react with the epitope on the antigen to which it was raised, not to perform in a particular way with sheep red blood cells in a man-made system. In other words, data derived with an immunoassay system is a better measure of the individual's response to exposure to an infectious organism than that obtained by either VN or HI techniques (see Morris, Chapter 2 and Hatfield *et al.*, p. 309, this volume). For this reason, it is most important that titres obtained by ELISA should *not* be converted to either VN or HI equivalents. The Editors are of the unanimous opinion that such a conversion will only further confuse the interpretation of the results and this can only be avoided by the early acceptance of data reported as ELISA titres.

REFERENCES

LANA, D. P., MARQUARDT, W. W. & SNYDER, D. B. (1983) Comparison of whole blood dried on filter paper and serum for measurement of the temporal response to avian infectious bronchitis virus by enzyme-linked immunosorbent assay. *Avian Diseases*, **27**, 813–821.

MALLINSON, E. T., SNYDER, D. B., MARQUARDT, W. W., RUSSEK-COHEN, E., SAVAGE, P. K., ALLEN, D. C. & YANCEY, F. S. (1985) Presumptive diagnosis of subclinical infections utilizing computer-assisted analysis of sequential enzyme-linked immunosorbent assays against multiple antigens. *Poultry Science*, **64**, 1661–1669.

MARQUARDT, W. W., SNYDER, D. B. & MALLINSON, E. T. (1982) ELISA and flock profiling in management and disease control. Pages 480–481 in Proceedings of the 86th Annual Meeting of the US Animal Health Association, Nashville, TN.

SNYDER, D. B., MARQUARDT, W. W., MALLINSON, E. T., SAVAGE, P. K. & ALLEN, D. C. (1984) Rapid serological profiling by enzyme-linked immunosorbent assay. III: Simultaneous measurements of antibody titers to infectious bronchitis, infectious bursal disease, and Newcastle disease viruses in a single serum dilution. *Avian Diseases*, **28**, 12–24.

SNYDER, D. B., MARQUARDT, W. W., MALLINSON, E. T., ALLEN, D. C. & SAVAGE, P. K. (1985) An enzyme-linked immunosorbent assay method for the simultaneous measurement of antibody titer to multiple viral, bacterial or protein antigens. *Veterinary Immunology and Immunopathology*, **9**, 303–317.

SESSION III

Food Applications

10
Recent Developments in Meat Speciation

S. J. JONES and R. L. S. PATTERSON
AFRC Institute of Food Research, Langford, Bristol, UK

Work on the identification of the species origin of meat using ELISA was first described in the 1983 Symposium (Patterson & Jones, 1985). The reason for undertaking research on meat speciation at the time was to develop good analytical procedures for use by trading standards and law enforcement agencies in their attempts to combat increasing problems of adulteration in the national meat supply. Instances of illegal species meats like horse or kangaroo had been finding their way into the meat chain and were causing much concern. Now more emphasis is applied to the detection of 1 or 2% of otherwise quite legal, acceptable 'meats' being found in batches which had been declared to be derived from a 100% pure single species, due to accidental contamination rather than deliberate adulteration. These problems came to light as a result of enforcement of the trading standards and labelling regulations. The elimination of confusing cross-reactions which could lead to erroneous conclusions has improved accuracy.

Meat can be presented in a variety of forms, each offering, to a greater or lesser extent, opportunities for adulteration and/or contamination. For example, whole meat can be in the form of carcasses, sides, quarters, primal joints or domestic joints; in such circumstances there are few problems as most species are still anatomically recognisable. Deboned meat, which is popular for wholesale supply because of its space- and (refrigeration) energy-saving advantage, is usually boxed or vacuum packed in plastic bags for storage and distribution in the frozen state. Opportunities for adulteration of the supply are now possible, especially since much of the material is used for product manufacture directly from the frozen state without thawing. Alternatively meat can be diced, cubed, chopped or minced, and is usually in bulk or on trays. Obviously the composition of such material can be extremely variable and the physical nature lends itself to easy adulteration.

Different sampling procedures must be applied to these situations: for whole meats, selection of pieces or cut samples, as many as required, is satisfactory; for frozen material, a wood-boring auger is a convenient and effective method of removing 'cores' of meat from the interior of solid frozen masses; for boxed meat, five one-inch cores in a 'domino-5' pattern are the minimum necessary; for comminuted material, several samples (100–300 g) must be taken from the bulk and each thoroughly mixed before analysis.

From the analysts' point of view, the composition of the animal 'body' can be quite complex. It contains muscle—the normal (voluntary) striated type which, after rigor, is called meat; also present are blood, fat, skin, bone, tendon, membranes, organs, intestines, etc. The principal meat components are the proteins of the muscle, blood and other connective tissue, lipids, small quantities of free amino acids, enzymes, carbohydrates and minerals.

For species identification purposes, the proteins provide most options. Besides the immunochemical procedures described in this chapter, the standard biochemical methods of electrophoresis and isoelectric focussing, and variants of these procedures, have been used to good effect in speciation, principally where single species (of either meat or fish) have been concerned; they are less effective where mixtures of more than one species are involved (see review by Jones, 1985).

The blood proteins are the easiest to extract, but they are not muscle-specific and their presence in a sample does not necessarily denote the presence of the corresponding species meat. For example, liver which contains high levels of serum albumin and is edible is classed as offal and not meat. Nevertheless, the serum albumins were the basis of the early speciation tests. Muscle proteins such as myosin, actin, titin, troponin, myoglobin, etc., can be used as antigens to raise antisera (Warnecke & Saffle, 1968; Hayden, 1977, 1979) but generally this approach has been restricted to the work of specialist laboratories. Even then the resultant anti-species antisera are not always fully species- nor muscle-specific.

Heat processing of meat causes denaturation of the protein and alters its immunoreactivity, thus rendering its detection impracticable by antisera raised originally to the native albumins (see review by Hitchcock & Crimes, 1985). Research laboratories are now turning their attention to the study of thermally stable and muscle-specific antigens. When the temperature of heat treatment exceeds 80°C, most proteins coagulate, precipitate and become insoluble in water, although some components can be extracted with saline or phosphate-buffered saline. Application of harsher conditions, e.g. use of either urea or guanidinium salts with mercaptoethanol, can achieve more complete solubilisation; after 'renaturing' dialysis, certain enzymes (adenylate kinase and creatinine kinase) can be shown to retain much of their activity (King, 1984) and possibly be effective as antigens. A similar renaturation of the disordered structural proteins, which still retain their primary peptide structure, may restore some of the secondary and tertiary structural characteristics of the original molecules and hence antigenic integrity. This has already been demonstrated in the case of soya protein analysis by ELISA (Hitchcock *et al.*, 1981). Although there is a risk of hybrids being formed during renaturation, such reformed materials may prove to be useful as antigens for production of antisera suitable for speciation of all heat-treated meat products (Manz, 1983, 1985).

Polyclonal antisera to serum proteins can be rendered species-specific by circulating them through chromatography columns containing the appropriate immobilised heterologous (unwanted) antigens. The desired species-specific antibodies can then be trapped by a further immunosorbent column containing the immobilised albumin of the species of interest. This acts as both a purification and a concentration step. An advantage of this procedure is that the columns are re-usable after regeneration, even although they are expensive to set up initially.

A simple modification has recently been introduced which renders many antisera more species-specific without incurring this expense, or the necessity of *de novo* production of more specific antisera (Jones & Patterson, 1986). The novel stage in this modified assay (see Fig. 1) is the addition to the diluted anti-species antiserum of heterologous antigens (serum albumins) at a concentration of 1 mg/ml PBST; unwanted cross-reactions then occur in solution rather than on the walls of the microtitration plate, where they would subsequently give rise to false positive results. These antibodies must be of sufficiently high affinity to preclude subsequent dissociation of the antigen–antibody complex. This blocked antiserum is then used in a conventional indirect ELISA format in which the sample extract has been adsorbed to the walls of the microtitration plate. The effectiveness of this blocking procedure can be seen in Fig. 2. Results of blocking three anti-species antisera (anti-cow, anti-horse and anti-pig albumins) with the respective heterologous serum albumins show marked decreases in cross-reaction for most of the other species, even with, in two cases, a small increase in the corrected optical

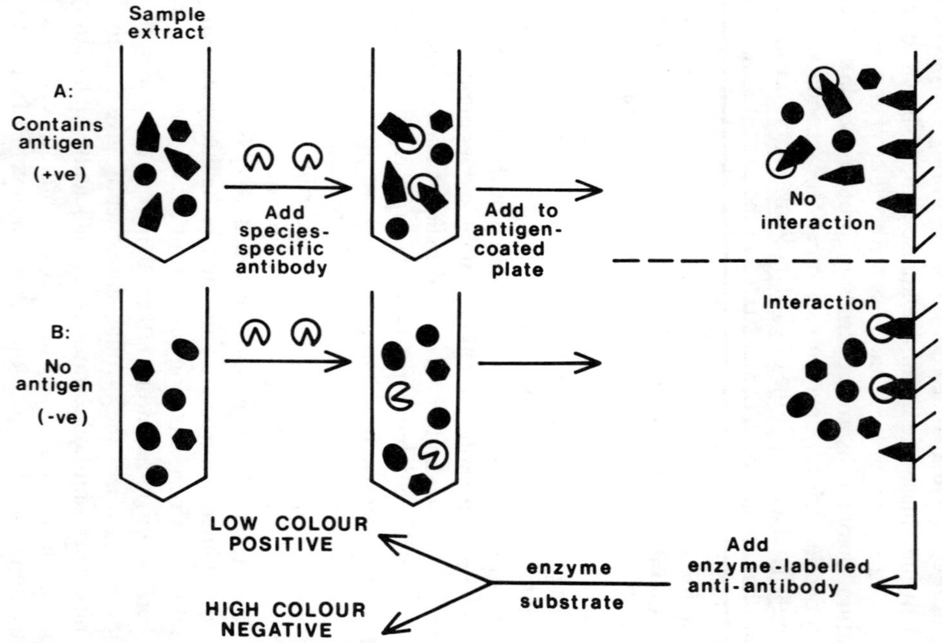

Fig. 1. Competitive ELISA for meat species identification. Species-specific antigen (♠) is pre-coated on the plastic plate surface.

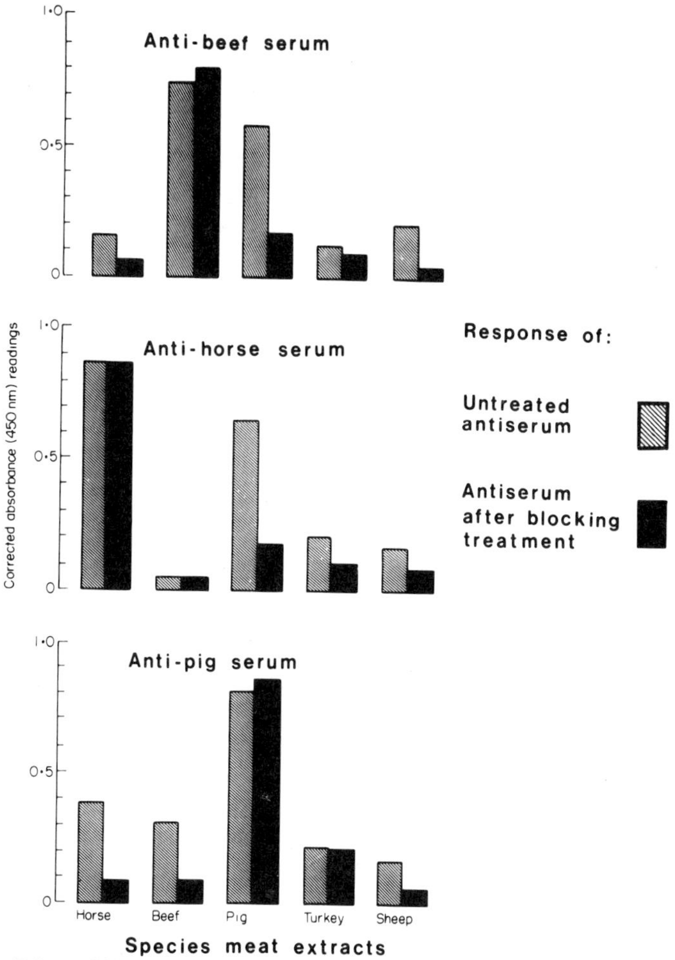

Fig. 2. Effect of blocking typical anti-species albumin antisera (not fully species-specific) with heterologous albumins. Treated antisera were used in a simple, indirect ELISA (soluble meat proteins are plate-bound) with improved species specificity.

density readings for the homologous species (beef and pig); this arises because of reduced background interference (colour).

The possible application of monoclonal antibodies to meat speciation should not be overlooked. However, it is felt that with the current developments in the methodology for polyclonal antisera the investment required for monoclonal antibody production would not be justified at present until truly muscle-specific, thermally stable antigens of good quality are available.

REFERENCES

HAYDEN, A. R. (1977) Detection of chicken flesh in beef sausages. *Journal of Food Science*, **42**, 1189–1192.

HAYDEN, A. R. (1979) Immunochemical detection of ovine, porcine and equine flesh in beef products with antisera to species myoglobin. *Journal of Food Science*, **44**, 494–500.

HITCHCOCK, C. H. S. & CRIMES, A. A. (1985) Methodology for meat species identification: a review. *Meat Science*, **15**, 215–224.

HITCHCOCK, C. H. S., BAILEY, F. J., CRIMES, A. A., DEAN, D. A. G. & DAVIS, P. J. (1981) Determination of soya proteins using an enzyme-linked immunosorbent assay (ELISA) procedure. *Journal of the Science of Food and Agriculture*, **32**, 157–165.

JONES, S. J. (1985) In: *Biochemical Identification of Meat Species*, Patterson, R. L. S. (ed.), Proceedings of the EEC Seminar, Brussels, Elsevier Applied Science Publishers, London, p. 193.

JONES, S. J. & PATTERSON, R. L. S. (1986) A modified indirect ELISA procedure for raw meat speciation using crude anti-species antisera and stabilised immunoreagents. *Journal of the Science of Food and Agriculture*, **37**, 767–775.

KING, N. L. (1984) Species identification of cooked meats by enzyme staining of isoelectrofocusing gels. *Meat Science*, **11**, 59–72.

MANZ, J. (1983) Detecting heat-denatured muscle proteins by means of enzyme-linked immunosorbent assay. Determining kangaroo muscle proteins. *Fleischwirtschaft*, **63**, 1767–1769.

MANZ, J. (1985) Detecting heat-denatured muscle proteins by means of ELISA. Determining bovine and porcine muscle proteins. *Fleischwirtschaft*, **65**, 497–498.

PATTERSON, R. L. S. & JONES, S. J. (1985) Species identification of meat in raw unheated meat products. In: *Immunoassays in Food Analysis*, Morris, B. A. & Clifford, M. N. (eds), Elsevier Applied Science Publishers, London, pp. 87–94.

WARNECKE, M. O. & SAFFLE, R. L. (1968) Serological identification of animal proteins. 1. Mode of injection and protein extracts for antibody production. *Journal of Food Science*, **33**, 131–135.

11

Overcoming Unwanted Interactions in Immunoassay, as Illustrated by an ELISA for Gliadin in Food

H. WINDEMANN

Department of Biochemistry, University of Berne, Switzerland

INTRODUCTION

The alcohol-soluble proteins (prolamines) from wheat, rye, barley and oats produce the harmful effects of coeliac disease or gluten-sensitive enteropathy in humans by causing characteristic changes in the intestinal mucosa. The patients so affected have to avoid eating these cereals, which are replaced by rice, maize, millet, soya, potatoes, etc. Many gluten-free foods are produced industrially and several immunoassays have been developed for the determination of wheat gliadin in supposedly gluten-free food (Ciclitira *et al.*, 1985; Fritschy *et al.*, 1985; Skerrit, 1985). This paper discusses a number of problems associated with such assays.

ENDOGENOUS ANTIBODIES

At the beginning of this development of an ELISA for wheat gliadin the problem of endogenous antibodies to gliadin in normal animal sera was encountered; these antibodies could be developed in animals being fed a normal laboratory diet, usually containing wheat, oats and barley. Pre-immune rabbit sera were therefore tested for binding to cereal prolamines. The results are shown in Fig. 1 for one group of seven rabbits. These results are typical of those obtained in our laboratory. Endogenous antibodies to cereal prolamines were found in all cases, more strongly to oats, rye and barley, and less so to wheat and maize. Taking into consideration the antibody concentration in the coating solution, the binding of the pre-immune sera was not very high in animals 2–7 and it is not considered to

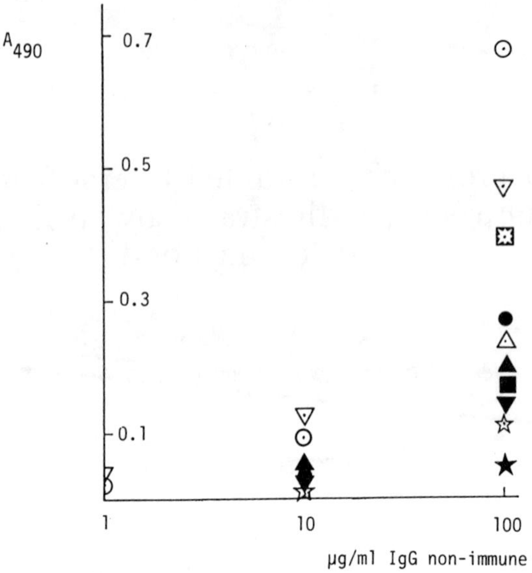

Fig. 1. Binding of pre-immune rabbit sera to cereal prolamines. Rabbit 1: ▽, wheat; △, rye; ⊙, oats; ⊠, barley; ☆, maize. Pool 1 (rabbits 2–7): ▼, wheat; ▲, rye; ●, oats; ■, barley; ★, maize. Conditions: coat, 5 μg/ml prolamine; antibody detection, protein A–HRP.

be a cogent reason to keep the rabbits out of contact with cereals or cereal straw. However, rabbit 1 was not used for subsequent immunisation. The presence of the endogenous antibodies has been confirmed by examination of the sera, at a dilution of 1:20, using the immunoblotting technique of Sutton *et al.* (1982) (Fig. 2). The resulting immunoblots stained so faintly that they could not be shown as photographs. The binding of antibodies to all wheat gliadin components was clearly recognisable and there was again no binding to maize prolamines.

In contrast with these observations, Coombs *et al.* (1983) reported very high titred sera against wheat gliadin and maize prolamines in some non-immunised rabbits fed a normal laboratory diet. Recently, Skerrit *et al.* (1985) described a variable degree of cross-reactivity of labelled anti-mouse IgC antibodies raised in both rabbits and sheep, and used as the anti-species antibody. These latter workers therefore achieved antibody visualisation using the peroxidase–antiperoxidase system.

It is obvious that some laboratory animals, depending on their species, age, nutrition and, probably, also the state of their intestinal mucosa, can

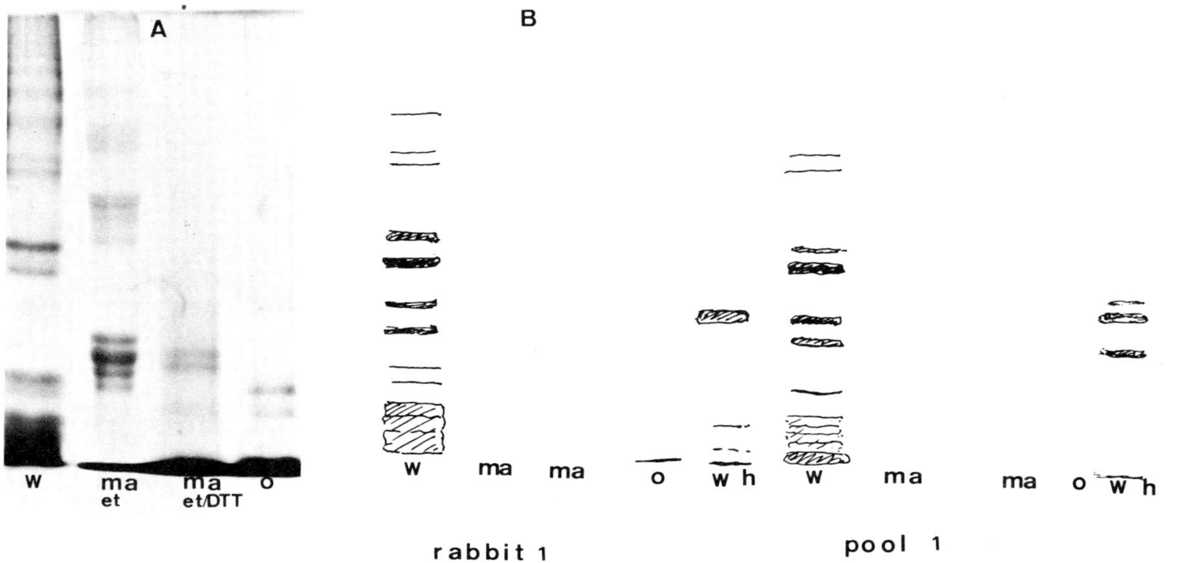

Fig. 2. SDS-PAGE electrophoresis (A) and subsequent Western blot (B) of cereal prolamines. The Western blot was incubated with non-immune rabbit serum 1 and a pre-immune pool of rabbit sera 1 at a dilution of 1:20. Antibody binding was detected with protein A–HRP conjugate. ma, Maize; o, oats; w, wheat; wh, wheat, heated; DTT, dithiothreitol; et, ethanolic extract.

develop remarkable amounts of antibodies against cereal proteins as a result of being fed these materials. The examination of the sera of potential antibody producers is essential prior to immunisation with wheat gliadin.

ASSAY CONDITIONS

The anti-gliadin antibodies so obtained were used to develop a non-competitive sandwich ELISA using the format Ab–Ag–Ab.E. Firstly, the influence of various buffers on the binding of ethanolic extracts of cereals to anti-gliadin antibodies was investigated. The binding values for wheat, maize and rice extracts are shown in Table 1. In PBS buffer high binding values for cereal extracts, gluten-containing and gluten-free, were generally obtained. They were not due to cereal peroxidase. The addition of the non-ionic detergent Tween 20 to PBS had no effect on the NSB whereas the addition of a protein such as BSA or gelatin to the PBS reduced the binding of rice and maize prolamines without affecting the binding of those of wheat. The addition of casein to the Tris/HCl diluent buffer significantly decreased

Table 1
Influence of Different ELISA Buffers upon Binding of Wheat, Maize and Rice Prolamines to Anti-gliadin Antibody as Determined by Sandwich ELISA

Coat	5 μg IgG/ml of specific antibody
Enzyme labelled antibody	HRP-labelled specific antibody
Peroxidase reaction time	20 min
Abbreviations:	
PBS	Phosphate-buffered saline (pH 7·3)
PBS–Tween 20	PBS containing 0·05% Tween 20
BSA	1% in PBS–Tween 20
Gelatin	0·2% in PBS–Tween 20
Casein	0·5% in Tris/HCl buffer (pH 7·5)

Sample diluent buffer	*Wheat (1:5 × 10⁴ dilution)*	*Maize (1:50 dilution)*	*Rice (1:50 dilution)*
PBS	0·50	1·0	0·9
PBS–Tween 20	0·50	1·3	1·1
BSA[a]	0·50	0·02	n.d.[b]
Gelatin	0·35	0·07	0·06
Casein	0·20	0·02	n.d.

[a] Saturation with 3% BSA for 20 min prior to sample incubation.
[b] Not detectable.
Results: A_{490} values (means of quadruplicate determinations).

Table 2
Influence of Antibody Purification upon Binding of Wheat and Maize Prolamines to Anti-gliadin Antibody as Assessed by Sandwich ELISA
(assay conditions as indicated in Table 1)

Antiserum	*Wheat*	*Maize*
Non-treated	0·80	0·16
Affinity purified	0·60	0·13
Adsorbed with maize prolamine	0·75	0·12

Wheat extract at $1{:}5 \times 10^4$ dilution.
Maize extract at 1:10 dilution.
Results: A_{490} values (means of quadruplicate determinations).

the binding of all prolamines, including that of wheat. After the addition of BSA (1%) to the samples and the saturation of antibody-coated plates with BSA, the assay was specific for wheat and it has been used successfully in the analysis of food. However, some undesirable cross-reaction of maize prolamines with the anti-gliadin antibody remained, as a consequence requiring dilution of the food extracts by at least 1:50 to avoid false positive results. Due to the high sensitivity of the assay, it was possible nevertheless to detect 0·1% wheat flour in a mixture. This interference however was the limiting factor in cases in which the highest sensitivity would be necessary (as, for example, detection of gliadin in blood).

Attempts were made to purify the anti-gliadin antisera by affinity chromatography and by adsorption of the sera with maize prolamines. As demonstrated in Table 2, these treatments failed to remove the cross-reacting component. In order to obtain more information about the reaction with maize, the antisera were examined by an immunoblotting technique (Sutton *et al.*, 1982). In this case, no binding of anti-gliadin antibody to maize prolamines was found, even after loading the gels with large amounts of these proteins. So it was assumed that there was at least some degree of non-specific reaction in the assay and attempts were made to minimise it. Table 3 shows the influence of conjugate type upon the binding values of wheat and maize extracts to anti-gliadin antibodies. It is evident that the alkaline phosphatase conjugate was superior to the HRP conjugate. This was especially true for some anti-gliadin–HRP conjugates which lost activity during storage, and those which contained free HRP. The most satisfactory results were obtained with alkaline phosphatase as label and enzyme amplification (Johansson *et al.*, 1986) for detection of

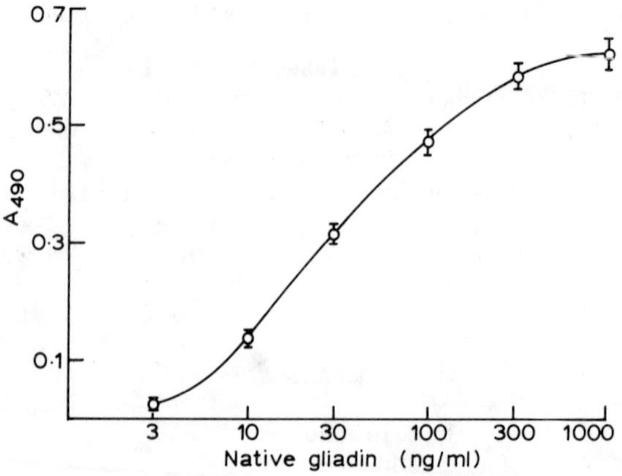

Fig. 3. Average standard curve for non-competitive sandwich assay for native wheat gliadin using alkaline phosphatase-labelled specific antibody and enzyme amplification. Conditions: coat, anti-wheat gliadin antiserum; label, specific IgG-alkaline phosphatase with enzyme amplification. ∯, standard deviation. Enzyme amplification was performed according to Johannsson *et al.* (1986) using 38 μg alcohol dehydrogenase and 1 U diaphorase/ml of amplifier buffer (100 μl added to each well). The absorbance values for calibration standards are corrected for NSB at zero gliadin concentration (mean, 0·19).

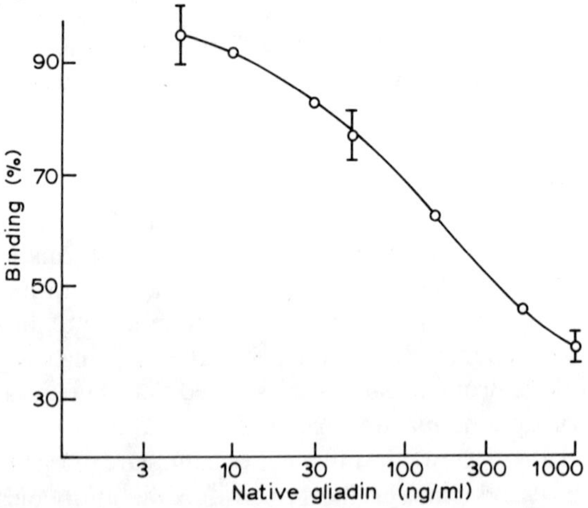

Fig. 4. Average standard curve for non-competitive indirect assay for native wheat gliadin. Conditions: coat, ethanolic extract of wheat flour; label, protein A–HRP. ∯, standard deviation. Antibody binding was detected with protein A–HRP conjugate. The binding values are expressed as percentages of maximum binding value (no antigen). The values of absorbance for calibration standards are corrected for substrate blank (mean, 0·02).

Table 3
Influence of Conjugate Type upon the Binding of Wheat and Maize Prolamines to Anti-gliadin Antibody as Assessed by Sandwich ELISA

Sample	*Immunoplate I (Nunc)*[a]	*Immunoplate I (Nunc)*[b]	*Immunoplate I (Nunc)*[c]
Wheat (1:5 × 10^4 dilution)	0·70	0·60	0·5
Maize (1:10 dilution)	0·20	0·15	n.d.[d]

[a] Anti-gliadin antibody labelled with HRP.
[b] Anti-gliadin antibody labelled with alkaline phosphatase.
[c] Anti-gliadin antibody labelled with alkaline phosphatase, enzyme amplification.
[d] Not detectable.
Results are A_{490} values and are means of quadruplicate determinations. Enzyme amplification was performed according to Johannsson *et al.* (1986) using the decreased concentration (10×) of alcohol dehydrogenase and diaphorase in amplifier buffer.

enzyme activity. There was no detectable binding of extracts of maize, rice, millet or soya at a dilution of 1:10. Figure 3 shows the corresponding standard curve for native gliadin using alkaline phosphatase as label and enzyme amplification.

The detection limit lies at 3 ng/ml (A_{490}, at zero antigen concentration plus 3 s.d.) and can be improved about five times by overnight incubation. In this way, the sensitivity of detection was increased at least 20-fold. In addition, the precision of the assay was superior to that obtained by classical ezyme detection with *p*-nitrophenylphosphate.

Another approach used frequently in food analysis, for example the detection of soya proteins (Crimes *et al.*, 1984), is the non-competitive, indirect ELISA with the format Ag–(Ag + Ab)–Protein A–HRP (see also Gould, Chapter 5).

In this particular assay variant the binding of extracts of maize, rice and millet at a dilution of 1:10 was hardly detectable. The assay has (Fig. 4) a detection limit of 30 ng gliadin/ml using a protein A–HRP conjugate for quantitation. However, in this laboratory the sensitivity of the sandwich assay was superior.

CHOICE OF IMMUNOGEN

The heat stability of wheat gliadin components is closely correlated with their content of sulphur-containing amino acids. The ω-gliadin, polypeptides lacking such amino acids, remain largely unaltered and alcohol-soluble after heat treatment (Schoffield *et al.*, 1983). The other gliadin components, particularly α- and β-gliadins, are involved in sulphydryl–disulphide interchange reactions and become insoluble on heating. These reactions can be reversed to some degree by including a reducing agent in the extractant (Schoffield *et al.*, 1983).

A comparison was made between antibodies against native and heated wheat gliadin (ethanolic extract of wheat bread) using ELISA and the immunoblotting technique.

Rabbits immunised with native wheat gliadin produced antisera of high avidity. As previously shown, the ELISA based on these antibodies is sensitive and specific for wheat gliadin. By immunodetection of electrophoretically resolved gliadin components, a dominant reaction with α- and β-gliadins was found (Windemann *et al.*, 1982). Using these antibodies the quantitative determination of gliadin is considerably affected by heat (Meier *et al.*, 1984) or by treatment with reducing agents, making quantitative determinations difficult with this antiserum. Only 2–5% of the original activity remains detectable after treatment with reducing agents. However, gliadin was detectable in heated samples containing wheat flour, even as an admixture at the 1% level.

Rabbits immunised with heated wheat gliadin (mainly ω-gliadins) produced antisera of low avidity. The sensitivity of the ELISA based on these antibodies is significantly decreased compared with that using

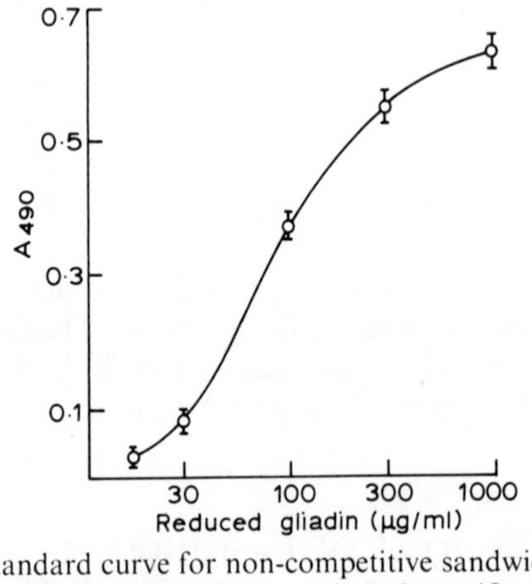

Fig. 5. Average standard curve for non-competitive sandwich assay for reduced wheat gliadin using alkaline phosphatase-labelled specific antibody as enzyme labelled primary antibody and enzyme amplification. See Fig. 3 for extra details. Conditions: coat, anti-heat-treated gliadin antiserum: label, specific IgG-alkaline phosphatase, enzyme amplification. ∮, standard deviation.

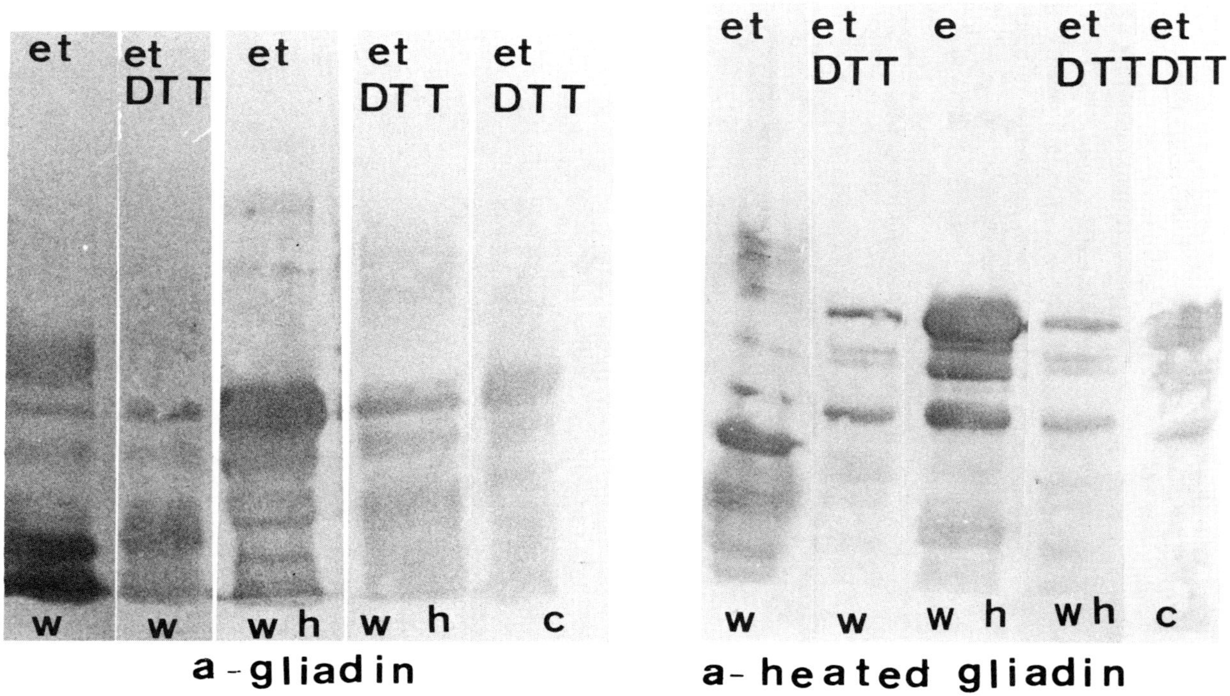

Fig. 6. Western blots (after SDS/PAGE) of ethanolic extracts of unheated and heated wheat flour prepared in the presence and absence of a reducing agent, dithiothrietol (DTT) and incubated with antisera to either native wheat gliadin or heated wheat gliadin. Abbreviations: w, unheated wheat flour; wh, heated wheat flour; c, control.

antibodies raised against native wheat gliadin (Fig. 5). The anti-heated gliadin antibodies react more strongly with reduced gliadin than with unreduced forms and the effect of heat treatment is far less pronounced (Fig. 9). These antibodies cross-react with prolamines from rye.

The comparison of both antisera by the immunoblotting technique revealed more similarities between antisera than differences (Figs 7 and 8). Moreover, the differences have a quantitative character (intensity and sharpness of bands) rather than a qualitative one. Both antisera bind to some prolamines from rye and barley. This is understandable in view of the large degree of homology in the amino acid sequences of prolamines of wheat, rye and barley (Wieser *et al.*, 1982).

It is obvious that the reactivity for native gliadin in the ELISA is

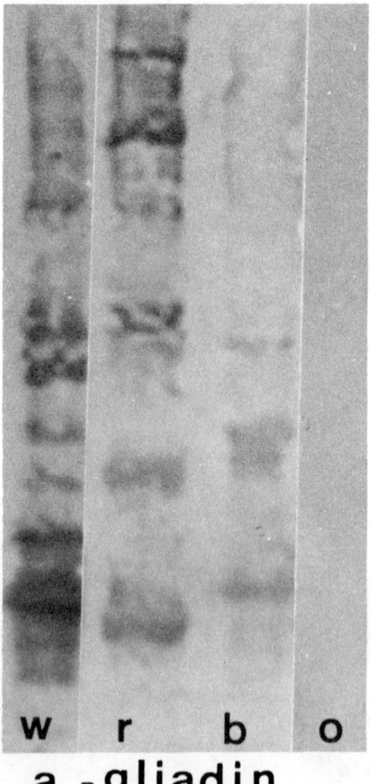

Fig. 7. Western blot of cereal prolamines (after SDS/PAGE) which was incubated with antibody against native wheat gliadin at a dilution of 1:2000. Antibody binding was detected using protein A–HRP conjugate. Abbreviations: w, wheat; r, rye: b, barley; o, oats.

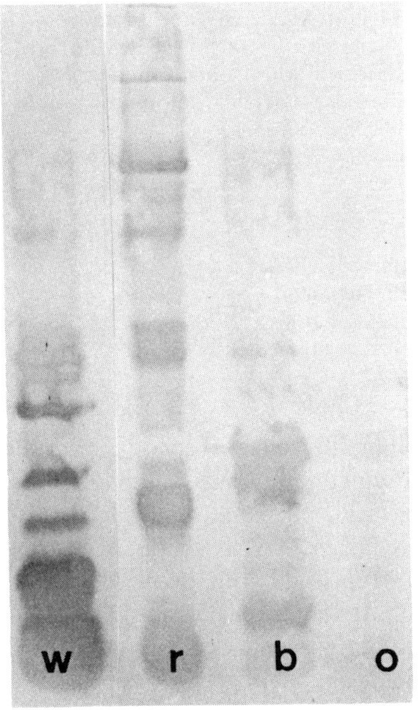

Fig. 8. Western blot of cereal prolamines (after SDS/PAGE) which was incubated with antibody against heated wheat gliadin at a dilution of 1:800. Antibody binding was detected using protein A–HRP conjugate. Abbreviations: see Fig. 7.

controlled by the high affinity antibodies in the antiserum. Usually the influence of antibody affinity is not so important in non-competitive sandwich assays (see Gould, Chapter 5), which use excess antibody. However, the use of labelled species-specific antibody as the second antibody may enhance the observed effect.

EXTRACTION FROM FOOD

A defined amount of wheat flour was added to a variety of foods. The gliadin was subsequently extracted with 70% ethanol and the recovery was determined by ELISA. The recoveries were satisfactory with the exception of foods containing phenols (see Table 4).

Table 4
Recovery of Gliadin Added as Wheat Flour from Food Containing Phenols by Extraction with 70% Ethanol
(samples contain 1% wheat flour, an additive as indicated and a complementary amount of starch)

Sample	*Gliadin* ($\mu g/g$)	*Normalised recovery* (%)
Wheat, starch	340	100
Wheat, starch, 40% cocoa[a]	88	26
Wheat, starch, 10% tea	65	19
Wheat, starch, 20% hops	82	24
Wheat, starch, 5% tannic acid	170	50

[a] Soluble cocoa powder.

To exclude any inhibitory effect of cocoa extract on the binding of gliadin in ELISA, a set of standard dilutions was made using a 1:50 dilution of the ethanolic cocoa extract in phosphate buffer. No matrix effect of cocoa could be detected. Moreover, nor was gliadin found by HPLC analysis of ethanolic extracts from food containing wheat flour and cocoa (Windemann *et al.*, 1985). It was assumed that gliadin remains in the ethanol-insoluble residue, and that this was due to interaction with cocoa phenols. The binding mechanisms involved in these reactions may be hydrogen bonding, hydrophobic and electrostatic interactions as well as covalent bonding in some circumstances. The use of 70% ethanol as extractant may favour the effect of phenols. As shown in Table 4, addition of other

Table 5
Improved Recovery of Gliadin from Food Containing Cocoa by Addition of Competing or Releasing Component and Extraction with 3 M Urea in 70% Ethanol
(samples contain 1% wheat flour, 40% cocoa (except where shown otherwise), an additive as indicated and a complementary amount of starch)

Additive	*Gliadin* ($\mu g/g$)	*Normalised recovery* (%)
Wheat, no cocoa, no additive	360	100
Wheat + cocoa + starch	88	26
+ 10% casein	295	82
+ 10% gelatin	274	76
+ 5% polyethylene glycol	252	70
+ 10% SDS	180	50

components known to be rich in phenols also decreases the recovery of gliadin. To avoid this interaction, the simultaneous addition of competing proteins, as well as urea, to the extractant was necessary. The results are shown in Table 5.

As recently reviewed by Clifford (1986), the affinity of proteins for phenols, and particularly for tannins, is attributed to a relatively large proline content as found in gliadin and gelatin, which has been used as a competing protein. This could also explain why a relatively large amount (10%) of competing protein is necessary. The role of casein is less obvious (Clifford, 1986). However, during analysis of gliadin and casein proteins by reversed-phase HPLC, which resolves the proteins on the basis of their differences in surface hydrophobicity, both proteins elute under very similar conditions (Windemann *et al.*, 1985). The formation of hydrophobic bonds between phenols and gliadin, favoured by the polar solvent, may perhaps contribute to the effect of casein. The anionic detergent SDS (10% of sample, 1% in ethanol) is less effective in preventing this interaction than polyethylene glycol.

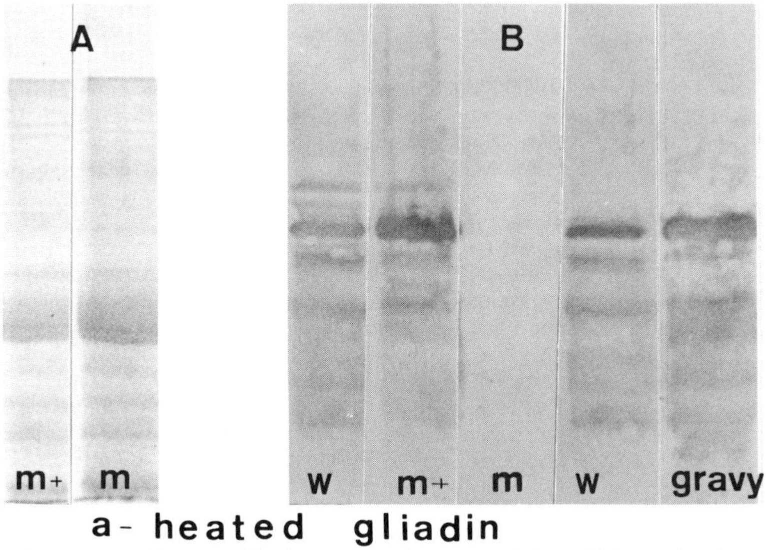

Fig. 9. Western blot (B) of food samples (after SDS/PAGE) which was incubated with antibody against heated wheat gliadin at a dilution of 1:800. Antibody binding was detected with protein A–HRP conjugate. The electrophoretic patterns (SDS/PAGE) of the meat samples (stained with Coomassie Brilliant Blue R 250) are shown in A. Abbreviations: m+, fried minced meat containing wheat flour; m, fried minced meat; w, wheat.

COMPLEMENTARY ANALYSIS

The two-dimensional immunoblotting technique was used to confirm the results of ELISA, as well as to obtain more information about antigen characteristics. This is shown in Fig. 9. Furthermore, a sample of fried minced meat (beef) containing wheat flour and a sample of gravy, both of which were positive in the ELISA, were tested by the immunoblotting technique (Fig. 9B). Fried minced meat without wheat flour was used as control. After blotting and visualisation with antibody, the stained gliadin patterns were clearly recognisable in the meat containing wheat flour and gravy, whereas no bands were detectable in the control meat sample. The electrophoretic patterns of both meat samples are also shown (Fig. 9A).

REFERENCES

CICLITIRA, P. J., ELLIS, H. J., EVANS, D. J. & LENNOX, E. S. (1985) A radioimmunoassay for wheat gliadin to assess the suitability of gluten-free foods for patients with coeliac disease. *Clinical and Experimental Immunology*, **59**, 703–708.

CLIFFORD, M. N. (1986) Phenol–protein interactions and their possible significance for astringency. In: *Interactions of Food Components*, Birch, G. G. (ed.), Elsevier Applied Science, London, pp. 43–64.

COOMBS, R. R. A., KIEFFER, M., FRASER, D. R. & FRAZIER, P. J. (1983) Naturally developing antibodies to wheat gliadin fractions and to other cereal antigens in rabbits, rats and guinea pigs on normal laboratory diets. *International Archives of Allergy and Applied Immunology*, **70**, 200–204.

CRIMES, A. A., HITCHCOCK, C. H. S. & WOOD, R. (1984) Determination of soya protein in meat products by an enzyme-linked immunosorbent assay procedure: collaborative study. *Journal of the Association of Public Analysts*, **22**, 59–78.

FRITSCHY, F., WINDEMANN, H. & BAUMGARTNER, E. (1985) Quantitative determination of wheat gliadins in foods by enzyme-linked immunosorbent assay. *Zeitschrift für Lebensmittel-Untersuchung und -Forschung*, **181**, 379–385.

JOHANNSSON, A., ELLIS, D. H., BATES, D. L., PLUMB, A. M. & STANLEY, C. J. (1986) Enzyme amplification for immunoassays. *Journal of Immunological Methods*, **87**, 7–11.

MEIER, P., WINDEMANN, H. & BAUMGARTNER, E. (1984) Determination of α-gliadin content of heated food, containing and free of gluten. *Zeitschrift für Lebensmittel-Untersuchung und -Forschung*, **178**, 361–365.

SCHOFFIELD, J. D., BOTTOMLEY, R. C., TIMMS, M. F. & BOOTH, M. R. (1983) The affect of heat on wheat gluten and the involvement of sulphydryl-disulphide interchange reactions. *Journal of Cereal Science*, **1**, 241–253.

SKERRIT, J. H. (1985) A sensitive monoclonal antibody-based test for gluten detection: quantitative immunoassay. *Journal of the Science of Food and Agriculture*, **36**, 987–994.

SKERRIT, J. H., DIMENT, J. A. & WRIGLEY, C. W. (1985) A sensitive monoclonal antibody-based test for gluten detection: choice of primary and secondary antibodies. *Journal of the Science of Food and Agriculture*, **36**, 995–1003.

SUTTON, R., WRIGLEY, C. W. & BALDO, B. A. (1982) Detection of IgE- and IgG-binding proteins after electrophoretic transfer from polyacrylamide gels. *Journal of Immunological Methods*, **52**, 183–194.

WIESER, H., SEILMEIER, W. & BELITZ, H.-D. (1982) Comparative investigations of partial amino acid sequence of prolamines and glutelins from cereals. *Zeitschrift für Lebensmittel-Untersuchung und -Forschung*, **174**, 374–380.

WINDEMANN, H., FRITSCHY, F. & BAUMGARTNER, E. (1982) Enzyme-linked immunosorbent assay for wheat α-gliadin and whole gliadin. *Biochimica Biophysica Acta*, **709**, 110–121.

WINDEMANN, H., MEIER, P. & BAUMGARTNER, E. (1985) Detection of wheat gliadins in heated foods by reversed-phase high-performance liquid chromatography. *Zeitschrift für Lebensmittel-Untersuchung und -Forschung*, **180**, 467–473.

12

The Specific Analysis of Methanogenic Bacteria used in the Fermentation of Food Waste

H. A. Kemp, D. B. Archer and M. R. A. Morgan

AFRC Institute of Food Research, Norwich, UK

INTRODUCTION

Wastes from the food processing industry are costly to dispose of as effluent because they are generally soluble, dilute and produced in large volumes. Treatment of this waste by anaerobic digestion on-site can be a way of reducing these costs. Anaerobic digestion of organic wastes by bacteria occurs naturally in environments such as intestinal tracts and sediments. However, anaerobic digestion can be used, in a digester, to treat industrial and agricultural waste, thus reducing pollution and simultaneously producing a useful fuel, methane, which can be a valuable byproduct.

The degradative steps involved in methanogenesis from waste, irrespective of its composition, involve four major metabolic stages (Fig. 1). However, because of the complexity of the process, involving a culture of many different microbes, detailed knowledge of methanogenesis in a digester is lacking. Monitoring and adjusting the process is very difficult, because the system is sensitive to disturbances which can lead to poor performance and failure. The last stage is the source of most problems, i.e. the degradation to methane of volatile fatty acids such as acetic, propionic and butyric acids (Archer, 1983). The acetogenic bacteria metabolise volatile fatty acids to produce substrates, including acetic acid, CO_2 and H_2, for the methanogens. Production of methane from these substrates is slow and is particularly susceptible to low pH. Acidification is a common cause of digester failure. A slight fall in pH (below 6) will inhibit the methanogenic bacteria, resulting in further acidification as the acetic acid is not metabolised (Archer, 1983). Acidogenic bacteria are less sensitive to low pH. Monitoring of the microbial flora, especially the methanogens, would

Complex organic waste

↓ Hydrolysis

Monomeric compounds

↓ Acidogenesis

Organic acids

↓ Acetogenesis

Acetic acid H_2/CO_2

↓ Methanogenesis

CH_4

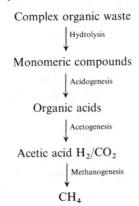

Fig. 1. The stages involved in methane production from organic waste.

greatly assist our understanding and control of the digestion process. It would also facilitate the development of rationally-based control procedures designed to ensure a stable process.

Methanogenic bacteria are distinguished from eubacteria by several factors: the absence of peptidoglycan cell walls, the presence of unusual membrane lipids, and the occurrence of unique transfer RNA and 5S ribosomal RNA. There are over thirty known species of methanogens and new ones are being constantly isolated and identified. Species of the two genera *Methanosarcina* and *Methanothrix* are known to produce methane from acetic acid. Most of the other methanogenic species utilise H_2 and CO_2 to form methane and many of these species, particularly *Methanobacterium* spp., are found in anaerobic digesters (Archer & Kirsop, 1988).

Enumeration of methanogenic species in digesters is difficult by standard microbiological techniques (Kirsop, 1984). The usual method of counting colonies on solid media or by serial dilution is unsuitable, because methanogens usually exist in clumps of cells or in biofilms in association with surfaces in the digester. In addition, the counts of methanogens may be a factor of 10–100 times lower than other organisms.

A number of indirect methods have been evaluated for the identification and enumeration of methanogens. These methods include assay of polyether lipids, use of fluorescent antibody labelling and assay of methanogen-specific coenzymes, such as coenzyme F_{420} (Archer & Kirsop, 1988).

Antibodies have been raised against methanogens for use in identification (Conway de Macario *et al.*, 1982; Macario & Conway de Macario, 1985) and have been shown to be specific. Enzyme-linked immunosorbent assays (ELISAs) developed in the Institute of Food Research (Norwich Laboratory) (IFRN) using polyclonal antisera were sensitive and genus-specific (Archer, 1984). However, cross-reactions with other methanogen species in anaerobic digester samples meant that antibodies of greater specificity were required.

DEVELOPMENT OF ELISAs FOR METHANOGENS

In this study, both polyclonal and monoclonal antibodies have been raised against *Methanosarcina mazei* strain S6 (DSM 2053) and *Methanobacterium bryantii* strain FR-2 (DSM 2257). Whole cells were used as the immunogen in Freund's adjuvant, injected intradermally into rabbits and intraperitoneally into rats. Monoclonal antibodies were produced by fusing rat spleen cells with rat myeloma cells (YB2/3: DAg 20, Galfré & Milstein, 1981). High titre antisera were produced in both rabbits and rats to both immunogens. Figures 2 and 3 show binding of two of these antisera to microtitration plates coated with whole cells. The polyclonal antiserum raised against *Ms. mazei* was genus-specific and did not show appreciable

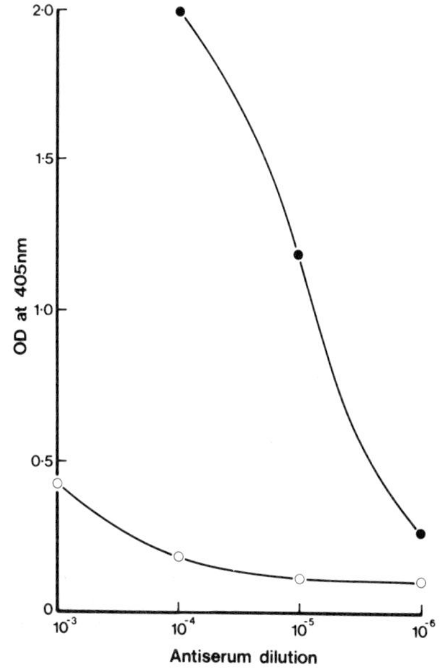

Fig. 2. Titration curves for a rabbit polyclonal antiserum (R135b_1) raised against *Ms. mazei* on a plate coated with *Ms. mazei* cells (●) and on a plate coated with *Mb. bryantii* cells (○).

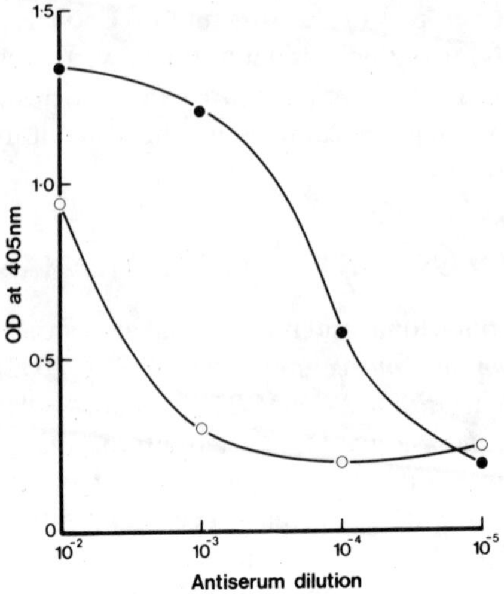

Fig. 3. Titration curves for a rat polyclonal antiserum (Rat $16b_1$) raised against *Mb. bryantii* on a plate coated with *Mb. bryantii* cells (●) and on a plate coated with *Ms. mazei* cells (○).

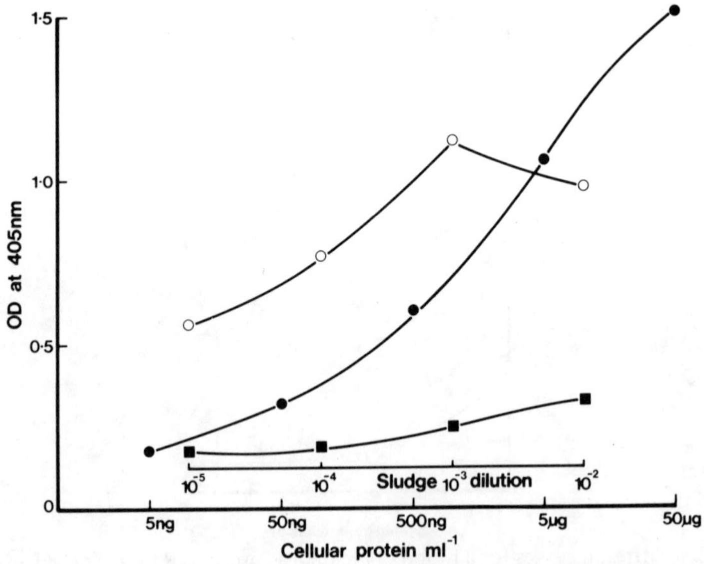

Fig. 4. Standard curve for *Ms. mazei* (●) in the two-site ELISA and dilutions of sludge samples rich in *Ms. mazei* (○) and poor in *Ms. mazei* (■).

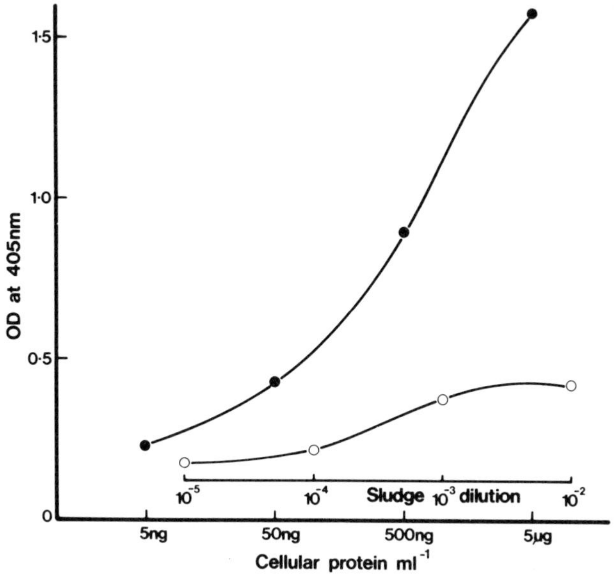

Fig. 5. Standard curve for *Mb. bryantii* (●) in the two-site ELISA and dilutions of sludge (○).

binding to *Mb. bryantii*. The polyclonal antiserum to *Mb. bryantii* did exhibit some binding to plates coated with *Ms. mazei* cells. Several hybridomas secreting antibodies to *Ms. mazei* were obtained, and monoclonal antibodies from one hybridoma cell line (IFRN-10), which showed no cross-reaction with *Mb. bryantii*, were chosen for use in the assay.

Sandwich, or two-site, ELISAs were developed for the enumeration of cells (Voller *et al.*, 1976). Microtitration plates were coated with rabbit polyclonal antibodies. After the cells had been allowed to react with the immobilised antibody, a second primary antibody was added; rat monoclonal anti-*Ms. mazei* antibody or rat polyclonal anti-*Mb. bryantii* antibody as appropriate. Specific binding of rat antibodies was detected with alkaline phosphatase-labelled anti-rat IgG conjugate.

Both assays had a limit of detection for cellular protein of 10 ng/ml (Figs 4 and 5), calculated by adding 2 SD to the zero value. Neither assay showed any cross-reaction with *Desulfovibrio desulfuricans* or *Escherichia coli*, two bacteria which can also be involved with methanogenesis and which are used in a model system at IFRN. The *Mb. bryantii* assay showed no cross-reaction with *Ms. mazei*. Similarly, the *Ms. mazei* assay showed no cross-reaction with *Mb. bryantii* or another methanosarcina, *Ms. barkeri* strain MS (DSM 800).

Two digester sludges were analysed in the *Ms. mazei* assay (Fig. 4). One which was rich in *Methanosarcina* spp. (judged microscopically) gave a response curve between 10^{-3} and 10^{-5} dilutions parallel to the standard curve. This suggested that over this range there was no interference in the assay from the other bacterial cells present. From this dilution curve, a value of 10 mg *Ms. mazei* protein/ml digester sludge was calculated. However, at a lower dilution of 10^{-2} cells, the binding in the assay was considerably reduced, probably due to the amount of cellular protein present. As there are approximately 10^9 total bacterial cells/ml in a digester sludge (Archer & Kirsop, 1988), there would be 10^6 cells per well at this dilution. The second sludge which contained levels of *Methanosarcina* spp., undetectable by microscopy, showed little reaction in the ELISA over the range of dilutions examined.

A sample of sewage sludge analysed in the *Mb. bryantii* ELISA (Fig. 5) gave a slight increase in binding at dilutions of 10^{-2} and 10^{-3}. An average value for cellular protein of 35 μg/ml was calculated from these readings. Furthermore, it did not recognise *Ms. barkeri* strain MS, a closely related methanogen of the same genus. This specificity was probably attributable to the use of a monoclonal antibody in the two-site assay. The ELISA for *Mb. bryantii* utilised two polyclonal antisera, but still showed no cross-reaction with *Ms. mazei.* Further work should elucidate the species specificity of this assay.

Since the assays can be used to quantify individual species of methanogenic bacteria in digester samples, they show potential for fast and reliable methods of monitoring anaerobic digester status.

ACKNOWLEDGEMENTS

The authors wish to thank Katy Hamand for technical assistance. This work was funded in part by the Ministry of Agriculture, Fisheries and Food.

REFERENCES

Archer, D. B. (1983) The microbiological basis of process control in methanogenic fermentation of soluble wastes. *Enzyme and Microbial Technology*, **5**, 162–170.

Archer, D. B. (1984) Detection and quantitation of methanogens by enzyme-linked immunosorbent assay. *Applied and Environmental Microbiology*, **48**, 797–801.

Archer, D. B. & Kirsop, B. H. (1988) The microbiology and control of anaerobic digestion. In: *Modern Anaerobic Technology*, Wheatley, A. D. & Cassell, L. (eds), Blackwell Scientific, Oxford, in press.

Conway de Macario, E., Macario, A. J. L. & Kandler, O. (1982) Monoclonal antibodies for immunochemical analysis of methanogenic bacteria. *Journal of Immunology*, **129**, 1670–1674.

Galfré, G. & Milstein, C. (1981) Preparation of monoclonal antibodies: strategies and procedures. In: *Methods in Enzymology*, Langone, J. J. & Van Vunakis, H. (eds), Academic Press, London, **73** (Part B), Immunochemical Techniques, pp. 3–46.

Kirsop, B. H. (1984) Methanogenesis. *CRC Critical Reviews in Biotechnology*, **1**, 109–159.

Macario, A. J. L. & Conway de Macario, E. (1985) A preview of the uses of monoclonal antibodies against methanogens in fermentation biotechnology: significance for public health. In: *Monoclonal Antibodies Against Bacteria*, Volume 1, Macario, A. J. L. & Conway de Macario, E. (eds), Academic Press, New York, pp. 269–286.

Voller, A., Bidwell, D. E. & Bartlett, A. (1976) Enzyme immunoassays in diagnostic medicine: theory and practice. *Bulletin of the World Health Organization*, **53**, 55–56.

13

The Use of Saliva to Measure Potato Steroidal Alkaloids in Humans

M. H. HARVEY, M. MCMILLAN

Department of Chemical Pathology, Lewisham Hospital, London, UK

B. A. MORRIS and V. MARKS

Division of Clinical Biochemistry, Department of Biochemistry, University of Surrey, Guildford, UK

INTRODUCTION

Potato Glycoalkaloids

The common potato (*Solanum tuberosum*) is one of the world's major agricultural food products. Its annual production ranks third behind wheat and rice, and it provides a versatile addition to a wide variety of processed foods. Nutritionally, it is a good source of protein, carbohydrate and minerals, as well as providing many vitamins, especially vitamin C.

Minor constituents of the potato include the steroidal glycoalkaloids, which are important because of their reputedly toxic properties. These alkaloids have been implicated in the causation of poisoning both in animals (Clarke & Clarke, 1975) and man (McMillan & Thompson, 1979). In humans, acute poisoning results in gastrointestinal, neurological and other disturbances; potato alkaloid levels of 41 mg/100 g (Harris & Cockburn, 1918) and 50 mg/100 g (Wilson, 1959) have been found in these cases. It has been postulated that these alkaloids might have a role in the aetiology of neural tube defects (Renwick, 1972).

In commercially available potato tubers, 95% or more of the total glycoalkaloid (TGA) fraction consists of α-solanine and α-chaconine (Pasechnichenko & Guseva, 1956). The glycosides are derivatives of the aglycone solanidine, with sugar residues attached to the A ring (Fig. 1). Intermediate forms, β- and γ-solanine and -chaconine, also occur with two

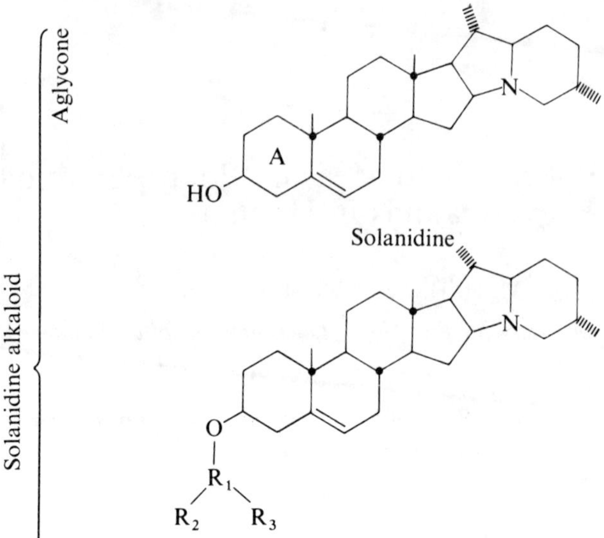

Glycosides

α-Solanine
R_1 = D-galactose
R_2 = D-glucose
R_3 = L-rhamnose

β-Solanine
R_1 and R_2 only

γ-Solanine
R_1 only

α-Chaconine
R_1 = D-glucose
$R_2 = R_3$ = L-rhamnose

β-Chaconine
R_1 and R_2 only

γ-Chaconine
R_1 only

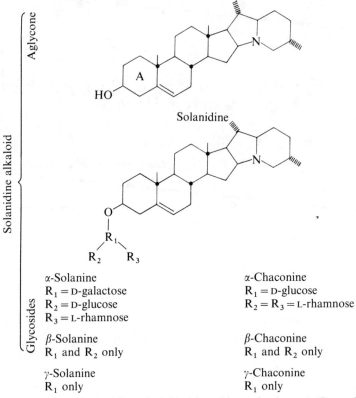

Fig. 1. Structure of solanidine alkaloids (glycosides and aglycone). (Reproduced with permission from McMillan & Thompson, 1979; courtesy Oxford University Press.)

and one sugar residues per mole respectively. The alkaloids have the 27-carbon skeleton of cholesterol, with nitrogen incorporated in the molecule. Glycoalkaloids are found in most tissues of the potato plant, the highest levels being found in the sprouts, flowers, fruit, leaves and stem (Table 1), and poisoning has sometimes resulted from their consumption. The major portion of the tuber TGA fraction is found in the peel and in areas of high metabolic activity, such as the eye, with relatively low levels in the flesh (Maga, 1980). Under certain conditions, alkaloid levels increase and concentrations can reach 80 mg TGA/100 g fresh weight of tuber with much higher levels in the peel. Cooking and other types of potato processing do not appear to reduce potato TGA levels (Bushway & Ponnampalam, 1981). The concentration of glycoalkaloids in the tuber is

Table 1
Distribution of Glycoalkaloids in the Potato and Potato Products

Potato part	*mg TGA/100 g fresh weight of tuber*
Sprouts	200–400
Flowers	300–500
Stems	3
Leaves	40–100
Whole tuber	1·2–20
Peel	30–60
Flesh	1·2–5·0
Bitter tuber	
Peel	155–220
Flesh	25–80
Potato product	*mg TGA/100 g equivalent fresh weight*
Powder	3·9–13·5
Crisps	3·2–18·4
Chipped	1·9–5·8
Oven chips	2·7–8·6
Canned	2·9–9·9

dependent on cultivation factors, post-harvest treatment, storage conditions and genetic background of the tuber (Jadhav *et al.*, 1981). New genetic varieties of potatoes are checked for their glycoalkaloid content before being introduced to the commercial market. It has been generally agreed that the TGA content of commercially available tubers should not exceed a level greater than 20 mg TGA/100 g fresh weight of tuber (Sinden & Deahl, 1976). As the toxic dose in man is not known, this limit is primarily governed by flavour properties; tubers of a high alkaloid content tend to have a bitter taste.

Recent surveys in the UK, Australia and the USA have shown that the majority of commercially available tubers have TGA concentrations below the recommended limit (Sinden & Webb, 1972; Davies & Blincow, 1984; Morris & Peterman, 1985). In Sweden, however, TGA concentrations ranged from 2 to 30 mg TGA/100 g (Johnsson & Hellenas, 1983). Nine of the 111 samples of new potatoes had levels above 20 mg TGA/100 g, the highest being in new potatoes collected before mid-July, when 76% had an elevated TGA content (Johnsson & Hellenas, 1983).

Salivary Steroids

Clinical assays for the measurement of steroids in serum have been in use for some time. More recently, assays have been described for the

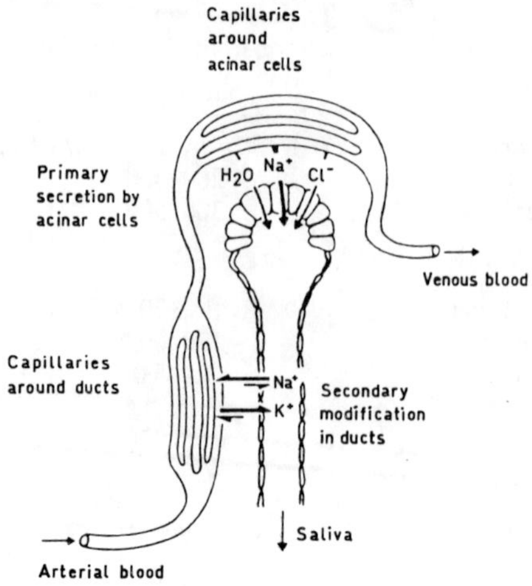

Fig. 2. Diagrammatic representation of the electrolyte and water movement in the parotid gland. (Reproduced with permission from Davenport, 1971; copyright © 1978 by Year Book Medical Publishers, Inc., Chicago.)

measurement of steroids in saliva (Read *et al.*, 1984), and because the potato glycoalkaloids have a similar structure, similar analytical methods have been developed.

The use of saliva as an alternative to serum for measurement of such analytes has the advantages of being a cheap, non-invasive technique providing an easy method of multi-sampling and patient self-collection. It has proved a useful index of the unbound plasma concentrations of a number of steroids, such as progesterone and testosterone (Vining & McGinley, 1984), and drugs, such as phenytoin and digoxin (Landon & Mahmod, 1984).

The salivary glands produce a mixed secretion consisting mainly of water, ions and mucins. Sodium is actively pumped from blood to saliva and water flows between the acinar cells under osmotic pressure, with bicarbonate and chloride ions following to maintain the ionic balance (Fig. 2). As the saliva moves down the ductal system, sodium is exchanged for potassium. This is a limited mechanism and with increased flow rate, sodium concentration in saliva increases, as consequently does chloride, bicarbonate and pH. The variation in bicarbonate concentration with flow rate can alter the pH from 6·5 at low flow rates to 8·0 at high flow rates.

The structure of the salivary gland allows for three main mechanisms by which molecules can enter saliva from the blood (Landon & Mahmod,

1984): active transport, ultrafiltration and intracellular diffusion. Drugs such as lithium have a saliva/plasma ratio of more than 2, indicating an active secretory mechanism. Small water-soluble molecules can pass into saliva via the tight junctions between the acinar cells, but these tight junctions prevent the passage of substances with molecular weights greater than 300 daltons.

Sucrose, molecular weight 342 daltons, is only present in saliva at 1% of its plasma concentration. This is also shown by lipid-insoluble conjugated steroids whose only route of entry is also ultrafiltration and which appear in saliva at approximately 1% of the unbound plasma concentrations (Vining & McGinley, 1984).

The major method of entry of drugs and steroids into saliva is intracellular diffusion through the capillary and acinar cell membranes. These compounds diffuse down a concentration gradient from the free fraction in the plasma, lipid-soluble non-ionised molecules of small molecular weight diffusing most rapidly. The salivary concentration of this type of compound is independent of flow rate. Hydrophilic molecules or lipid-soluble compounds which have subsequently been metabolised to glucuronides or sulphates are largely unable to enter saliva by intracellular diffusion. Ionisation of certain acidic or basic compounds can be influenced by salivary pH (depending on their pK_a) and hence levels are altered with salivary flow rate.

The advantages of salivary measurements must be balanced against the limitations involved. Contamination of saliva must be considered when measuring salivary analytes. The presence of drug or food in the mouth when sampling can falsely increase salivary concentrations, as can contamination from handling the compound. Blood in the saliva, caused by vigorous brushing of teeth, or plasma exudate, i.e. gingivitis, also leads to falsely increased salivary concentrations.

A strict protocol for the collection of saliva must be maintained (Table 2). In order to avoid these sources of contamination, the mouth should always be thoroughly rinsed with water prior to collecting the sample, a period of 30 min being allowed to elapse before beginning the collection so as to allow equilibration to be restored. In the case of potato alkaloid measurement, saliva was collected in the morning before lunch; a blood sample was also collected. Subjects were asked to rinse the mouth 30 min before sampling to remove any food. The presence of mucins in saliva cause difficulties in handling. These are removed by freezing and thawing centrifugation of the saliva which breaks down the mucins to remove any epithelial cells and leave a clear supernatant for assay.

Table 2
Collection of Saliva for Glycoalkaloid Assay

(1) Specimens collected before lunch. Blood sample taken immediately before or after saliva collection.
(2) Subject to rinse mouth with water 30 min prior to sample. No further food or drink to be taken.
(3) Mixed saliva (5 ml) collected in a universal container.
(4) Sample frozen, thawed and spun. Supernatant removed and stored at −20°C until assay.

Measurement of Potato Glycoalkaloids

A wide variety of methods has been developed for measurement of steroidal glycoalkaloids in the potato (Coxon, 1984). Historically, colorimetric methods have been most widely used, but more recently HPLC, RIA and ELISA have proved advantageous. The analysis of body fluid concentrations of potato alkaloids has been made possible by the development of RIAs, employing a tritiated solanidine label and an antiserum raised to a solanine–BSA conjugate synthesised by the periodate cleavage method (Butler & Chen, 1967). The RIA was initially used to quantify serum solanidine in a group of hospital patients (Matthew *et al.*, 1983) and in a group of healthy volunteers (Harvey *et al.*, 1985*a*).

The antiserum cross-reacted 100% with solanidine, α-solanine and α-chaconine, but did not cross-react with structurally related endogenous steroids. Method specificity for solanidine was achieved by prior extraction of the sample with chloroform, leaving α-solanine and α-chaconine in the aqueous layer. Direct analysis of the serum produced a measure of the total alkaloid concentration, i.e. solanidine, α-solanine, α-chaconine and any cross-reacting metabolites.

The lower levels of analytes in saliva compared with the levels in serum warrant the development of assays with greater sensitivity. Salivary alkaloids were measured by adaptation of the serum assays, using an increased sample volume (Harvey *et al.*, 1985*b*) and a recently produced antiserum of increased avidity (G/S/RG14, 23.10.85). The salivary assays did not exhibit the matrix effect seen in those using serum, where standards needed to be diluted in alkaloid-free serum prepared by affinity chromatography. The detection limit and assay precision were improved for both solanidine and total alkaloid in saliva (serum solanidine detection limit = 1·3 nmol/litre, salivary solanidine = 1·0 nmol/litre; serum total alkaloid detection limit = 1·0 nmol/litre, salivary total alkaloid = 0·5 nmol/litre).

STUDIES OF SALIVARY GLYCOALKALOIDS

Salivary alkaloid concentrations have been measured in a group of healthy volunteers from the UK and in a group from Sweden (Harvey *et al.*, 1985*b*). The UK subjects consisted of 18 males and 15 females eating their normal diet during the summer months. The Swedish group included seven subjects eating their normal diet and three who ate potatoes known to be high in glycoalkaloids, Ulster Chieftain (20–30 mg TGA/100 g) and a new Swedish variety, SV72118 (18–30 mg TGA/100 g). The high alkaloid intake group ate 200–300 g of cooked, unpeeled potato daily for one week before sampling. Although the subjects noted a bitter taste when eating the potatoes, no toxic effects were observed. Saliva and blood samples were collected 12–14 h after the last meal.

The results of the study are shown in Fig. 3. Serum and salivary solanidine and total alkaloid concentrations are shown for all subjects, UK subjects, Swedish subjects and Swedish subjects minus the ones with high alkaloid intake. The mean and median serum total alkaloid concentrations are higher than the serum solanidine. The mean ratio of 2·7:1 for total alkaloid to solanidine in the serum is much lower than in the potato, suggesting possible glycoside metabolism.

The range and mean of the serum solanidine and total alkaloid concentrations are higher than the salivary values in each group. As salivary values are thought to reflect the free unbound concentration of the serum, the above findings are to be expected.

Linear regression analysis of the results (Table 3) shows a significant correlation between serum and salivary solanidine as well as serum and salivary total alkaloid content. The mean serum solanidine, 14·5 nmol/litre, is nearly a third of the mean total alkloid, 38·5 nmol/litre. This difference is not reflected for saliva, where solanidine represents about 20% of the serum mean but salivary total alkaloid only about 10%. Levels of the mean

Table 3
Linear Regression Data for Serum and Salivary Solanum Alkaloid Concentrations

	n	*Mean*	*Median*	*Range*	*Regression line*	*r*	*t*	*P*
Solanidine (nmol/litre)								
Serum (X)	42	14·5	5·0	2·5–92·5	$Y = 0{\cdot}094X + 1{\cdot}86$	0·734	5·72	<0·001
Saliva (Y)	42	3·2	2·4	0·6–10·8				
Total alkaloids (nmol/litre)								
Serum (X)	42	38·5	27·5	3·3–125	$Y = 0{\cdot}812X + 0{\cdot}123$	0·892	12·15	<0·001
Saliva (Y)	42	3·7	2·3	1·3–12				

(Reproduced with permission from Harvey *et al.*, 1985*b*; courtesy The Macmillan Press Ltd.)

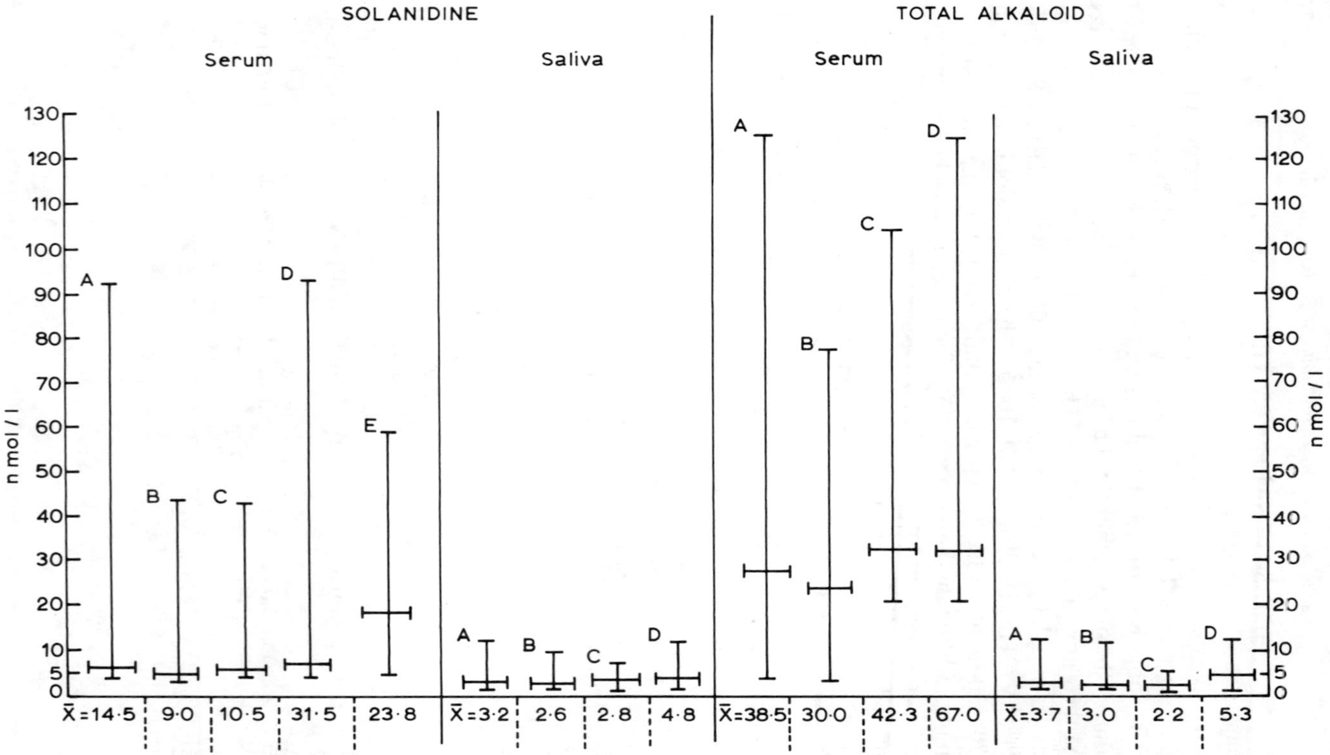

Fig. 3. Summer solanidine and total alkaloid concentrations in serum and saliva: A, all subjects ($n = 43$); B, UK subjects ($n = 33$); C, all Swedish subjects ($n = 10$); D, Swedish subjects minus the three subjects on high alkaloid diets ($n = 7$); E, winter UK concentrations ($n = 57$); $\bar{X}$, mean; ⊤, range; |—|, median value.

Table 4
Comparison of Alkaloid Concentrations in Swedish Subjects on a High Alkaloid Diet with those in Swedish Subjects on a Normal Diet

	n	*Mean*	*Median*	*Range*	*t*	*P*
Serum solanidine (nmol/litre)						
Normal	7	10·5	6·8	2·5–42·5	−7·54	<0·001
High alkaloid	3	80·8	77·5	72·5–92·5		
Serum total alkaloid (nmol/litre)						
Normal	7	42·3	32·5	20·8–105	−4·62	<0·01
High alkaloid	3	125	>125	125–>125		
Salivary solanidine (nmol/litre)						
Normal	7	2·8	2·8	<0·25–2·0	6·173	<0·001
High alkaloid	3	9·4	10·3	2·9–4·3		
Salivary total alkaloid (nmol/litre)						
Normal	7	3·0	2·2	1·3–6·3	6·03	<0·001
High alkaloid	3	10·5	10·9	8·6–11·9		

(Reproduced with permission from Harvey *et al.*, 1985*b*; courtesy The Macmillan Press Ltd.)

salivary solanidine, 3·2 nmol/litre, and the mean salivary total alkaloid, 3·7 nmol/litre, are very similar.

The differences in serum and salivary alkaloids are further demonstrated by comparing the group of Swedish subjects on high alkaloid intake with the normal group (Table 4). The subjects on a high alkaloid diet have significantly higher serum solanidine and total alkaloid concentrations than the normal subjects, as would be expected. In both groups, the serum total alkaloid concentrations are higher than those of solanidine.

In saliva, alkaloid concentrations in the high intake group are again significantly higher than those for the normals. However, in both groups the salivary total alkaloid and the salivary solanidine levels are essentially equal. This would be expected from the nature of molecular entry into saliva, as discussed above.

Solanidine is very lipid-soluble, has a molecular weight of less than 400 daltons and should enter saliva easily by intracellular diffusion. The glycosides, α-solanine, and α-chaconine, have molecular weights greater than 800 and, more importantly, hydrophilic sugar residues which tend to exclude these compounds from saliva. Salivary total alkaloid should therefore be predominantly solanidine with a minor contribution from the smaller glycosides.

CONCLUSION

These results show the advantages and usefulness of salivary assays for measuring certain molecules. Solanidine has the ideal structure for entering saliva by intracellular diffusion and salivary concentrations show good correlation with serum. The solanidine glycosides have been shown to be largely excluded from saliva and represent compounds for which salivary analysis would be inappropriate. Whether salivary analysis will be useful to measure body burdens of other food components has yet to be discovered.

REFERENCES

BUSHWAY, R. J. & PONNAMPALAM, R. (1981) α-Chaconine and α-solanine content of potato products and their stability during several modes of cooking. *Journal of Agriculture and Food Chemistry*, **29**, 814–817.

BUTLER, V. P. Jr & CHEN, J. P. (1967) Digoxin-specific antibodies. *Proceedings of the National Academy of Science, USA*, **57**, 71–78.

COXON, D. T. (1984) Methodology for glycoalkaloid analysis. *American Potato Journal*, **51**, 169–183.

CLARKE, E. G. C. & CLARKE, M. L. (1975) In: *Veterinary Toxicology*, Clarke, E. G. C. & Clarke, M. L. (eds), Williams and Williams, Baltimore, pp. 359–360.

DAVENPORT, H. W. (1971) In: *The Digestive Tract*, Year Book Medical Publishers, Chicago, p. 87.

DAVIES, A. M. C. & BLINCOW, P. J. (1984) Glycoalkaloid content of potatoes and potato products sold in the UK. *Journal of Science of Food and Agriculture*, **35**, 553–557.

HARRIS, F. & COCKBURN, T. (1918) Alleged poisoning by potatoes. *Analyst (London)*, **43**, 133–136.

HARVEY, M. H., MCMILLAN, M., MORGAN, M. R. A. & CHAN, H. W.-S. (1985*a*) Solanidine is present in the sera of healthy individuals and in amounts dependent on their dietary potato consumption. *Human Toxicology*, **4**, 187–194.

HARVEY, M. H., MORRIS, B. A., MCMILLAN, M. & MARKS, V. (1985*b*) Measurement of potato steroidal alkaloids in human serum and saliva by radioimmunoassay. *Human Toxicology*, **4**, 503–512.

JADHAV, S. J., SHARMA, R. P. & SALUNKHE, D. K. (1981) Naturally occurring toxic alkaloids in foods. *CRC Critical Reviews in Toxicology*, **9**, 21–104.

JOHNSSON, H. & HELLENAS, K.-E. (1983) Total glycoalkaloid in Swedish potatoes. *Var Foda*, **35**, 299–314.

LANDON, J. & MAHMOD, S. (1984) Distribution of drugs between blood and saliva. In: *Immunoassays of Steroids in Saliva (Ninth Tenovus Workshop)*, Read, G. F., Riad-Fahmy, D., Walker, R. F. & Griffiths, K. (eds), Alpha Omega Publishing Ltd, Cardiff, pp. 47–55.

MCMILLAN, M. & THOMPSON, J. C. (1979) An outbreak of suspected solanine poisoning in schoolboys. *Quarterly Journal of Medicine*, **48**, 227–243.

MAGA, J. A. (1980) Potato glycoalkaloids. *CRC Critical Reviews in Food Science and Nutrition*, **12**, 371–405.

MATTHEW, J. A., MORGAN, M. R. A., MCNERNEY, R., CHAN, H. W.-S. & COXON, D. T. (1983) Determination of solanidine in human plasma by radioimmunoassay. *Food Chemistry and Toxicology*, **21**, 637–640.

MORRIS, S. C. & PETERMAN, J. B. (1985) Genetic and environmental effects on levels of glycoalkaloids in cultivars of potato. *Food Chemistry*, **18**, 271–282.

PASECHNICHENKO, V. & GUSEVA, A. R. (1956) Quantitative determination of potato glycoalkaloids and their preparative separation. *Biochemistry (USSR)*, **21**, 606–611.

READ, G. F., RIAD-FAHMY, D., WALKER, R. F. & GRIFFITHS, K. (eds) (1984) *Immunoassays of Steroids in Saliva (Ninth Tenovus Workshop)*, Alpha Omega Publishing Ltd, Cardiff.

RENWICK, J. H. (1972) Hypothesis; anencephaly and spina bifida are usually preventable by avoidance of a specific but unidentified substance present in certain potato tubers. *British Journal of Preventative and Social Medicine*, **26**, 67–88.

SINDEN, S. L. & DEAHL, K. L. (1976) Effect of glycoalkaloids and phenolics on potato flavour. *Journal of Food Science*, **41**, 520–523.

SINDEN, S. L. & WEBB, R. E. (1972) Effect of variety and location on the glycoalkaloid content of potatoes. *American Potato Journal*, **49**, 334–338.

VINING, R. F. & MCGINLEY, R. A. (1984) Transport of steroids from blood to saliva. In: *Immunoassays of Steroids in Saliva (Ninth Tenovus Workshop)*, Read, G. F., Riad-Fahmy, D., Walker, R. F. & Griffiths, K. (eds), Alpha Omega Publishing Ltd, Cardiff, pp. 56–63.

WILSON, G. S. (1959) A small outbreak of solanine poisoning. *Monthly Bulletin of Ministry of Health (London), Public Health Laboratory Service*, **18**, 207–210.

14

An Immunochemical Method for the Measurement of Mould Contamination in Tomato Paste

A. ROBERTSON, D. UPADHYAYA, S. OPIE

Campden Food Preservation Research Association, Chipping Campden, Glos, UK

and

J. SARGEANT*

Lord Rank Research Centre, High Wycombe, Bucks, UK

INTRODUCTION

The Howard Mould Count (HMC), developed some 75 years ago (Howard, 1911), is the officially recognised method for assessing, and thus controlling, the amount of decayed fruit incorporated into comminuted tomato products. The technique relies upon the microscopic examination of non-homogenised juice, or suitably diluted paste, on a slide specifically designed for the purpose. A defined field of view (1·332 mm) is inspected for mould filaments and counted as positive if any present are greater than one-sixth of the field diameter, as measured using an ocular graticule, or if the sum of up to three mycelial fragments in the field is estimated to be greater than this length. Generally, on a single tomato paste sample, two slides are counted and the result expressed as percentage positive fields. Up to four more may be counted if the result is close to the acceptance/rejection limit. Percentage positive fields are related to the amount of rotten fruit incorporated into the product. This relationship, however, is only semi-quantitative due to the nature of mould growth. The presence of extra filaments in a positive field is ignored such that an individual filament can be as significant to the HMC as a large clump of mould.

* Present address: Beeches Biotech, Beeches Farm, Buckland St Mary, Chard, Somerset, UK.

To date, the occurrence of mould in tomatoes has not been associated with the presence of substances injurious to human health. However, incorporation of rotten fruit into pastes and juices does result in a loss of quality and 'wholesomeness' of the products. It is not permitted to import or to use tomato paste in the UK which has an HMC of 50% or above. Restrictions on the import and use of substandard tomato paste are imposed in numerous other countries throughout the world, with the United States having direct legislation based on an HMC of 40% positive fields.

The subjectivity of the HMC technique results in large inter-laboratory variation and even intra-laboratory variation between different operators. The method is therefore dependent upon highly trained staff, is laborious and, depending on the number of slides counted, can be extremely time-consuming. Furthermore, recent processing techniques have caused changes in the degree of comminution which affects the accuracy of the method. Homogenisation in the case of tomato juice, to provide a cloud-stable product, has resulted in such severe mould filament damage as to render the HMC impossible. Finally, the method does not take account of the size and amount of mould within a field to allow it to be fully quantitative.

Alternative approaches to the visual measurement of mould have therefore been the subject of numerous studies. Many have been indirect measurements based on chemical changes effected by mould growth. Damage by other causes or the high levels of fungal growth required to facilitate such changes have contributed to their lack of success. A direct method based on the level of chitin, the major component of fungal mycelial walls, has been suggested (Jarvis, 1977). The method involves acid hydrolysis of chitin to glucosamine followed by colorimetric or gas chromatographic determination. This procedure is both tedious and the results subject to inaccuracies due to variation in the glucosamine content between mould genera and possible contamination of products by insect fragments. The production of ergosterol, a fungal metabolite, has been studied (Seitz *et al.*, 1977) in grain samples. Once again, the method is tedious and the result affected by only some fungi producing the metabolite in some circumstances. Recently near infrared reflectance spectroscopy (NIR) has been used to detect mould in tomato paste, both directly by correlation with fungal weight and indirectly by correlation with percentage rotten fruit (Davies *et al.*, 1987). It is considered that this method may be useful for the rapid screening of tomato paste.

Immunoassays have also been used for the detection of fungal mycelia

(Casper & Mendgen, 1979). The detection of mould contamination in heat-preserved foods, however, presents special problems. For a quantitative assay to be reliable and reproducible, the antibody must be mould-specific and not cross-react with the growth substrate. Furthermore, it should react with a fungal component or components which are not subject to large variations as a result of growth rate, substrate or age. It would be ideal, although not essential, if the antigenic site(s) was common to all mould genera, although this factor could be overcome by use of mould 'cocktails' in the preparation of the antibodies. More importantly, the antigenic sites of moulds should be unaffected by the heat treatments to which processed foods, and specifically comminuted tomato products, are subjected.

Recently two reports (Notermans & Heuvelman, 1985; Lin *et al.*, 1986), one specifically concerning tomato paste, have recognised the potential of an immunochemical technique for the measurement of mould. Both groups have shown that heat treatment does not destroy the antigenic sites of mould. However, neither have used mould cocktails as the immunogen. The level of cross-reaction has not been high enough between mould genera to make an EIA assay useful in commercial tomato paste where different mould compositions may be found according to the growth location of the original fruit.

This chapter reports the production of antibodies to both heated and unheated mould 'cocktails', and to each individual mould in these preparations, to test cross-reactivity. The development of an EIA for the qualitative assessment of mould in commercial tomato pastes is also reported.

MATERIALS AND METHODS

Choice and Culture of Fungi

Alternaria alternata, *Botrytis cinerea*, *Fusarium solani*, *Mucor piriformis* and *Rhizopus stolonifer*, representing 90–95% of the fungal spoilage organisms found on tomatoes, were used to prepare an immunogen 'cocktail'. To eliminate substrate effects on fungal morphology, moulds were initially grown on tomato broth prepared from salt-free tomato paste. When this was found to have little affect on antibody production, synthetic media (malt extract broth, Oxoid CM57) was substituted to minimise any cross-reaction with tomato solids. All cultures were incubated at 22°C and the mycelium harvested after 6 and 10 days, depending on growth.

Preparation of Immunogens

Method 1

Individual fungal cultures were filtered under vacuum through sterile filter paper (Whatman No. 1). Samples (2 g) of each were weighed into each of two universal bottles to give a total of 10 g mixed mycelia. Sterile distilled water (10 ml) was added to each sample. Tomato paste pasteurisation conditions were simulated by steaming one sample at 100°C for 6 min followed by rapid cooling in cold water. The other sample remained unheated. Both heated and unheated samples were then washed five times by centrifugation using 100 ml aliquots of sterile distilled water. The washed mycelia were finally freeze-dried and the resultant material ground under liquid N_2 using a mortar and pestle. The remaining liquid N_2 was allowed to boil off and the mycelial powder quickly placed into stoppered glass vials, which were stored in a vacuum desiccator at room temperature until required.

Preparation of insoluble and soluble immunogen fractions. 100 mg of the heated and unheated mixed fungal powders were suspended in 5 ml of phosphate-buffered saline with Tween 20 (PBST), pH 7·6, containing $Na_2HPO_4.12H_2O$ (2·9 g), KH_2PO_4 (0·2 g), KCl (0·2 g), NaCl (8 g) and Tween 20 (0·5 ml) in 1 litre water. The suspension was sonicated in an ultrasonic bath for 5 min and centrifuged at 3000*g* for 5 min. The supernatant representing the soluble mycelial fraction was dialysed against two changes of deionised water for 24 h at 4°C. Protein concentrations (Lowry *et al.*, 1951) of the dialysates of the unheated and heated fungal mixtures were found to be 0·9 and 0·8 mg/ml respectively. The two dialysates were freeze-dried and the lyophilisate stored in a vacuum desiccator at −20°C.

The pellets representing the insoluble fungal fractions were washed ten times by centrifugation, using 5 ml aliquots of PBST. The final pellets were resuspended at 20 mg/ml in PBS without Tween 20 and frozen as a stock suspension at −20°C.

In addition, the moulds were cultured on synthetic medium, to reduce the risk of any cross-reaction of the antiserum with tomato solids. It was considered unnecessary to heat the moulds prior to immunisation, nor was it thought important to separate the soluble and solid mycelial fractions.

Whole cryoground mycelia were therefore emulsified in Freund's complete adjuvant prior to injection. Solutions of the lyophilised soluble fractions were prepared in PBS without Tween 20 and were emulsified with

Freund's complete adjuvant (1:1 v/v) to give a final protein concentration of 0·5 mg/ml. The insoluble fungal suspensions were emulsified with Freund's complete adjuvant (1:1 v/v), containing 10 mg/ml mould mycelia solids.

The emulsified soluble and insoluble preparations (0·5 and 1·0 ml, respectively) were injected subcutaneously into different New Zealand white rabbits. The animals were boosted twice at monthly intervals, and again six months after priming.

Method 2

Fungal cultures were washed by centrifugation as described in Method 1. The individual and mixed mould preparations were then freeze-dried and stored in a vacuum desiccator at −20°C until required. Prior to immunisation, the freeze-dried preparations were emulsified in Freund's adjuvant as previously described. These preparations (20 mg) were used directly for immunisation, as described in Method 1. Similarly 2, 10, 50 and 100 mg aliquots of the mixed mould preparation were also injected into separate rabbits.

Purification of the Antisera

The antisera were dialysed overnight against two changes of PBS (5 litres) and the dialysates centrifuged at 20 000*g* for 10 min to remove insoluble material. IgG was isolated using protein A-sepharose according to the method of Hjeln *et al.* (1972).

Conjugation of IgG with Peroxidase

The IgG fraction of each antiserum was labelled with HRP (Sigma Chemical Company) at a ratio of approximately 2 mole peroxidase per mole antibody using periodate condensation (Wilson & Nakane, 1978).

Immunofluorescence Microscopy

Mould material (2 mg) or 0·2 ml tomato paste diluted to 1·345°Brix (1°Brix = 1% w/w sucrose) was washed twice by centrifugation at 3000*g* for 1 min with 5 ml aliquots of PBST. The final pellets were resuspended in PBST (0·75 ml), to which was added antibody (5 μl) prepared by Method 1. After gentle mixing, the suspension was incubated for 30 min at ambient temperature. The suspension was then washed twice by centrifugation, using 4 ml aliquots of PBST to remove unreacted antibody. The pellet was resuspended in PBST (0·75 ml) and 10 μl FITC-labelled anti-rabbit IgG (Miles–Yeda) added. The suspension was incubated for 30 min at ambient temperature, followed by two washes with PBST (4 ml) to remove any unreacted second antibody. The final pellet was resuspended in PBST (1 ml). A drop of this suspension was placed on a microscope slide, covered with a coverslip and viewed under a Reichard Polyvar microscope fitted with an epi-illumination fluorescence module.

Indirect Enzyme Immunoassays

(a) Sequential Assay
Aliquots (100 μl) of mould suspension or tomato paste diluted to 1·345°Brix were added to PBST (0·75 ml) contained in 15 ml neoprene conical centrifuge tubes. After gentle mixing, 5 μl of the protein A-purified anti-mould cocktail antibody preparation were added and the mixture incubated at 30°C with shaking. Unreacted antibody was removed by successive washing with 4 × 4 ml aliquots of PBST using centrifugation at 3500*g*. The final pellet was resuspended in PBST (0·75 ml), 10 μl HRP-labelled anti-rabbit IgG (Sigma) added and the mixture incubated as previously for 30 min. The unreacted second antibody was removed by successive washing with PBST as already described. The final pellet was resuspended in PBST (0·5 ml) and 50 μl used for the peroxidase assay using 2,2′-azino-bis-3-ethyl benzothiazoline-6-sulphonic acid (ABTS) as substrate (Childs & Bardsley, 1975).

(b) 'One-step' Assay
The above method was followed closely except that the protein A-purified anti-mould cocktail antibodies (1 μl) and peroxidase-labelled anti-rabbit IgG second antibodies (10 μl) were added simultaneously. The incubation and washing procedures were carried out as above.

Direct Enzyme Immunoassay
The HRP-labelled anti-mould cocktail antibody (5 μl) was added to the diluted mould suspension or tomato paste. All other stages of the assay were similar to those already described.

RESULTS AND DISCUSSION

Antibody Production and Performance
Immunofluorescence microscopy was performed to visually assess the antisera raised to mixed mould immunogen cocktails prepared from insoluble and soluble fractions of heated and unheated fungal mycelia. Antibodies from all the rabbits reacted with the antigens used for im-

munisation. Antisera raised to the soluble fraction of the mould cocktail were of much higher titre than those raised to the insoluble mycelial material. However, it was not quantifiable using this techinque. There appeared to be little difference in the titre of antibodies raised to heated and unheated moulds, indicating that mycelial antigenic sites are not significantly changed by heat treatments simulating those used in the production of tomato paste. Figure 1(a) shows a typical immunofluorescence micrograph of a single mould used in the cocktail (*A. alternata*). Similar micrographs were obtained for the other moulds used. The higher intensity of fluorescence at the mycelial wall would suggest that even though the antibody used in this instance was that raised to the soluble mycelial fraction, the antigenic sites are situated at the surface of the mycelial filament. The antigens, therefore, are most likely removed by damage, such as that occurring during cryo-grinding of freeze-dried mycelia, combined with PBST extraction. It is unlikely that the fungal wall antigens will also be present naturally in soluble form within the mycelia.

Figures 1(b) and 1(c) show mould from contaminated processing machinery and from the fruit visualised by immunofluorescence. It was considered that this application of immunochemistry could be combined with image analysis systems now available to provide an automated Howard Mould Counting technique with much of the operator subjectivity removed. Such a technique would be analogous to the direct epifluorescence filter technique (DEFT) for mould reported by Pettifer *et al.* (1985; Pettifer, 1986).

The EIA technique, however, offers advantages of low cost equipment as well as a method which is objective, simple, sensitive, specific, rapid and, most of all, quantitative. An EIA has therefore been developed for use with commercial pastes. On the basis of the information obtained from the work reported so far, a second series of antibodies were produced. Maximum animal response to this series was achieved after ten weeks with the 50 mg injection of antigen providing optimum antibody titre.

Antisera were also raised to the individual mould genera used in the cocktail. The results given in Table 1 show the percentage cross-reaction of these with each of the other moulds used in the cocktail. It can be seen that the highest interactions were generally found between moulds and their own antibodies. The exception was *Fusarium solani*, where the antibody showed the lowest immunoreactivity towards its own antigen. These results suggest that there are common fungal antigens which, when produced by the methods described in this paper, provide antibodies capable of cross-reaching with moulds of other genera. The data also indicate that the levels

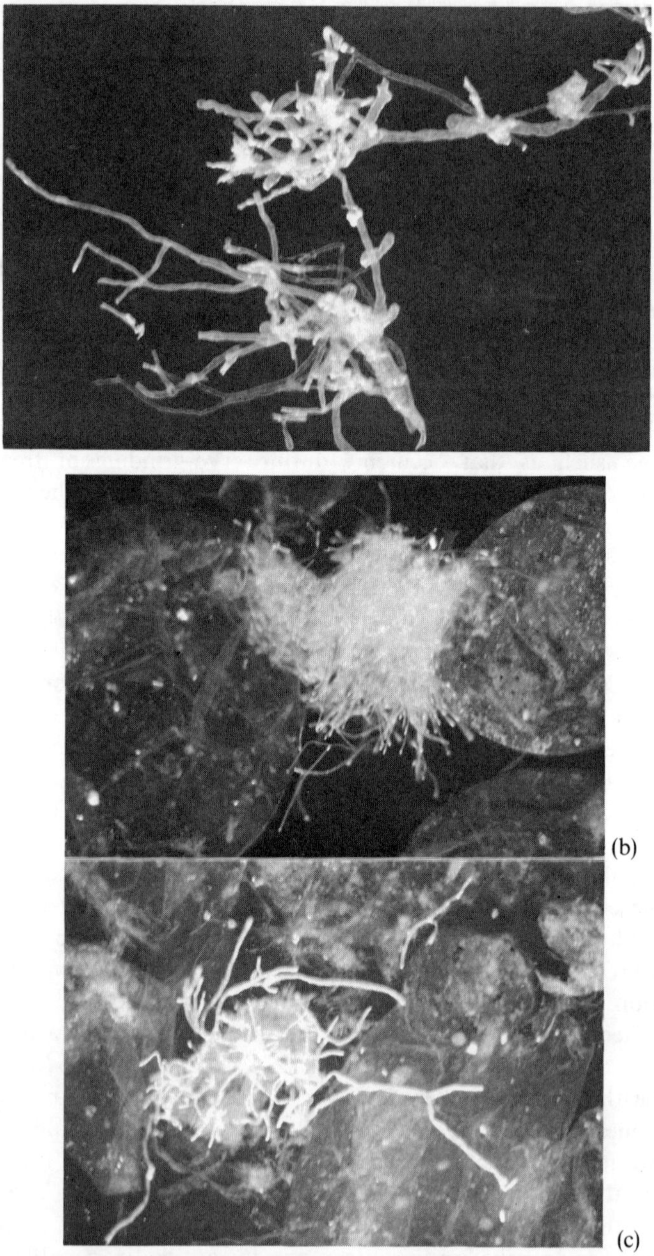
(a)
(b)
(c)

Fig. 1. (a) Typical immunofluorescence micrograph of a single mould used in the cocktail (*A. alternata*); (b) mould from contaminated processing machinery and (c) that from the fruit visualised by immunofluorescence.

Table 1
Cross-reactivity of Individual Antisera with other Genera in the Mould Cocktail

Antibody	*Antigen*				
	Alternaria	*Mucor*	*Rhizopus*	*Fusarium*	*Botrytis*
Alternaria	100	120	73	86	88
Mucor	70	100	88	96	75
Rhizopus	52	82	100	41	51
Fusarium	174	135	138	100	104
Botrytis	91	60	50	54	100

The reaction of the antisera with its own antigen was expressed as 100% and cross-reactions are relative to this.

of reaction and cross-reaction of the antibodies with whole or large intact areas of fungal mycelia are possibly more dependent on the configuration of mould surface, and therefore the availability of the antigenic sites along the mycelial surface, than on the abundance of sites or antibody titre.

Development of an EIA

For such a method to be quantitative in tomato paste, where the number and ratio of mould genera may vary depending upon the origin of the fruit, some knowledge is required of the response of the anti-cocktail antiserum to unit weight of the individual moulds. The fluorescein-labelled anti-rabbit IgG second antibody used for immunofluorescence microscopy was therefore substituted by a similar antibody conjugated with HRP. Figure 2 shows the effect of increasing the concentration of the anti-mould cocktail antiserum whilst maintaining the weight of each mould constant and the HRP-conjugated anti-rabbit IgG second antibody in excess. This effectively provides an estimate of the binding capacity of each of the moulds with the anti-mould cocktail antiserum which, as already mentioned, is perhaps a function of the combined effect of the abundance and availability of antigenic sites. Steric hindrance between antibody molecules, as antigenic sites become saturated, may therefore also contribute to the plateau effect observed. The graph shows that there are significant differences in the binding capacities of the mould genera which would affect results on tomato pastes of very different mould compositions. However, if the anti-mould cocktail antiserum is held at limiting concentrations, in the early linear area of the graph, it should have little effect on assay response.

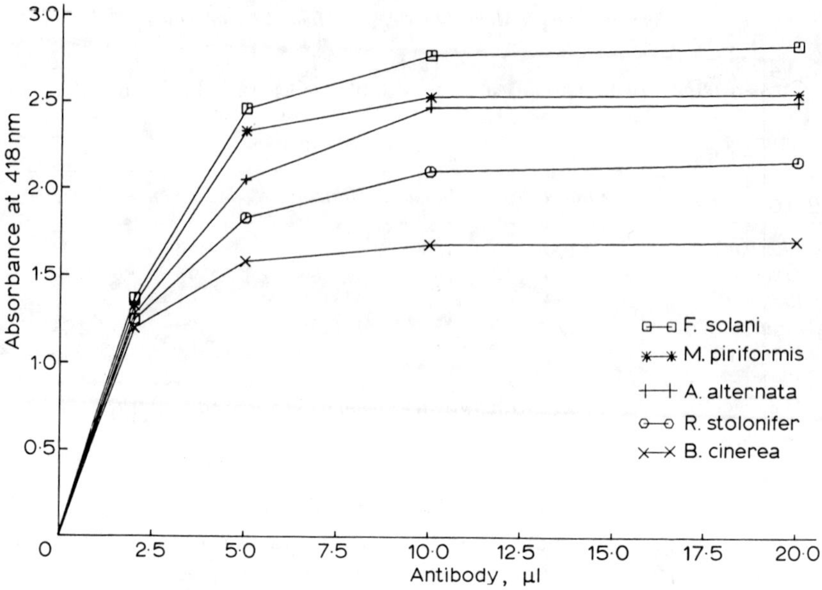

Fig. 2. First antibody saturation curve with individual moulds. Antibody raised against unheated soluble mould fraction; crude antiserum used neat.

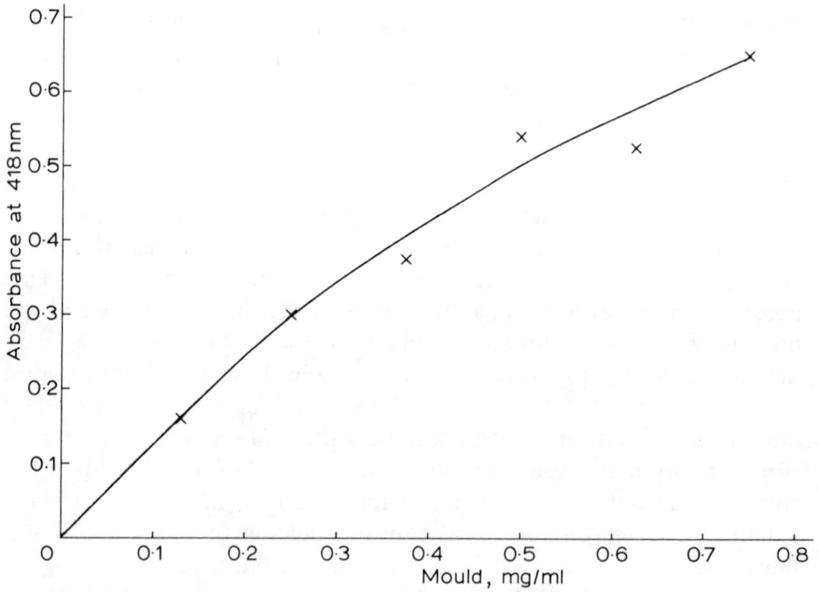

Fig. 3. Standard curve using anti-mould cocktail antiserum. Antibody raised against unheated soluble mould fraction.

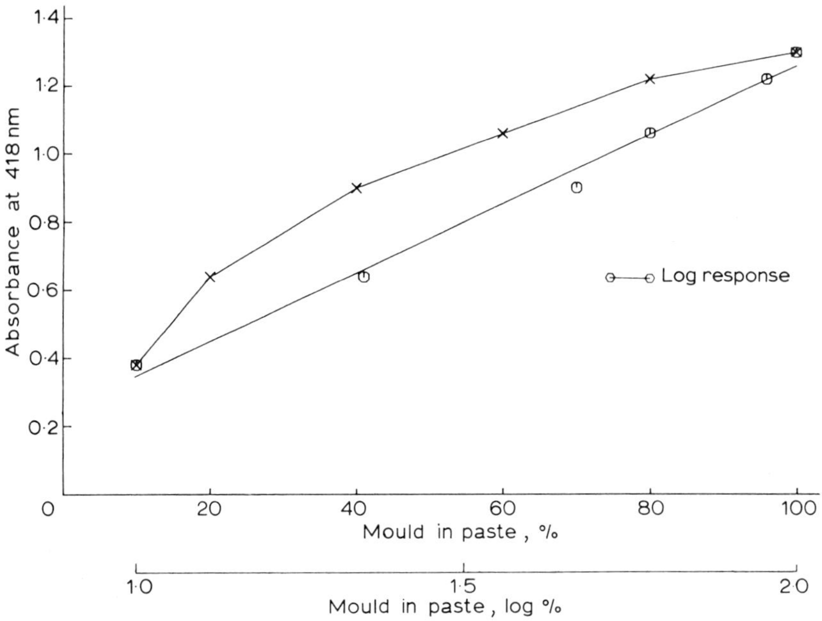

Fig. 4. Standard curve using dilutions of a tomato paste having 98% HMC.

Figure 3 shows the EIA response with increasing amounts of the five cocktail moulds, mixed in equal concentrations. Under the limiting anti-mould cocktail antiserum levels, as defined above, the response was curved over the range 0·1 to 0·8 mg/ml mould. Similar results were obtained using a tomato paste of 98% HMC diluted to cover a range of mould counts nominally between 10 and 100% (Fig. 4), although a logarithmic plot gave reasonable linearity. Linearity of the assay over the entire mould count range was best achieved at low concentrations of first antibody, although assay sensitivity was also low. It could not be improved by increasing the levels of either the first or second antibodies, although assay sensitivity could be extended (Fig. 5). As the concentration of the anti-mould cocktail antiserum was increased, available antigenic sites were filled to a level which was clearly dependent on the ratio of mould to concentrations of first antibody.

This relationship was not straightforward. Doubling of the first antibody concentration, as shown in Fig. 5, neither gave linearity with higher mould concentrations nor did it provide proportional increases in binding, as measured using the HRP-labelled anti-rabbit IgG second antibody. It was

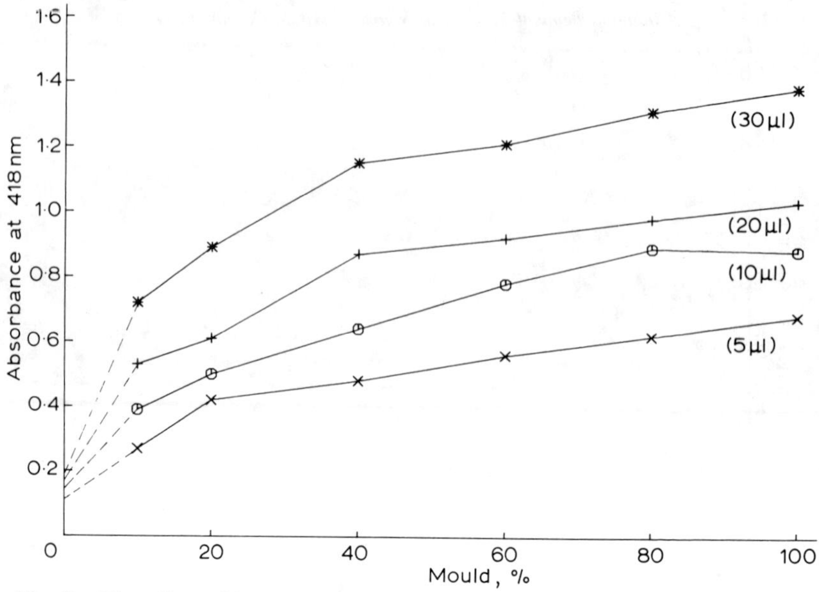

Fig. 5. The effect of increasing mould concentration on absorbance at 418 nm using various concentrations of mixed first antibody in the sequential assay format.

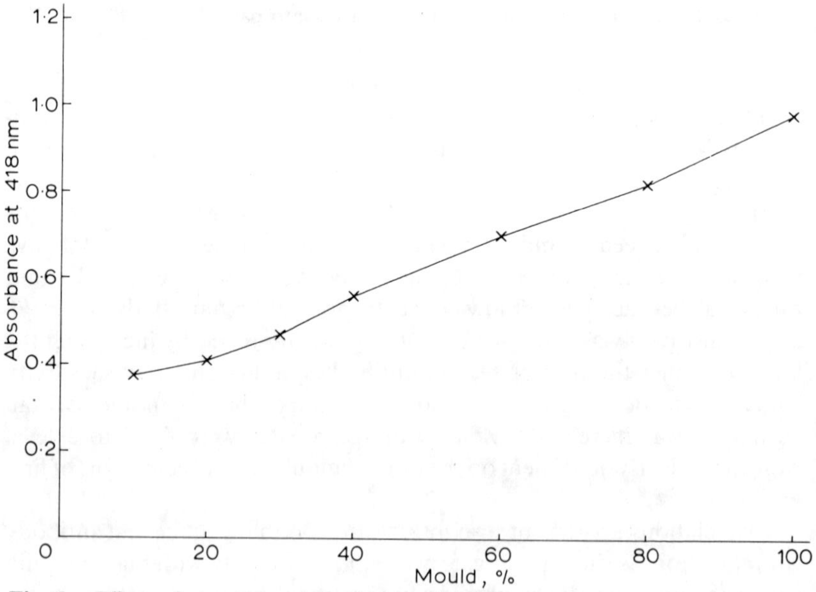

Fig. 6. Effect of simultaneous addition of first and second antibodies on the standard curve.

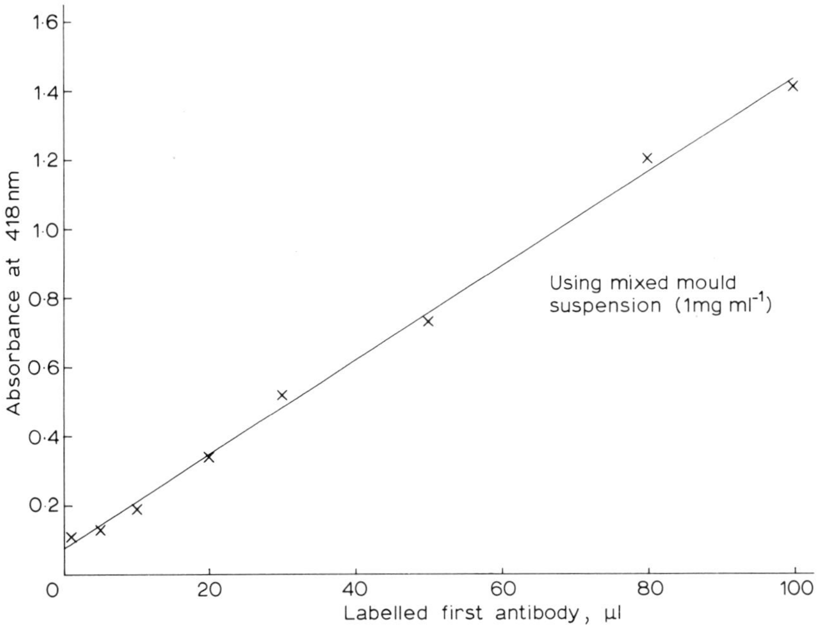

Fig. 7. Effect of increasing the concentration of the labelled first antibody.

deduced that the abundance and configuration of the antigenic sites along a mycelium surface might be important factors affecting both assay linearity and sensitivity. The steric hindrance of either or both of the antibodies might be causing many of the problems in the assay.

In an attempt to assess whether the binding of the first or the second antibody was being impaired by steric hindrance, both antibodies, at ratios previously shown not to produce insoluble complexes, were added to the assay simultaneously to encourage complexing of the two before the first antibody reacted with the antigenic determinants at the mould surface.

A linear response was achieved over the whole assay range, as shown in Fig. 6. The best sensitivity was achieved at anti-mould cocktail antiserum concentrations much lower than those used in the sequential addition assay. This would suggest that, in a two-stage assay, it was the binding of the labelled second antibody which was sterically hindered.

The direct EIA using HRP-labelled anti-mould cocktail antibodies was found to be similarly free from problems due to steric hindrance. Figure 7 shows a linear response with increasing concentration of labelled first antibody and constant concentration (1 mg/ml) of mixed moulds. A highly

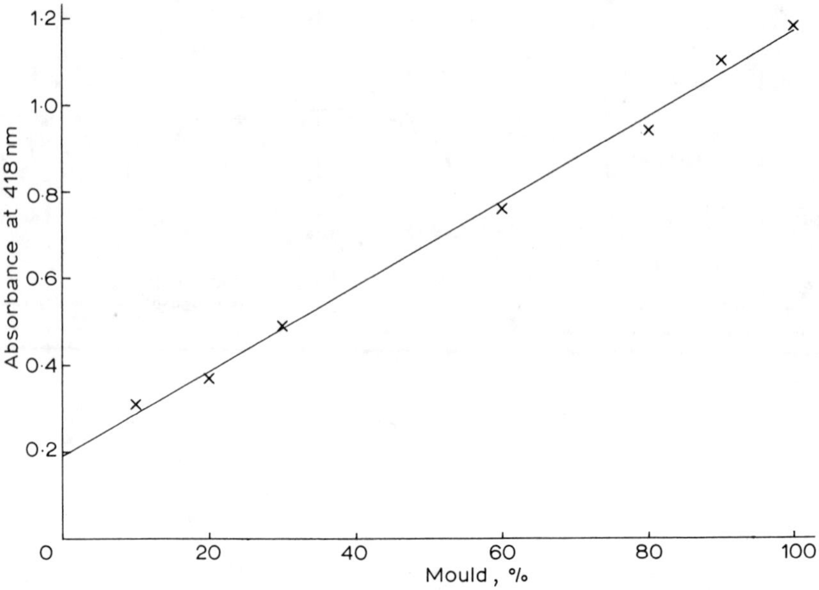

Fig. 8. Effect of increasing mould concentration at constant labelled first antibody.

sensitive linear response (Fig. 8) was obtained with increasing mould concentration in tomato paste and constant (5 μl) HRP-labelled first antibody. To produce this curve a 98% HMC paste was diluted to provide a nominal range of mould concentration from 10 to 100%, but in doing so the tomato solids were also diluted. However, to ensure that the EIA response was not due to cross-reaction with tomato solids, a low HMC paste, with a solids content equivalent to that of the 98% HMC sample, was also assayed. This gave a low EIA response showing that antibody binding was occurring specifically with mould and not the tomato solids.

Relationship between HMC and EIA

At best the HMC is only a semi-quantitative method. The method makes no allowance for the presence, in fields of vision, of mould clumps which will be counted as positive fields in the same way as those containing only a single mycelium. Mould clumps are commonly found in commercial pastes and are the result of contamination from either processing machinery or the tomato fruit itself. Both may be seen in Figs 1(b) and 1(c). An EIA method would measure quantitatively any mould as a function of mycelial

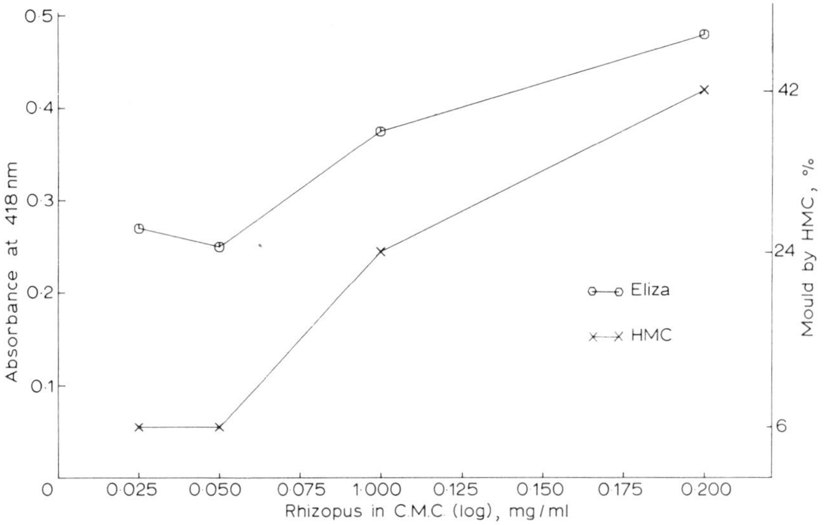

Fig. 9. Comparison of results from EIA and HMC.

antigen concentration and consequently any relationship between the HMC and the immunoassay will be influenced by the relative abundance of clumps and free mycelia in a sample.

A reasonable relationship should, however, be observed where mould is evenly distributed as single filaments. Although this may never occur in practice, a series of experimental samples of differing mould concentrations were prepared by resuspending gently homogenised mould mycelia in 1% carboxymethyl cellulose (CMC) of the correct density to maintain a stable suspension. HMCs were then performed on these in parallel with the EIA method. The similar results of both assays are shown in Fig. 9. The HMC is capable of producing quantitative results, providing mould is evenly distributed and can be counted unambiguously. It can therefore be compared directly to the EIA.

The correlation between the direct EIA and the HMC obtained by analysing a number of commercial tomato paste samples is shown in Fig. 10. Samples were counted only twice using the HMC but analysed in duplicate by EIA. It can be seen that in general there was very good agreement between the two methods, but one sample measured by HMC at 60% positive fields resulted in low EIA readings. This sample is being inspected carefully and the clump distribution and mould type studied. Some variation in EIA duplicates is also noticeable and considered to be

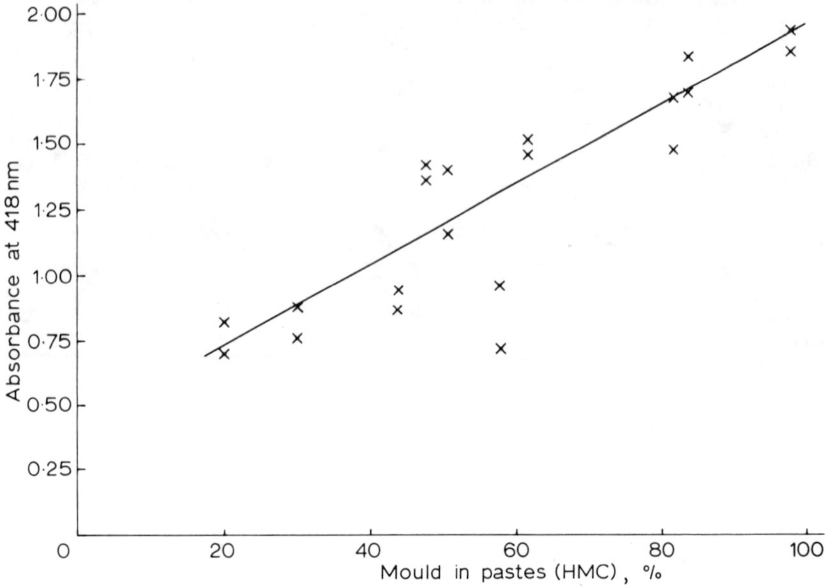

Fig. 10. Correlation between direct EIA and HMC.

due primarily to mould distribution and sampling problems, which can probably be overcome by gentle homogenisation of the tomato paste before sampling. The results obtained so far suggest that this direct EIA provides a quantitative alternative to the tedious and difficult to standardise HMC. The direct EIA method can clearly be applied also to homogenised products such as juices, and the same assay philosophy should be applicable to other mould genera and/or other products. Work is continuing with the identification of the mould antigens, particularly those common to many genera.

ACKNOWLEDGEMENTS

The authors gratefully acknowledge the Ministry of Agriculture, Fisheries and Food for funding this work. Thanks are also due to Mr M. Hall for performing the Howard Mould Count on tomato paste samples, and to Dr S. Alcock and Mr K. Brown for culturing the fungi used in this work. We are grateful to the AFRC Institute of Food Research, Norwich, for providing the initial fungal cultures, and to the Liverpool Port Health Authority for providing samples of tomato paste.

REFERENCES

CASPER, R. & MENDGEN, K. (1979) Quantitative serological estimation of hypoparasite: detection of *Verticillium lecanii* in yellow rust infected wheat leaves. *Phytopathologie Zeitschrift*, **94**, 89.

CHILDS, R. E. & BARDSLEY, W. G. (1975) Steady state kinetics of peroxidase with 2,2′-azino-di-3-ethyl benzothiazoline-6-sulphonic acid as chromogen. *Biochemical Journal*, **145**, 93–103.

DAVIES, A. M. C., DENNIS, C., GRANT, A., HALL, M. N. & ROBERTSON, A. (1987) Screening of tomato purée for excessive mould content by near infrared spectrometry: a preliminary evaluation. *Journal of the Science of Food and Agriculture*, **37**, 349–355.

HJELN, H., HJELN, K. & SJOQUIST, J. (1972) Protein A from *Staphylococcus aureus*—its isolation by affinity chromatography and its use as an immunosorbent for the isolation of immunoglobin. *FEBS Letters*, **28**, 73–76.

HOWARD, B. J. (1911) Tomato ketchup under the microscope with practical suggestions to ensure a clean product. Circular 68, Bureau of Chemistry, US Department of Agriculture, Washington, DC.

JARVIS, B. (1977) A chemical method for the estimation of mould in tomato products. *Journal of Food Technology*, **12**, 581–591.

LIN, H. H., LISTER, R. M. & COUSIN, M. A. (1986) Enzyme-linked immunosorbent assay for detection of mould in tomato purée. *Journal of Food Science*, **51**, 180–183.

LOWRY, O. H., ROSEBROUGH, N. J., FARR, A. L. & RANDALL, R. J. (1951) Protein measurement with the Folin phenol reagent, *Journal of Biological Chemistry*, **193**, 265–275.

NOTERMANS, S. & HEUVELMAN, C. J. (1985) Immunological detection of moulds in food by using the enzyme-linked immunosorbent assay (ELISA): preparation of antigens. *International Journal of Food Microbiology*, **2**, 247–258.

PETTIFER, G. L. (1986) The direct epifluorescence filter technique. *Journal of Food Technology*, **21**, 535–546.

PETTIFER, G. L., WILLIAMS, R. A. & GUTTERIDGE, C. S. (1985) An evaluation of possible alternative methods to the Howard Mould Count. *Applied Microbiology*, **1**, 49–61.

SEITZ, L. M., MOL, H. E., BURROUGHS, R. & SAUER, D. B. (1977) Ergosterol as an indicator of fungal invasion of grains. *Cereal Chemistry*, **54**, 1207–1217.

WILSON, M. B. & NAKANE, P. K. (1978) *Immunofluorescence and Related Staining Techniques*, Knapp, W., Holuber, K. & Wick, G. (eds), Elsevier/North-Holland Biomedical Press, Amsterdam, p. 215.

SESSION IV

Problems and Strategies in Immunoassay Application

15

Problems Associated with Developing Food Immunoassays

J. C. Allen
North East Wales Institute, Deeside, Clwyd, UK

INTRODUCTION

Many of the problems of kit development are common to the development of any ELISA, whether destined for food analysis or clinical diagnosis. However, there are specific difficulties associated with the multiplicity of ways in which the analyte can be presented in a food sample. Clinical samples are usually blood, urine or cerebrospinal fluid, and may have a known history and be uniform in character. In contrast, foods may be pastes, liquids, gels or solids; raw or cooked, frozen or commercially sterilised. Any analytical procedure devised should ideally be able to measure the analyte in any product or, at the very least, the limits of applicability of a particular procedure must be fully explored and defined.

Preceding chapters have shown that a competent research group with a facility to raise its own antibodies can produce an ELISA system which will work in its hands, and will be acceptable within the limits of its needs for as long as the supply of antibody lasts. It is quite a different matter to develop a robust, rugged and reliable assay kit, with sufficient stocks of stable and calibrated reagents, suitable for use by relatively inexperienced staff and appropriate in its application to a wide range of food samples.

Some of the procedures employed to develop such kits and the problems encountered will now be examined.

SPECIFICITY OF ANTISERA

A good antibody is the key to a good immunoassay. It must bind avidly and specifically with the analyte, and ideally must not cross-react with anything else likely to be present. Sufficient stocks must be produced to maintain standardisation between production runs of kits over an extended period of time. Other chapters and poster presentations have referred to the advantages of raising antisera in the larger animals and/or producing monoclonal antibodies. There are research papers that have reported values for 'typical' assays, but requests for details have revealed that the results were in fact obtained from a minute amount of the best antiserum produced. Such a method cannot possibly become the basis of a commercial kit.

It is important to know how specific the antibody is. For instance, a soya protein antiserum raised by using 'renatured' soya protein as the immunogen was found to be least reactive towards glycinin, the 11S component of soya protein. However, some immunoreactivity was observed towards glycinin which had been denatured by boiling in 10M urea for 30 min: it would appear that the action of the urea was able to expose common or new antigenic determinants. This same antiserum cross-reacted at a low level with urea-denatured casein but not with native casein (Fig. 1). This unexpected cross-reactivity could, however, be removed by affinity chromatography of the antiserum on a denatured casein–sepharose column. To circumvent such unexpected cross-reaction requires a thorough knowledge of the composition of foods that a customer might wish to analyse for a particular analyte. A further illustration of this point came from our work with an antiserum to bovine casein (Fig. 2). This antiserum did not cross-react with α-lactalbumin or β-lactoglobulin, the principal proteins of whey, but there was some cross-reactivity with whole whey protein. Table 1 illustrates this further and also shows the reduction in

Table 1
Cross-reactivities of Sheep Anti-casein Antisera

Sample	*Cross-reactivity (%)*	
	Crude anti-casein antiserum	*Affinity-purified anti-casein antiserum*
Whey protein concentrate (cheddar)	28·0	2·5
Whey protein concentrate (acid)	40·4	12·5
Whey protein (DMV)	40·4	3·8
α-Lactalbumin	3·5	2·8
β-Lactoglobulin	5·3	4·5
κ-Casein	39·1	5·8
Calcium caseinate	81·8	92·5

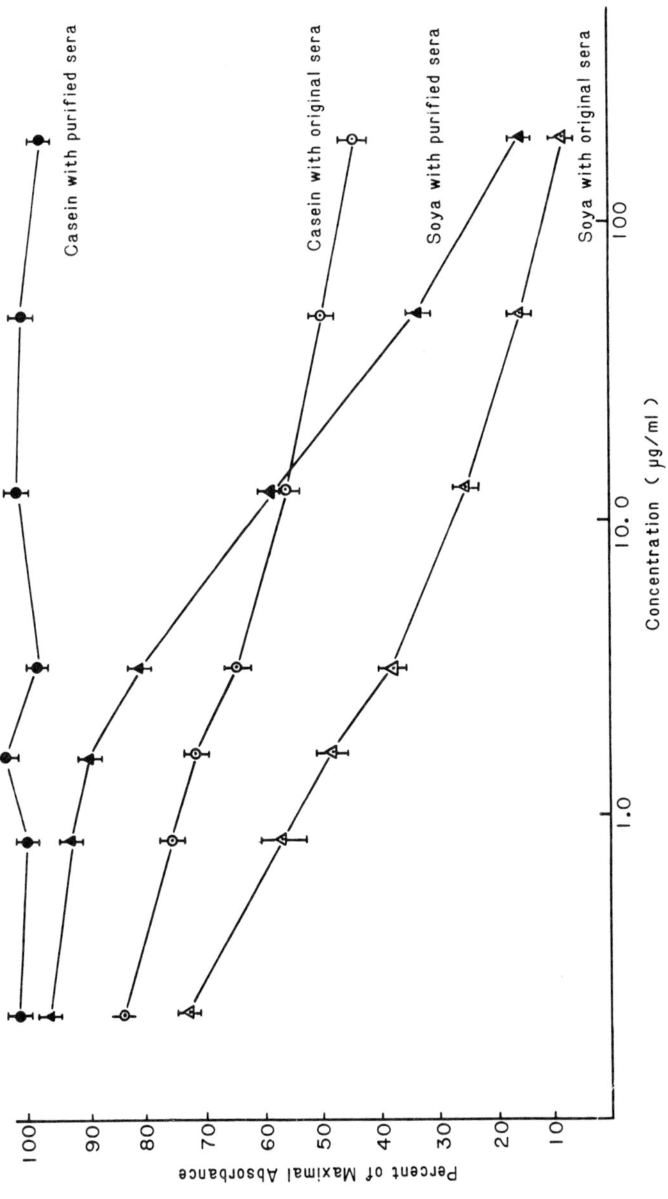

Fig. 1. Cross-reactivity of denatured proteins in the soya protein ELISA. An antiserum raised in sheep against denatured soya protein was used in a competitive ELISA. Cross-reactivity of the antiserum with denatured casein was removed by affinity chromatography on a denatured casein-sepharose column.

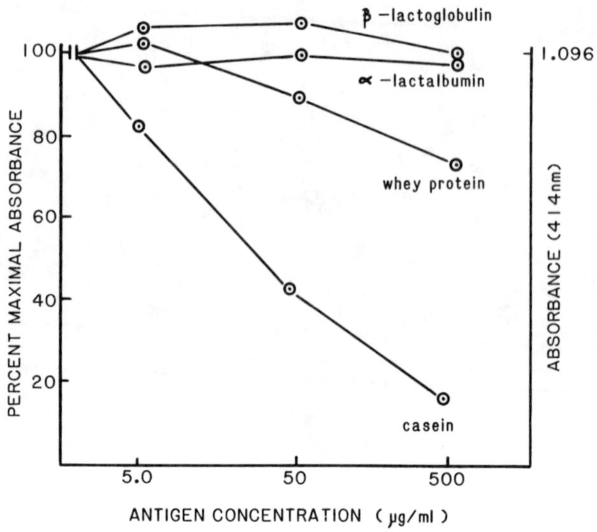

Fig. 2. Cross-reactivity of sheep anti-bovine casein with whey protein in an indirect competitive ELISA. The cross-reactivity was not due to α-lactalbumin or β-lactoglobulin.

cross-reactivity following affinity chromatography of the anti-casein antiserum on a casein–sepharose column. It was initially thought that the reason for the cross-reactivity stemmed from the presence, and immunological recognition, of the glycomacropeptide which is released from κ-casein to the whey during the rennetting process. However, subsequent work did not substantiate this, and it is now believed that the cross-reactivity with the whey derives not from the glycomacropeptide itself but from other peptides split off from the casein during cheesemaking, and which correspond to epitopes on the casein and are thus recognised even by the affinity-purified antiserum (Morris, 1985).

Cross-reactivity problems can also occur in antisera produced for testing meat species. Although commercial antisera may be acceptable for the immunoprecipitation and immunodiffusion tests for which they were designed, they can exhibit marked cross-reactivity in ELISA systems (see Lumley *et al.*, p. 285, this volume) unless they are affinity-purified (see also Patterson & Jones, 1985; Johnston *et al.*, 1985).

CHOICE OF ASSAY VARIANT

There are many ingenious variants of the microtitration plate ELISA system. The kit manufacturer must choose an assay system that will ensure

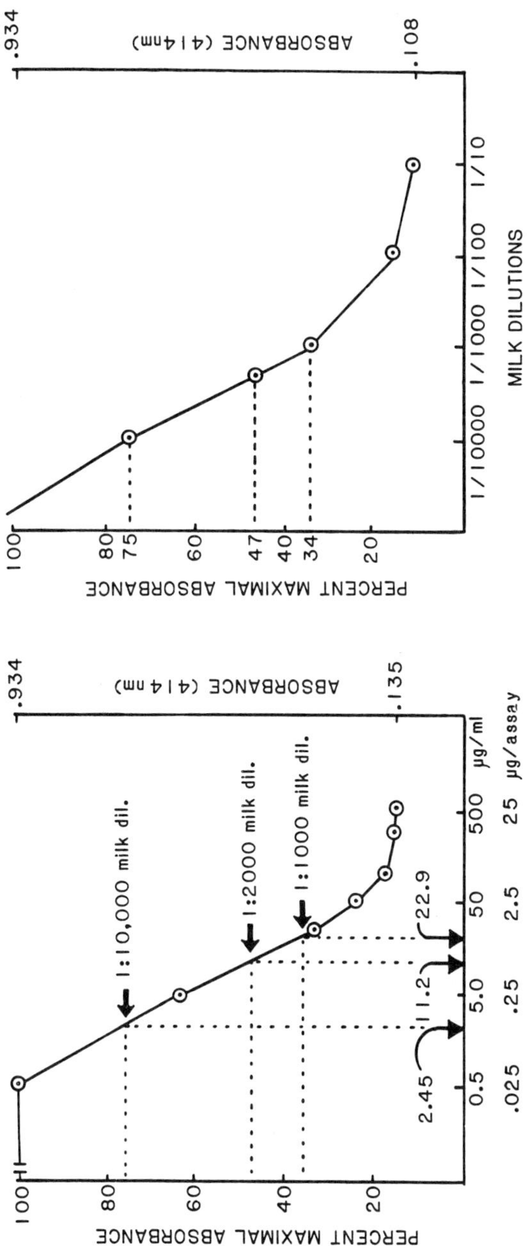

Fig. 3. Casein determination in whole pasteurised milk by direct competitive ELISA.

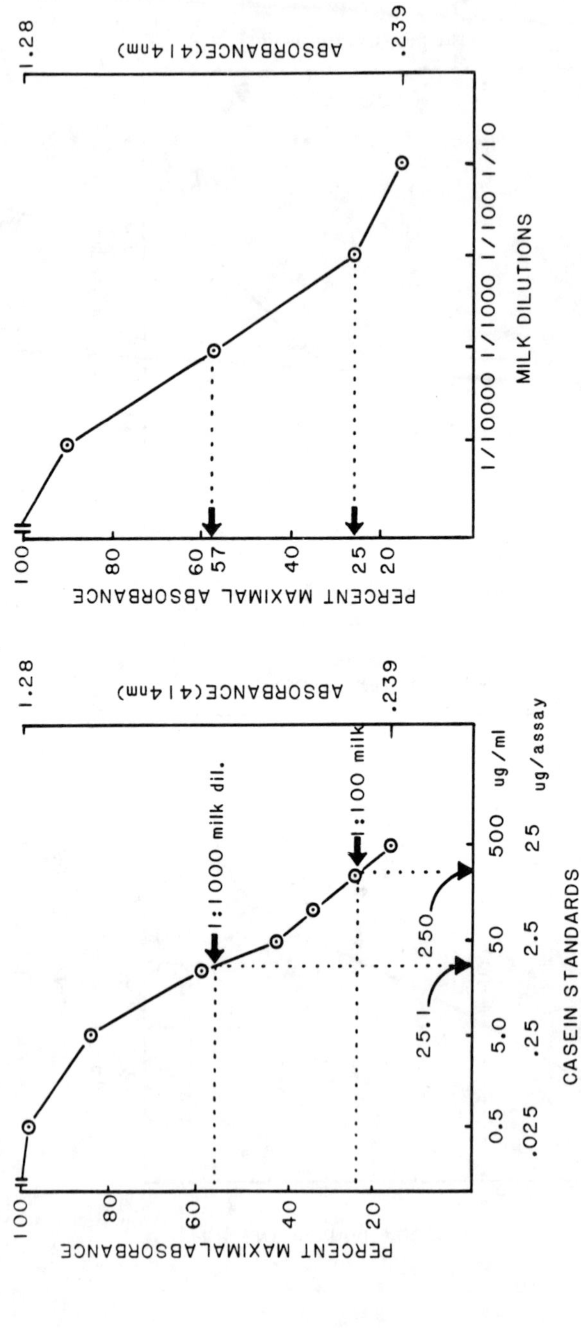

Fig. 4. Casein determination in whole pasteurised milk by indirect competitive ELISA.

that the kit will be reliable and robust while using as few expensive reagents as possible and employing a minimum number of manipulations, each one of which is potentially error-producing, especially in relatively unskilled hands. How this choice can affect the characteristics of the assay is illustrated by our experiences with a direct competitive ELISA (Fig. 3) and an indirect competitive ELISA (Fig. 4) for assaying bovine casein.

Either assay might eventually be destined to determine casein levels in liquid milk, in which it is a major component, or to detect casein employed at relatively minor concentrations as a meat extender. The results from both assay variants gave satisfactory dose–response curves but spanned different casein concentration ranges. The direct method using an enzyme-labelled primary antibody was so sensitive that, to determine casein in liquid milk, a dilution of 1:1000 or even 1:10 000 was necessary; this was not easy to do accurately and was the step most likely to produce error in the whole process. Despite requiring an additional step the indirect ELISA was no more difficult to perform and required only a 1:100 or 1:1000 dilution of the sample; it was generally more reproducible. In addition, the direct assay required the antiserum to be affinity-purified before being used to coat the plate, thus entailing some loss of activity. One millilitre of serum sufficed for 30 000 wells in the indirect assay but only 10 000 wells in the direct, thus giving the indirect assay a cost advantage.

NON-SPECIFIC BINDING

Non-specific binding is due to non-covalent binding of molecules to the walls of the microtitration plates or to each other by an interaction which does not derive from antigen–antibody complementarity.

A common method to counteract this effect is to block the free binding sites on the plate with BSA. To do this, dilute the antibody in coating buffer, add it to the well and leave overnight at 4°C. The following morning empty the wells, wash with buffer, add a solution of BSA and incubate. The wells are then emptied and dried. The BSA fills the unoccupied sites and thereby reduces NSB. The blocking of unoccupied sites is further discussed by Morris (1985) and Sauer *et al.* (1985).

SAMPLE PREPARATION

The problems discussed so far are common to the development of any immunoassay. The challenge to those working on assays for food analysis is

Table 2
Recovery of Soya Protein from 'Spiked' Meat Samples

Meat	*Added soya protein* (%)	*Recovery* (%)	*CV* (%)
Beef mince	3·15	101 ($n = 10$)	10·3
Beef mince	7·0	91·4 ($n = 10$)	8·8
Economy sausage	2·3	94 ($n = 5$)	9·5

Soya protein isolate PP500E was added as a hydrolysate prepared by mixing 1 part isolate, 5 parts water and 0·02 part sodium pyrophosphate. The percentage soya protein refers to the total amount of soya protein added as a percentage of the weight of the meat.

that of prior sample preparation, which stems from the range of different matrices in which the analyte is likely to appear. A reliable immunoassay thus depends not only on the immunoassay procedure itself but on the development of a sample preparation procedure which gives complete, or at least consistent, extraction of analyte from all foods containing it. Painstaking work is necessary at this stage to ensure the robustness and reliability of the final assay kit, but the problem is by no means insuperable. Soya protein can be incorporated in foods in a variety of forms, for example as isolates, full-fat flours, defatted flours, concentrates and texturates, which differ not only in their technological but also their immunological properties. In order to reduce the soya protein to a comparable state for ELISA, the soya protein assay kit which has been developed demands that the sample of food be homogenised, extracted into urea/dithiothreitol at 100°C and finally 'renatured' before being assayed. This process has been

Table 3
ELISA of Soya Protein in Meat Products

Product	*% Soya protein (wet weight)*		
	From specification	*By ELISA*	*% Expected*
Pork and beef sausage	1·30	1·28 ($n = 17$)	98
Mince with added soya	3·15	3·29 ($n = 28$)	104
Pork luncheon meat	1·80	1·76 ($n = 2$)	98
Economy sausage	1·48	0·69 ($n = 6$)	47
Liver sausage	1·17	1·24 ($n = 2$)	106
Beef sausage	0·98	0·92 ($n = 2$)	94

Table 4
Precision of Soya Protein ELISA

Sample	*Soya protein* (%)	*Intra-assay*		*Inter-assay*	
		n	*CV* (%)	*n*	*CV* (%)
Mince	3·15	10	6·5	10	10·3
Sausage	1·3	10	6·7	6	7·2

shown to give a consistent extraction of soya protein in the same molecular form, whatever its origin.

It was also essential to investigate the reproducibility of the method and the recovery of soya protein from 'spiked' meat samples. Further comprehensive work was necessary before a procedure could be established which was both straightforward and consistent in its extraction of soya protein from various foods, as illustrated in Table 2.

Some assay results for soya protein in meat products are given in Table 3. With one exception, these are close to the manufacturer's specification, and give an indication of the potential reliability and accuracy of the assay kit. The exception, a sample of 'economy sausage', is probably due to the fact that the specification was from a general formulation provided by the manufacturer rather than an individual batch formulation. It is therefore quite possible that this particular batch contained less soya protein than would normally have been the case.

Table 4 shows the precision of the soya protein ELISA, both inter- and intra-assay. Coefficients of variation for the commercial kits are now well within the ranges common in clinical diagnostics.

KIT STABILITY AND PRESENTATION

Commercial ELISA kits, like foods themselves, are perishable. They therefore need to be clearly labelled with a 'best before' date. All the plates, buffers, reagents, standards and controls need careful checking for compatibility, and for stability against both chemical and microbiological deterioration. This again requires a great deal of essential but relatively routine work. The objective of commercial immunoassay kits is to provide the end-user with standardised reagents that are ready to use.

CONCLUSIONS

Enzyme-linked immunoassays are by no means a panacea for the food analyst. Nevertheless, for many analytes, the commercial assay kits now appearing offer the easiest, fastest, most accurate and least expensive method currently available. It is fully expected that their use will gain acceptance by public analysts, and that they will assume a significant role in the range of techniques now available for food analysis.

REFERENCES

JOHNSTON, L. A. Y., TRACEY-PATTE, P. D., PEARSON, R. D., HURRELL, J. G. R. & AITKEN, D. P. (1985) Identification of the species of origin of meat in Australia by radioimmunoassay and enzyme immunoassay. In: *Immunoassays in Food Analysis*, Morris, B. A. & Clifford, M. N. (eds), Elsevier Applied Science Publishers, London, pp. 95–110.

MORRIS, B. A. (1985) Principles of immunoassay. In: *Immunoassays in Food Analysis*, Morris, B. A. & Clifford, M. N. (eds), Elsevier Applied Science Publishers, London, pp. 21–51.

PATTERSON, R. L. S. & JONES, S. J. (1985) Species identification of meat in raw, unheated meat products. In: *Immunoassays in Food Analysis*, Morris, B. A. & Clifford, M. N. (eds), Elsevier Applied Science Publishers, London, pp. 87–94.

SAUER, M. J., FOULKES, J. A. & MORRIS, B. A. (1985) Principles of enzyme immunoassay. In: *Immunoassays in Food Analysis*, Morris, B. A. & Clifford, M. N. (eds), Elsevier Applied Science Publishers, London, pp. 53–72.

16

The Problems of Using ELISAs for Food Analytes in Support of Litigation

N. M. Griffiths

Meat and Livestock Commission, Milton Keynes, UK

The use and potential of immunological methods in the analysis of food is only just beginning to be realised. Until recently, factory and control laboratories' experience of immunological methods has been with simple immunodiffusion based on commercial antisera to whole blood proteins specific to a given species. ELISAs have recently been finding favour in food analysis because in the main these assays do not require expensive equipment; they are robust and suitable for screening purposes; and they are objective, sensitive and can be semi-automated. In food control laboratories these assays are being applied with some success to the determination of soya protein in meat products, meat species recognition, residue detection in meat, taints in meat, enzymes and aflatoxins. The realisation that these assays only depend on the availability of relevant antibodies produces an exciting new field for research scientists to pursue in the application of these assays to the food industry. The use of two of these assays will be reviewed, i.e. the determination of soya protein in meat products and the identification of meat species, with particular reference to their use in litigation.

Before discussing the assay for soya protein in meat products it is important to realise why soya protein needs to be determined by food control laboratories. The Meat Product and Spreadable Fish Product Regulations 1984 came into effect on 1 July 1986 and require meat products which are ready for delivery to the consumer to carry a declaration stating either the minimum meat content or the maximum added water content. In order to ascertain which declaration to place on the label, or to check that the declaration on the label is correct, the manufacturer or enforcement authority must, in many cases, resort to analytical techniques. In both the maximum added water and minimum meat declarations the analyst is required to determine the meat content of the sample. In order to ascertain this, he must consider the definition of meat contained within the Regulations, namely 'Meat is the flesh, including fat, and the skin, rind, gristle and sinew in amounts naturally associated with the flesh used, and includes permitted parts of the carcase'. Novel proteins such as soya protein are not meat and as such are not allowed to count towards any declared meat content.

In order to determine meat content, the analyst resorts to the traditional Stubbs and Moore procedure involving the determination of moisture, fat, protein and ash. The protein content is calculated from the total nitrogen figure multiplied by 6·25. Fat-free meat is calculated by assuming an average percentage of nitrogen in fat-free meat for each species, and relating this to the percentage of nitrogen found in the sample. Fat is then added to give the total meat content in the meat sample. This calculation assumes, however, that no nitrogen-containing ingredient, other than meat, is present in the product. In a sausage or beefburger, however, material such as cereal and soya protein (flour, grit, texturate or isolate) contribute to the nitrogen content of a sample, and in order to arrive at the nitrogen due to meat, non-meat nitrogen must be subtracted from the total nitrogen determined.

For added soya products the inhibition ELISA procedure, as suggested by Hitchcock *et al.* (1981), proved to be the best method available in terms of cost, time and accuracy (Griffiths *et al.*, 1981), and the assay was tested collaboratively in 22 UK and Irish laboratories in 1984 (Crimes *et al.*, 1984).

The author's involvement, together with Unilever Research, in the setting-up and running of this trial demonstrated the work required in transferring a research assay to an assay which could be used practically in 22 laboratories. The transfer from in-house-generated anti-soya protein antibodies to those which were commercially available and the generation of detailed protocols and training workshops were some of the problems which had to be tackled and overcome. The trial concluded that the repeatability and reproducibility of the method was such that low levels of soya flour or textured concentrate added to meat products could be confidently identified and quantified. It must be pointed out, however, that the recipe values quoted for comparison were corrected for the response factors of the soya material used in this particular trial. Recoveries from defatted flours were found to vary from 74·4 to 83·9%, isolates from 92·6 to

118·1%, concentrates from 70·2 to 88·2% and exudates from 52·4 to 166·2%, when compared to a common standard (Unisol).

It is clear that without a knowledge of the type of soya material used in the product the assay can be subject to considerable errors. These errors should and must be taken into account when the result of the assay is used in court. However, there have been court cases where this has not been done, and this indicates a lack of understanding of the idiosyncrasies of the method by those analysts involved in the cases concerned.

The next example to be considered is that of meat speciation. In applying legislation covering meat unfit for human consumption and the labelling of meat and meat products, it is necessary for the enforcement authorities to test for the species of meat present. They are seeking to protect the consumer against the unwitting consumption of horse and kangaroo meat and meat products described as being of one species but containing meats other than that declared. Meat product manufacturers and retailers also need to check on the species of their bought-in supplies.

Current methods of identifying the species of meat rely on tests using antibodies to the proteins present in blood serum. These tests are sensitive in that they provide a positive result if only a small quantity of protein of a particular species is present. However, Griffiths & Billington (1984) showed quite clearly that these tests do not give an accurate estimate of the amount of the particular species of meat present. The response of 24 joints of beef in a similar ELISA procedure to that mentioned earlier was compared to a standard reference sample of meat. Responses varied from 51·2 to 159·3%. This variation in response is due primarily to the variation in blood and thus antigen content from one cut of meat to another. It is, however, also influenced by the corresponding variation in fat content, the history and age of the sample, and the reproducibility of the extraction procedure. When analysing suspected mixtures the antibody specificity must be known, and account must be taken of possible batch to batch variations. These points are further discussed elsewhere in this volume (see Allen, Chapter 15 and Lumley *et al.*, p. 285, this volume).

Although new techniques, almost certainly ELISAs, will hopefully be commercially available shortly, speciation at present is performed largely by simple qualitative immunodiffusion techniques, and these will remain in use for some time.

However, there have been many court cases where prosecution for the analysts using qualitative procedures have stated quantitative levels of pork, for example in a product described as minced beef, when it is clear that quantification is not possible. As fines are normally set at the level of adulteration observed, this has obvious consequences.

Again this appears to be the result of a lack of understanding of the techniques being used. Furthermore, blood and soluble proteins occur in exudate from meats; and so, for example, if mincing equipment is not cleaned thoroughly between batches, the exudate from one species being minced can contaminate the next batch. This can lead to the false-positive identification of the species in a subsequent batch of a different species.

All of these problems have led to pressure for the development of assays which rely on antibodies to a less variable and insoluble antigen in meat, for example an antigenic determinant which is part of the myofibrillar protein.

In conclusion, although the potential of ELISAs in food analysis is beyond dispute, their successful use in the fair and just enforcement of food law requires not only very careful design and testing of the complete assay procedure but also a thorough understanding of the assays' inherent limitations. Immunologists are well used to working within these limitations, but in general they are poor in communicating this information to the analytical chemists in the food control laboratories. If the immunologists wish to see the fruits of their research being used 'down line', then they must give further thought as to how best to develop assays and devote more time to dialogue with the user. This volume is a valuable start to this process.

ACKNOWLEDGEMENT

The material in this chapter is published with the kind permission of the Meat and Livestock Commission.

REFERENCES

CRIMES, A. A., HITCHCOCK, C. H. S. & WOOD, R. (1984) Determination of soya protein in meat products by an enzyme-linked immunosorbent assay procedure: collaborative study. *Journal of the Association of Public Analysts*, **22**, 59–78.

GRIFFITHS, N. M. & BILLINGTON, M. J. (1984) Evaluation of an enzyme-linked immunosorbent assay for beef blood serum to determine indirectly the apparent beef content of beef joints and model mixtures. *Journal of the Science of Food and Agriculture*, **35**, 909–914.

GRIFFITHS, N. M., BILLINGTON, M. J. & GRIFFITHS, W. (1981) A review of three modern techniques available for the determination of soya protein in meat products. *Journal of the Association of Public Analysts*, **19**, 113–119.

Hitchcock, C. H. S., Bailey, F. J., Crimes, A. D., Dean, D. A. G. & Davis, P. J. (1981) Determination of soya proteins in food using an enzyme-linked immunosorbent assay procedure. *Journal of the Science of Food and Agriculture*, **32**, 157–165.

17

A Strategy for Immunoassay Data Reduction

A. B. J. NIX
Department of Mathematical Statistics and Operational Research, University College, Cardiff, UK

and

G. V. GROOM
Tenovus Institute for Cancer Research, Cardiff, UK

INTRODUCTION

RIAs have gained wide favour in medical and research laboratories over the past 30 years. The availability of commercial kits for many assays has helped to simplify the technology and increase the reliability and confidence of the user in the results. In spite of the large sums of money paid for these reagents, and the sums previously committed to the development of the methods, little fundamental research has gone into the problem of processing the data from the assays. As non-isotopic assays begin to flourish, and automated systems increase the use of these techniques and introduce them into new areas of science, the potential errors of inappropriate data reduction will become more important, and perhaps one of the major sources of error in the assay. The various stages of immunoassay data reduction will be discussed, pointing out the pitfalls, and some strategies suggested that urgently need attention to avert a loss of confidence of users in the manufacturers of the assay reagents. Comparison of immunoassay methods to assess bias, perhaps of a new technique, may be invalid if curve-fitting procedures are not first resolved. Conversely, all the effort and cost of establishing specificity, sensitivity, precision and ruggedness in an assay may be lost unless curve-fitting is also considered.

PRELIMINARY SCREENING OF DATA FROM STANDARDS

Before one proceeds to establish a standard curve, there are a number of preliminary screening exercises that need to be performed on the data obtained from the standards.

Transformation of the Data

The analysis provided by most curve-fitting packages requires the replicate count data to be distributed in a Gaussian manner for each standard point if the interpretation of results is to be correct. It follows that serious attempts must be made to check the Gaussian assumption. If it is concluded that the data are non-Gaussian, then an appropriate transformation must be sought. It is not sufficient to use a particular transformation merely because others have found it acceptable in other circumstances. A general family of transformations which may be useful is expressed in the following equation, where the transformed variable Y is defined in terms of the original variable X by

$$Y = \frac{X^{\lambda} - 1}{\lambda}$$

λ is the parameter to be determined on some specified criterion, such as the coefficient of skewness of the transformed data, and should be zero. This transformation is fairly general as it can be shown to be equivalent to

$$Y = \log_e X \quad \text{as } \lambda \text{ tends to zero}$$

and

$$Y = X - 1 \quad \text{for } \lambda \text{ equal to unity.}$$

The authors are not suggesting that this is the only transformation to consider, but merely that it has all the power-type functions built in, with the popular logarithmic transformation being a particular extreme.

Whatever transformation has been used, the data should be re-checked for Gaussian character after the transformation has been applied. The difficulty in applying tests for Gaussian character in practice is that they need a fairly large database to be effective. As a result, data may have to be accumulated (if appropriate) as assays are performed, thereby necessitating a continual check on the Gaussian assumption. It should also be remembered that it may be necessary to use different transformations for different standards, particularly if the standard curve has asymptotes, as this usually causes skewness of the distributions in such regions.

Outliers

These are usually referred to as atypical values, but they require definition. If a value occurs which is extreme, relative to the main body of the data, then this may have occurred as a consequence of being a 'rare' event, or because of the influence of some unknown factor. In the latter case, the point may be justifiably ignored as an outlier. However, in the former case the point should be accepted since the consequence of not doing so would be to improve the apparent precision of measurement, leading to a false sense of security. Clearly, in practice the two possibilities are difficult to resolve and it is difficult to achieve an objective decision. If the user cannot resolve this problem, then neither can a statistical algorithm devised by that user. It is the view of the authors that statistical algorithms for outlier rejection should be used only as flagging devices, the decision to exclude the point or points being left to the assayist who may be aware of further information about the data points which will help resolve the issue. Whatever decision is made, the point should not be merely disregarded but should initiate a procedure to find possible explanations.

TYPE OF RESPONSE CURVE

Box & Hunter (1962) categorised the various curve-fitting techniques in two ways: (a) empirical or interpolatory methods and (b) theoretical or regression methods.

The use of empirical methods assumes that the function connecting the points is continuous and smooth, but does not assume any overall functional form. Thus a curve fitted in this way places complete reliance on the accuracy of the points, so that any lack of fit is attributed to the curve-fit procedure used. This confidence in the accuracy of the data points is questionable due to the known presence of response error, and the possibility of outlying results occurring. These weaknesses in the interpolatory approach are highlighted when using the simple spline function, since this particular form of empirical curve-fit passes through all of the data points.

Theoretical procedures, on the other hand, fit a given functional form or model to the data. This implies some knowledge of the underlying physical mechanism of the system. Some idea of the behaviour of the system can then be obtained by estimating the parameters of the model and their precision. These procedures, unlike the empirical methods, do not place so much reliance on the accuracy of the data points, and as such will probably be more robust. It is the view of the authors that some form of rigidity is essential in any curve-fitting situation to avoid erroneous oscillations in the fitted line. In addition, this rigidity should have its foundation in the physico-chemical formulation of the system under investigation. To put this into context, it is undesirable to have a standard curve that passes implicitly through every data point, no matter whether it is an erroneous point or not.

LEAST SQUARES FITTING PROCEDURE

The statistical technique used to estimate the parameters in a given model is usually the least squares procedure (LSP). This technique is illustrated in Fig. 1, where the observed responses are indicated.

The vertical distance of the ith point from the curve is called the ith residual and denoted by d_i. The total residual sums of squares (SS) is therefore

$$SS = d_1^2 + d_2^2 + d_3^2 + d_4^2 + d_5^2 + d_6^2$$

where it has been assumed that there are six standard responses. The LSP selects that curve which minimises SS. This is possibly a sensible fitting technique but should be used with care as unexpected problems can arise. Consider the two response curves shown in Fig. 2. Both curves pass through all the points and have zero residuals, but clearly the fit of curve B would be preferred to that of curve A. Thus minimising the residual SS, as performed

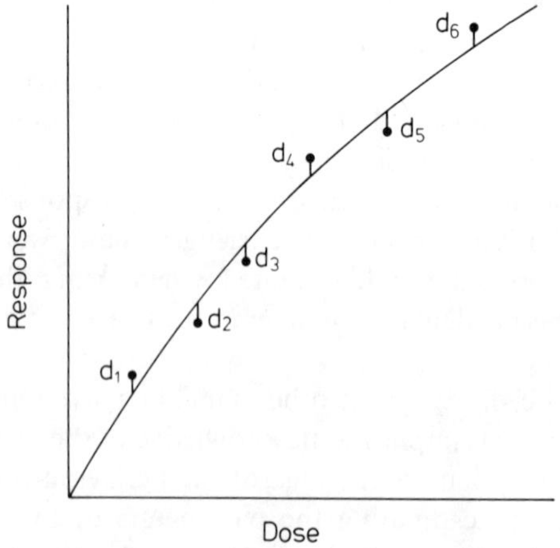

Fig. 1. Typical least-squares regression curve of response on dose. Residual errors of the six data points are shown as $d_1, \ldots, d_6$.

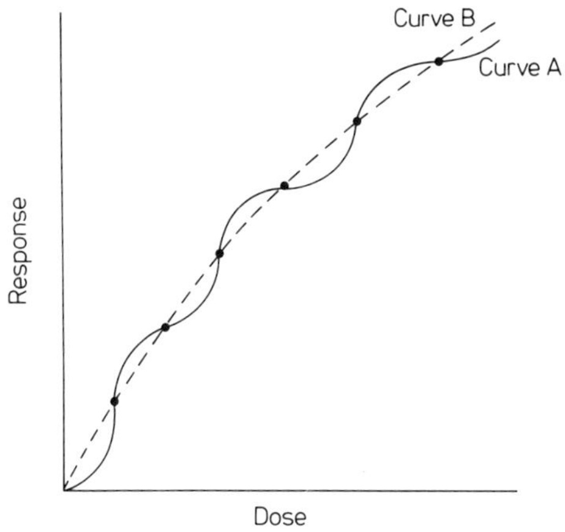

Fig. 2. Two regression curves, A and B, which both have zero residuals at all data points. Curve B would be preferred to curve A for assay calculation. Least squares is thus a fitting procedure and not an assessment criterion.

in the LSP, is desirable, but not a sufficient criterion by itself for assessing goodness of fit. It is recommended that the entire dose–response curve should be viewed as a high resolution plot before the curve is accepted. A table of residuals at the standard points is insufficient for this purpose. Curve assessment will be discussed again later.

STATISTICAL WEIGHTING

If we accept that all standard curve data points are not equally important in carrying out curve-fitting, then we must weight the points so that the more precise ones influence the curve-fitting most.

As an illustration of the possible effects of weighting, consider the diagrammatic representation of a typical response curve shown in Fig. 3. Curve A would be obtained from fitting a curve assuming equal precision (weight) for each data point. If the responses at the points X, Y and Z were known to be more precise than the others, then curve B may be obtained. The use of the weighted curve-fit would lead to a different bias than if the unweighted curve was used, and this bias may be positive or negative at different concentrations.

In *most* regression models, the weights are defined to be the reciprocals of the response variances. This being the case, the smaller the response variance the larger is the weight, so that the curve-fit routine is forced to pay

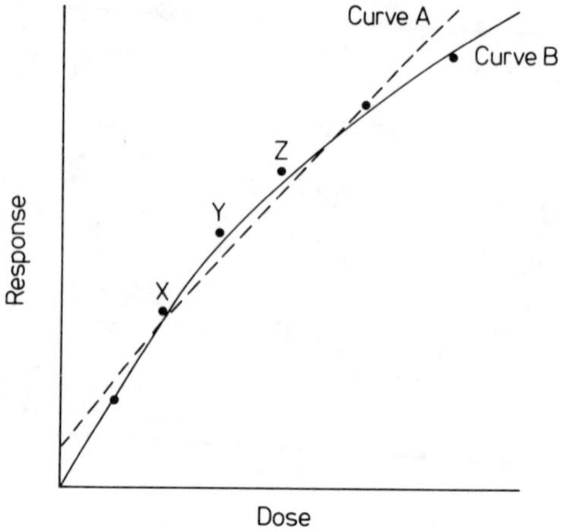

Fig. 3. Two regression curves fitted to six data points. In curve A each data point has equal weight. In curve B the points *X*, *Y* and *Z* have greater weight than the others.

more attention to those points on the calibration curve having greatest precision.

Another example of the effects of weighting is shown in Fig. 4, where a straight-line regression model has been fitted to the data using LSP, both with and without weighting. As can be seen, the observations near the zero are more precise than those more distant from it. The weighted and unweighted fits produce very different lines, the former passing closer to the points which are more precise. Appropriate weighting functions must be used in all curve-fit routines.

A number of consequences of the use of a weighting function now emerge.

(a) The appropriate weighting function must be established before it can be used, that is the response-error profile for the calibration data must be estimated. It is common practice to fit a smooth curve to the plot of standard deviation of response versus response. Since the weighting function requires the variance (the square of the standard deviation), variance versus response should be plotted. The difference in prediction between the two methods can be of the order of 3%. Care must be taken in selecting which plot is most appropriate, this being related to the subsequent use of the predictions.

(b) If standard curves are fitted to the *means* of replicate responses rather than to the individual points, then a weighting function is required when

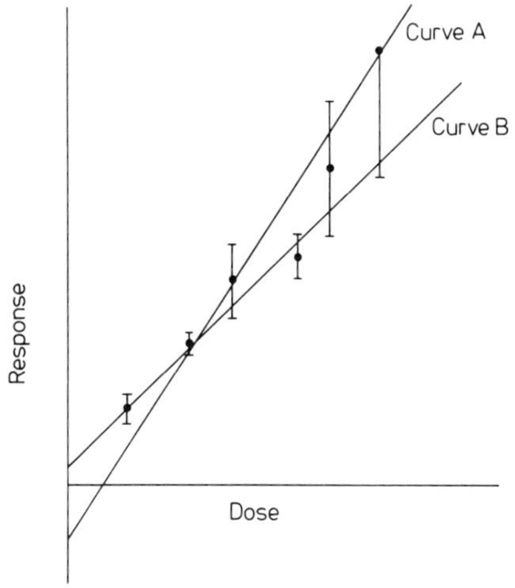

Fig. 4. The effect of weighting when fitting a straight line. Curve A is the unweighted fit, resulting in a negative intercept in this example. Curve B is the weighted fit, resulting in a positive intercept. The standard deviations associated with each data point are shown by vertical bars.

the orders of replication are different for different points. This situation would arise when equal replication is used but an outlier rejection rule is employed. Standard curves should always be fitted to the individual replicates and not the mean value, thus avoiding the need for a weighting function due to the use of different orders of replication.

(c) Data reduction packages currently available often offer the user a weighted and an unweighted curve-fit for any particular model, without requesting the appropriate weighting function to employ. Presumably the package either has an in-built functional form for the weighting function, or it estimates it from the standard replicates with very few degrees of freedom. In such situations, the user must make every effort to establish that the weighting function used is appropriate to the situation at hand. It is probably better to use an unweighted fit than an incorrect one, if there is no choice in the matter.

PRECISION PROFILES

The concept of the precision profile was suggested by Ekins (1981). The construction of this profile can either be geometrical (by hand) or analytical

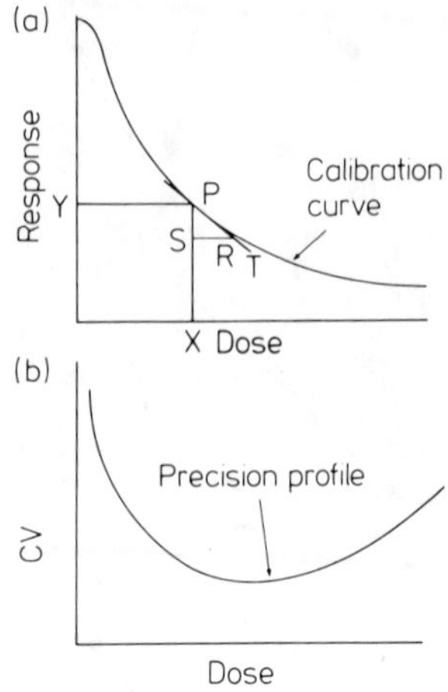

Fig. 5. Geometrical derivation of precision profile. The coefficient of variation is determined from (a) as described in the text and plotted against the dose to yield the precision profile shown in (b).

(by use of a computer), the two approaches being equivalent. For the purposes of this paper the geometrical approach will be described.

A calibration curve is fitted to the data obtained from the standards using appropriate statistical procedures as dealt with above. For each concentration, X, the calibration curve gives the corresponding response, Y (see Fig. 5(a)). A tangent to this curve, PT, is drawn at point P. From the point P, in the direction PX, a line PS is marked where S is chosen such that $PS = \sigma_y$, the response error at Y. A horizontal line is now constructed from S to meet PT at R. The distance SR then gives the standard error in the dose at the selected concentration level, X. In this manner the coefficient of variation (CV) is calculated and plotted against the corresponding dose

Table 1
Data Points for a Typical Assay Standard Curve Showing the Observed Count Rate and that Calculated, using a Commercially Available Data Reduction Package, from a Cubic Polynomial (excluding end-points) and a Four-parameter Logistic Curve-fitting Function
(the data points are plotted in Fig. 6)

Dose	*0*	*1·25*	*2·5*	*5*	*10*	*20*	*30*	*40*	*50*	*80*	*100*
Observed	10 004	9 373	8 872	7 997	6 662	5 024	3 953	3 385	3 002	2 408	2 171
Predicted logistic	9 945	9 432	8 913	7 994	6 606	4 946	4 021	3 439	3 043	2 375	2 132
Predicted cubic	—	9 239	8 843	8 105	6 826	4 968	3 870	3 320	3 108	2 395	—

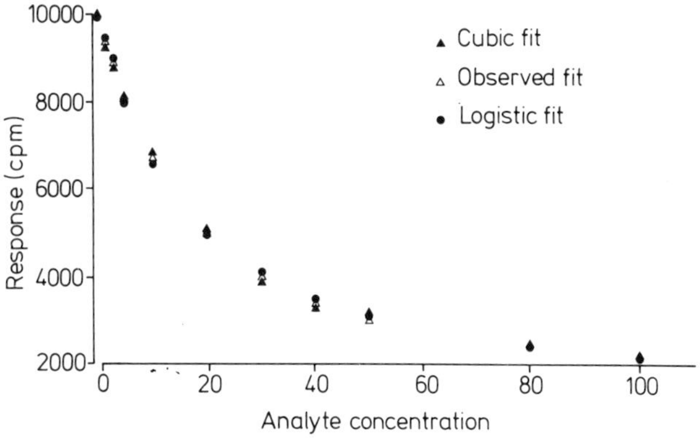

Fig. 6. Data points achieved using a cubic polynomial and a four-parameter logistic curve-fit model are plotted alongside the observed data points for a typical standard curve. The count rates are given in Table 1.

level to give the precision profile as shown in Fig. 5(b). The precision profile therefore represents the CV of the dose recorded as a function of that dose.

The suggested interpretation of the precision profile is that it is a measure of assay performance. However, while the assay procedure does contribute to the shape and position of the precision profile, it is not the only contributory factor. As an illustration of this point, consider the standard curve data shown in Table 1. Two alternative curve-fit procedures were used to obtain the standard curve, namely a simple cubic polynomial function and a four-parameter logistic function. The plotted values, together with the raw data, are shown in Fig. 6. Both curve-fits appear to be equally 'good' and quite close to all observed points. The derived precision profiles, using the same response-error relationships, are shown in Fig. 7. The most striking feature observed here is the way in which the precision profile peaks for the cubic fit. The reason for this is that a cubic calibration curve has a near plateau at this point, resulting in a very shallow gradient and hence an elevated value for imprecision. This example clearly illustrates the influence of curve-fit choice on precision profiles, a factor separate from technical assay performance. This problem is present particularly when polynomial curve-fit procedures are utilised where oscillations in the curve will lead to shallow slopes for imprecision calculation. However, it emphasises that curve-fitting should be an integral part of the establishment and validation of a new assay, and that changing the curve-fit may yield different precision profile performance characteristics, independent of the actual assay performance.

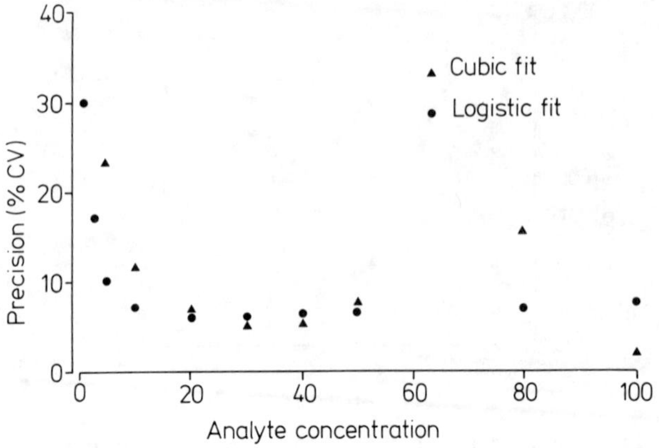

Fig. 7. Precision profiles derived from the cubic polynomial and the four-parameter logistic curve-fit used in Fig. 6. The profile for the cubic curve-fit peaks at the 80-unit point, but not for the logistic model.

The problems associated with interpreting precision profiles do not end with the choice of curve-fit used. The precision profile is an estimated quantity, since it relies upon the fitted standard curve, amongst other things, and as such has estimation error associated with it. To illustrate this point the following simulation exercise was performed. A computer was used to produce values equivalent to replicate count rates at 11 standard dose levels in such a way that the response-error profile was kept constant.

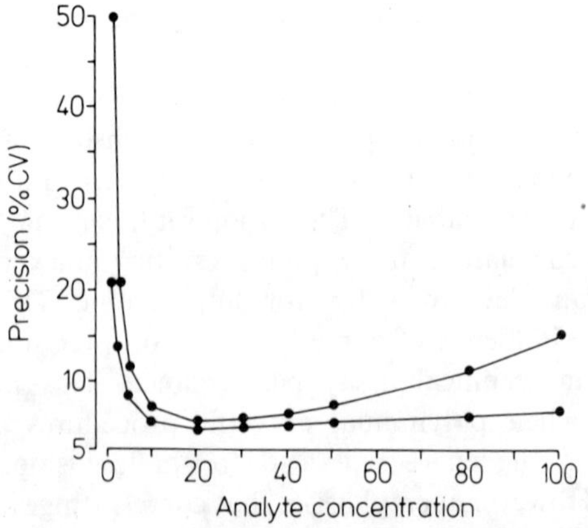

Fig. 8. The range of precision profiles achieved from computer simulation of 1000 assays, analysed using a four-parameter logistic curve-fit model, where *true* response-error profile was kept constant.

The four-parameter logistic function was then used to obtain a calibration curve, and hence a precision profile. This exercise was repeated 1000 times, thus simulating the running of 1000 assays, each having the same *true* precision profile. The envelope of all the obtained precision profiles is shown in Fig. 8. As can be seen, the error in estimating the precision profile, even from one curve-fit, is not insignificant and should be borne in mind when quoting precision levels.

Precision profiles are undoubtedly a very useful way of expressing estimated precision levels, but users must be aware of the technique's sensitivity to curve-fitting functions and its own estimation errors, so that odd shapes and changes in precision levels need not necessarily be associated with assay performance at all.

CONFIDENCE INTERVALS

It is common practice to indicate uncertainties in predictions by placing an error envelope about the standard curve and then to use this to derive confidence intervals for the true mean predicted dose. To construct these envelopes (see Fig. 9), a dose level, *X*, is selected and, from the standard

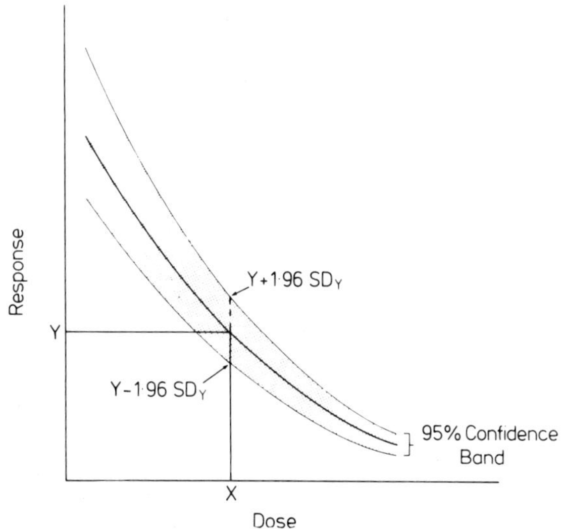

Fig. 9. 95% confidence interval bands about a standard curve. The bands can indicate the confidence interval of the mean *calculated* dose, but not of the *true* dose unless there is zero bias in the fitted curve across the entire dose range.

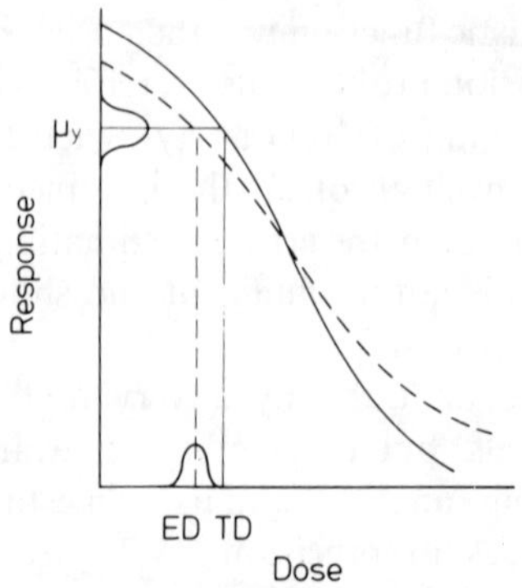

Fig. 10. Inappropriate use of errors in estimated dose (ED), interpolated for a given mean response (μ_y), to indicate errors in true dose (TD). The dashed line represents the fitted curve while the solid line is the true but unknown dose–response relationship. Bias in the fitted curve leads to bias in the confidence intervals of any estimate.

curve, the corresponding response, Y, is obtained. From the response-error relationship, the standard deviation SD(Y) may be found. These values now determine the interval $Y \pm 1{\cdot}96\,\text{SD}(Y)$, as shown in Fig. 9. If this is repeated for all response levels, the interval will define a band about the standard curve, which may be termed the 95% confidence band. Converting these confidence intervals into ones for dose values follows exactly the same procedure as that described above for precision profiles.

Deriving confidence intervals in this way will almost certainly not yield 95% confidence intervals for the true mean dose levels, but will provide the mean of the calculated dose levels from the standard curve. For them to relate to the true dose level, the curve-fit would have to have zero bias across the entire dose range and the positioning of the curve to be without any error. The derived confidence intervals have a role to play in a data reduction package, but their use and interpretation must be very clear.

The significance of this may be seen by reference to Fig. 10. Here the solid line represents the true, but unknown, dose–response relationship and the dotted line shows the fitted standard curve, assumed to be without any error at the moment. For a true mean response, μ_y, the true dose should be TD, while the actual reported estimated dose is ED. These are different because the curve is biased from the true points. If the response-error distribution is included, this will result in a distribution of reported doses as shown in Fig. 10. Thus the confidence intervals calculated refer to ED and not to TD as would be preferred. The variability of the standard curve increases the variability in the reported dose and so increases further the spread of reported results about ED. As a consequence of this, reported '95% confidence intervals' really have a much lower confidence coefficient, possibly as low as 80%. The effects of variability of the standard curve will be returned to later, this really being at the heart of curve assessment.

GOODNESS-OF-FIT TEST FOR THE STANDARD CURVE

After proceeding through the maze of the selection and fitting of a standard curve-fitting procedure and specifying the weighting function, the data reduction program usually provides some index as to the goodness-of-fit. The standard statistical approach for doing this, included in a number of commercially available data reduction packages, is to compare the 'lack-of-fit' sums of squares (SS), suitably normalised by its degrees of freedom, with the SS due to 'pure' error, i.e. the error within replicate estimates, again suitably normalised by its degrees of freedom. The 'lack-of-fit' SS is the difference between the residual SS, after the curve has been fitted, and the pure error SS. For a 'perfect' curve-fit, the normalised lack-of-fit SS and pure error SS will both estimate the same thing, i.e. both are unbiased estimates of the measurement error. If, on the other hand, the curve-fit is not correct, then the normalised lack-of-fit SS would be inflated by a term relating to the bias present in the model. The method then evaluates the ratio of the normalised lack-of-fit SS to pure error SS. If this ratio is too large, then the curve suffers from lack of fit.

Several points must be noted with this approach. Firstly, the critical point for deciding whether the ratio is too large usually relates to the 95th percentile of the appropriate F-distribution. The distributional properties of the ratio of the two SS requires the normality of the observations for it to be F-distributed. This can be a major cause for concern, particularly when considering tail percentiles, such as the 95th, which are sensitive to minor distributional changes.

Secondly, the test can be too sensitive and fail almost all assays if the within-replicate error is very small. The explanation for this, possibly undesirable, effect is simple and lies in the origins of the test. Whatever curve-fit is being used it will not express the *exact* relationship between response and dose. As such the residual SS, although possibly small for a 'good' curve-fit, will always be considerably in excess of the pure error. Therefore the ratio will be large and a lack-of-fit message will be issued. This problem is illustrated in Fig. 11, where curve (b) is seen to be a

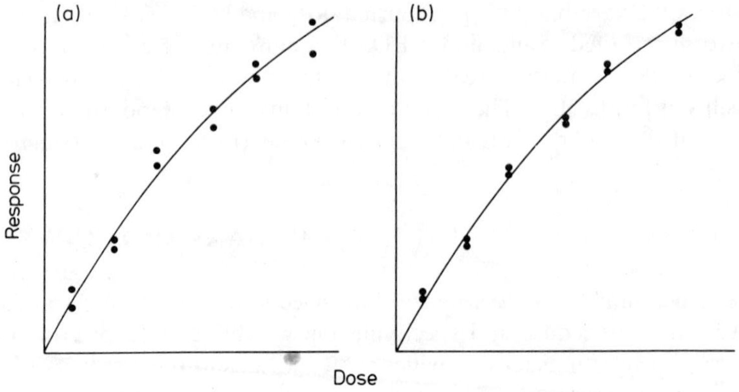

Fig. 11. (a) Regression curve with poor duplication and no lack-of-fit message. The lack-of-fit sums of squares are comparable to the within-replicate sums of squares, yielding a small F-ratio. (b) Regression curve with excellent duplication resulting in a lack-of-fit message. The lack-of-fit sums of squares are larger than the within-replicate sums of squares, yielding a large F-ratio.

reasonable compromise on the variation seen between the points, but would still be flagged for lack of fit because of high replicate precision, whereas a curve with poorer precision (a) would not be so flagged.

Such goodness-of-fit tests are therefore merely useful monitoring devices. The interpretation of 'lack-of-fit' messages must be made with care by laboratory managers who fully appreciate the theory behind the test. In inexperienced hands they can be confusing, if not completely fallacious.

THE PROBLEM OF DATA REDUCTION PACKAGES

We are sure that commercial companies approach the problem of software development for the data reduction of immunoassays in a conscientious manner. However, our observations suggest that the full importance of rigorously assessed curve-fitting packages has been missed. Several points lead us to this conclusion.

Often, particularly with the development of the new technologies, the software is contained in a sealed 'black box' that forms an integral part of the equipment which cannot be accessed by the user. This 'take-it-or-leave-it' approach can only invite criticism. It does not allow for independent assessment of the package.

The data reduction packages are more often than not assembled by a nominated employee, whose expertise lies neither in statistical methodologies nor numerical analytical techniques. This can lead to the use of inappropriate tests or techniques described above.

To cover all eventualities, some packages offer a glittering array of possible curve-fit routines. Unfortunately, they do *not* offer advice on how to choose the appropriate one for a particular assay. The user is left with making some arbitrary decisions, based either upon subjective ignorance or, perhaps more disastrously, upon inaccurate assumptions of how the package may operate.

It would also appear that the computer logic may not be what it is claimed to be. An exercise was carried out to determine the degree of between-laboratory error due to the use of different curve-fitting regimes, over and above the error due to the different reagents and assay techniques the participants used. Instead of distributing samples for assay by the laboratories, we distributed a piece of paper containing the count rates for a duplicate standard curve, plus the counts for three simulated quality control (QC) samples, to 250 hospital laboratories in the UK (Groom *et al.*, 1987). The laboratories were asked to create a curve from the standard points provided and interpolate concentrations for the three QC samples. They were asked to achieve this using graph paper and pencil, and also using any computer packages they had available. The curve-fits used, the computer, the source of the program, etc., were recorded. As expected, variation in the reported results was observed for users of *different curve-fit models* but also for users of any particular curve-fit model on hardware from *different manufacturers*. Most disconcerting was the finding of variation in results *within a particular instrument* from a particular manufacturer, where hardware/software updates had been introduced into later models of the machine. The variation of results in such situations was of the order of 1–4%, but occasionally in excess of 10%. These errors would be on top of any technical error (pipetting and other manipulations) by laboratory staff in carrying out an assay.

Finally, it cannot be over-emphasised that curve-fitting cannot overcome poor assay optimisation and can indeed exacerbate errors in assays which include standard points outside the working range of that assay. In such cases, the inclusion of such standard points can seriously distort the curve-fit, leading to very large unacceptable bias of interpolated results. Searching for an alternative, perhaps 'better', curve-fit model in this case is fruitless since it is the experimental design of the assay which is at fault and must be remedied.

SUGGESTED STRATEGY

It would seem that we are faced with the question of who or what can provide suitable data reduction packages to overcome these present problems.

It is unlikely that statisticians can help in such a situation because the statistician will produce a conventional solution to a conventional problem. He/she will not be aware whether the basic assumptions behind the tests are valid in the context of the immunoassayist, or what can be assumed about the functional forms of the error distributions involved. Available statistical packages will probably also incorporate assumptions which may be inappropriate to the assay in question.

Therefore a team comprising immunoassayists, statisticians, numerical analysts, computer programmers and representatives of any interested professions should be established. This team should be charged with producing a British Standard which would apply to all data reduction packages in use. Considerable research still remains to be done, but by combining the complementary expertise of the team a software package could be achieved in which the user (laboratory or kit manufacturer) would have confidence.

It is clear that a key feature of this problem is the choice of an adequate curve-fit model. Although easily stated, there is no agreed criterion upon which to compare curve-fits. The least squares procedure is commonly used but, as we have shown, should be considered a *fitting* criterion, not an *assessment* criterion, particularly when used, as it is in immunoassay, in a reverse sense to predict dose from response, although analytically that is a regressed response with each dose level. The following two assessment criteria for standard curves may be considered candidate procedures to overcome this problem.

Figure 12 illustrates the data points for a standard curve established from replicate determinations of a response variable, Y, obtained for a number of predetermined dose levels, X. The response-error profiles are shown for various dose levels and the standard curve would be fitted to the observed responses. An enlargement of part of this curve is shown in Fig. 13. For the given fixed mean response levels, the reported dose levels should be those of the standards. However, the actual reported dose levels are found by interpolation (see Fig. 13). The difference between the reported dose and the actual dose is then the error, and is the quantity which should be minimised to achieve the best fit. Note that this is *not* the residual (vertical) error associated with the least-squares approach. If a number of

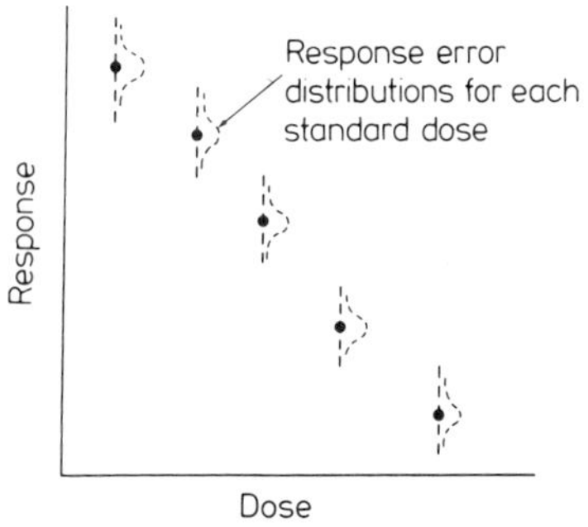

Fig. 12. Response-error profiles for each of a series of data points, assayed in replicate, to be used to produce a standard curve.

such standard curves were fitted to different observed standard responses, then the distribution of reported doses for each fixed response level might be as illustrated in Fig. 14. Thus there will be a bias associated with the reported dose, together with variation about the mean reported dose. An ideal curve-fit would have zero bias and zero variation. Both these factors need to be considered to assess the curve-fit suitability. A statistical function which brings together both of these components of error is the mean square error (MSE) and may be defined as

$$\text{MSE} = \text{variance of reported dose} + (\text{bias of reported dose})^2$$

An effective standard deviation can be found by taking the positive square root of the MSE. To completely simulate the use of a standard curve, the

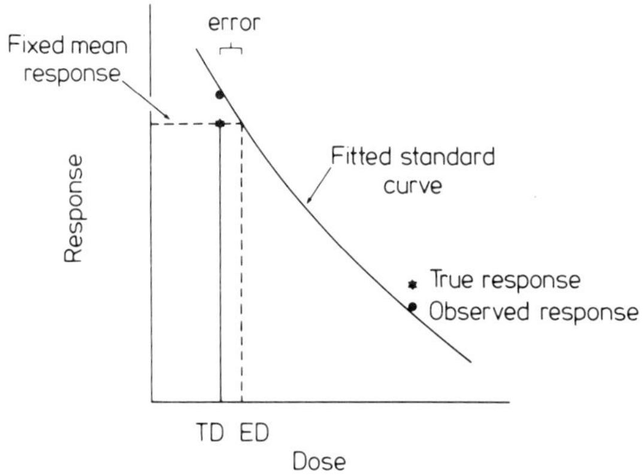

Fig. 13. The error (bias) between true and estimated reported dose of a standard data point for a fixed mean response. This bias must be minimised to achieve goodness of fit.

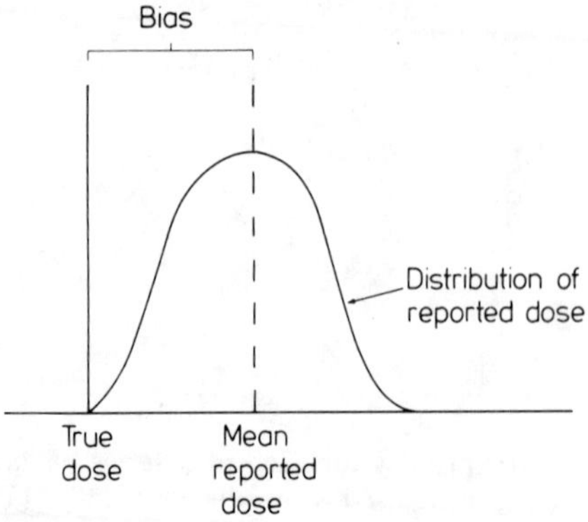

Fig. 14. The bias of true dose from the distribution of reported doses of a standard data point for each fixed response level. This variation in bias must be minimised to achieve goodness of fit.

fixed response levels need to be replaced by a response-error distribution for non-standard samples. This is illustrated in Fig. 15. The consequence of superimposing response-error is to add more variability to the reported dose rather than to change the bias.

It is now possible to assess, by simulation, the various components of error associated with the reporting of a dose value. These components are due to (a) variability of the non-standard response but keeping the standard curve fixed, (b) fixed non-standard response but variable standard curve (due to response-error in the standards), and (c) variability in both the non-standard response and standard curve factors.

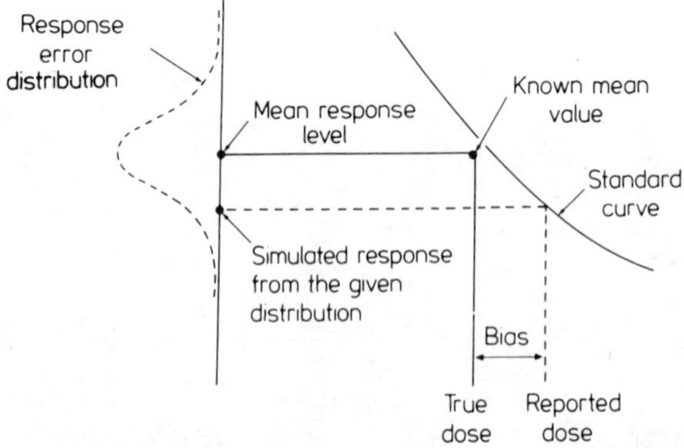

Fig. 15. The calculation of bias from true dose for reported doses of non-standard samples, when variation in both the response and the standard curve is considered.

Table 2

Comparison of Root Mean Square Error (RMSE) with Assessments of Error in Response or Curve for Three Curve-fit Models for a Prolactin Assay

(data were obtained by computer simulation of 1000 assays (see text))

Dose	*0·00*	*1·25*	*2·5*	*5*	*10*	*20*	*30*	*40*	*50*	*80*	*100*
Four-parameter logistic curve-fit											
Mean	0·31	1·38	2·60	4·9	9·8	19·4	30·9	40·8	51·8	78·2	96·9
Bias	0·31	0·13	0·10	−0·03	−0·2	−0·56	0·92	0·87	1·86	−1·76	−3·02
SD(a)	0·28	0·43	0·47	0·32	0·64	1·10	1·62	2·79	4·15	6·04	5·83
SD(b)	0·30	0·46	0·50	0·37	0·69	1·18	1·77	2·94	4·31	6·47	7·29
SD(c)	0·43	0·48	0·51	0·38	0·72	1·30	1·99	3·07	4·70	6·71	7·89
Amersham curve-fit											
SD(c)	0·41	0·48	0·51	0·38	0·71	1·30	2·03	3·17	4·79	6·80	7·98
Logit–log curve-fit											
SD(c)	0·37	0·43	0·52	0·56	0·97	1·58	3·38	4·08	5·18	7·31	12·69

SD(a), singleton, variable response error, fixed curve error (this is equivalent to precision profile figure).
SD(b), singleton, variable response error, variable curve error.
SD(c), effective SD for singleton using the RMSE.
Comparison of these three SDs for any given curve-fit model shows the magnitude of error unaccounted for if precision profile alone is used. Comparison of SD(c) for different curve-fits allows choice of best-fit model for a particular assay.

Such a simulation study has been performed on radioimmunoassays for different analytes using different curve-fitting routines (Kay *et al.*, 1986). A summary of the results for a human prolactin assay is given in Table 2. The interpretation of the relative performance of the different curve-fit models is carried out by considering a dose level, e.g. 5, and noting that the standard deviation (SD(a)) obtained from the usual construction of a precision profile is 0·32 in this case. This is compared with an increased standard deviation of 0·37 when the variability includes that from the standard curve (SD(b)) and finally with 0·38, which is the standard deviation including the bias term (SD(c)). Thus an increase in standard deviation of some 16 to 19% is seen over the simple precision profile value. These results clearly indicate that the conventional approach can seriously underestimate the true imprecision associated with an assay.

When the four-parameter logistic, Amersham and logit–log curve-fit models were compared using the above criterion (Table 2), effective standard deviations of 0·38, 0·38 and 0·56 were obtained at this concentration of 5 units. This indicates that, for this dose level, the logit–log function was inferior to the other two models, which were apparently equivalent. This must be repeated at the other doses to determine the best curve-fit for the assay. Each assay can be tested in this way during its validation so that the most appropriate curve-fit can be assigned and become as much an integral part of the assay as the reagent volumes and incubations.

It is hoped that this review of the problems confronting immunoassayists in the data reduction of their assays has highlighted the care required in this important stage of carrying out an assay. As much error can be imparted into the assay at this stage as during the reagent manipulation stages, while the commercial packages available at present offer little more than confusing 'black boxes' whose efficiency often cannot be checked. The establishment of a working team to determine adequate criteria for curve-fitting and provide a British Standard would considerably ease the confusion of kit reagent manufacturers, hardware manufacturers and, not least, the laboratory staff performing these immunoassays.

ACKNOWLEDGEMENTS

The authors would like to gratefully acknowledge Carole Kay for processing some of the data referred to in the text. The work was supported by the Department of Health and Social Security, the Welsh Office and the Tenovus Organisation.

REFERENCES

BOX, C. E. P. & HUNTER, W. G. (1962) A useful method for model building. *Technometrics*, **4**, 301–318.

EKINS, R. P. (1981) The 'precision profile': its use in RIA assessment and design. *SupraRegional Assay Service Newsletter*, **1**, 7–22.

GROOM, G. V., KAY, C. & NIX, A. B. J. (1987) The effect of curve-fitting on RIA bias and its influence on inter-laboratory assessments, in preparation.

KAY, C., NIX, A. B. J., KEMP, K. W., ROWLANDS, R. J., RICHARDS, G., GROOM, G. V., GRIFFITHS, K. & WILSON, D. W. (1986) Dose interpolation of immunoassay data: uncertainties associated with curve-fitting. *Statistics in Medicine*, **5**, 183–192.

18

Factors Influencing the Relative Costs of Immunoassays and Conventional Analyses of Food Constituents and Contaminants

M. R. A. MORGAN

AFRC Institute of Food Research, Norwich, UK

INTRODUCTION

Immunoassays offer the food analyst several advantages over conventional procedures. Immunoassays can be very specific and extremely sensitive, a combination that can result in sample preparation protocols that are much simpler and quicker than those for alternative procedures. In addition, immunoassays facilitate the routine handling of large sample numbers. It is not surprising, therefore, that an almost invariable feature of reports describing immunoassays for food constituents and contaminants are statements of the potential cost benefits available. Unfortunately, such statements are rarely based on objective comparisons because appropriate data are not available.

Cost is a major factor in deciding which type of analytical procedure should be performed in order to obtain a particular result. However, other factors, such as availability, speed and reliability of assay, may dominate under certain circumstances. The important elements in costing an analytical technique are listed in Table 1. The availability of an immunological approach may affect each of these.

ASSAY RAPIDITY (EXCLUDING LABOUR COSTS)

The cost of analysis of a food matrix may include storage costs incurred whilst waiting for the results; for example, delays of several days are not uncommon when monitoring for *Salmonella* contamination while conventional microbiological analysis is carried out. Immunoassays can

Table 1
Important Factors Contributing to Assay Cost

(i)	Consequences of delay whilst result is obtained
(ii)	Consequences of lack of assay reliability
(iii)	Equipment costs
(iv)	Labour costs
(v)	Reagent costs

cut these costs drastically by reducing assay time. Dipstick immunoassays or card tests, where a spot of sample is applied to a reagent-coated support, are not only rapid but simple too, although there may be problems with sample preparation for many food matrices. If quantitation of analyte is required, rather than a 'yes/no' answer, then procedures become slightly less simple. However, dramatic improvements can still be seen over conventional methodology, for example, in the analysis of *Clostridium botulinum* toxins by ELISA, where assay time is hours rather than days (Shone *et al.*, 1985; see Modi *et al.*, p. 325, this volume).

RELIABILITY

An assay may be cheap to perform, but unless it has suitable reliability it may give rise to considerable financial problems in the longer term. An extreme example would be the failure to detect a particular pathogen or toxin in a food product. At this early stage in the development of immunoassays for application to food matrices it is not possible to compare their reliability with conventional techniques in the hands of food analysts. In many instances, particularly those where conventional procedures are dependent on subjective judgement, it would be difficult to imagine immunoassays being less reliable (see Robertson *et al.*, Chapter 14).

EQUIPMENT

The equipment costs for immunoassays can vary considerably. The use of dipstick-type assays requires little expenditure other than that for sample preparation. The microtitration plate format appears at present to be the most useful general procedure. For qualitative food analysis in its most basic form, one pipette, one wash bottle and one pair of eyes may be all that is required. As the requirement for more accurate quantitation increases, automatic plate washers, plate readers, and sample and reagent dispensers and diluters are available from a number of manufacturers. Even at this level of sophistication the cost of equipment, bearing in mind its wide applicability, compares favourably with that required for alternative techniques.

LABOUR

Since immunoassays can be simpler and quicker than conventional procedures, assay costs can be reduced because staff at a more junior level can be employed to carry out more assays in a given time or redeployed on other duties. An example of this was observed in the analysis of some 50 potato samples for glycoalkaloid content by both a chemical method and by a microtitration plate ELISA in our laboratory (Morgan *et al.*, 1985). The chemical procedure used (Sanford & Sinden, 1972) was lengthy, required considerable analytical skill and utilised toxic reagents. Briefly, potatoes were Soxhlet-extracted for 16 h, and the glycoalkaloids concentrated and precipitated before colorimetric determination by reaction with antimony trichloride/concentrated hydrochloric acid reagent. The ELISA procedure used (Morgan *et al.*, 1983) required a simple 2-min aqueous extraction of glycoalkaloids from the potato sample, followed by dilution of extract and assay. Labour costs were 15 times greater for the chemical method than for the ELISA. This difference is not simply the result of the time taken for the actual assay procedure, but also the time required for sample preparation in the chemical method.

REAGENTS

Simplified sample extraction methods will reduce the solvent costs incurred in alternative procedures. Antibodies are the key reagents in immunoassays and it is their properties that enable simple methods employing simple equipment to be developed. The cost of antibody production is difficult to quantify. Polyclonal antisera having the desired avidity and specificity might be produced within six months or may take in excess of two years. Monoclonal antibodies can also be produced within six months, though the search for an antibody of the desired characteristics may take much longer and is labour-intensive.

Despite the costs, the search for an antibody preparation having the desired characteristics is well worth while, bearing in mind the potential benefits bestowed by an immunoassay. Thus recently described ELISAs for the analysis of aflatoxins may either employ simple solubilisation procedures (for example the work of Morgan *et al.* (1986) on peanut butter) or none at all (for example the work of Jackman (1985) on milk). Alternative methods are considerably more tedious and time-consuming.

CONCLUSIONS

Immunoassays are increasingly being regarded as realistic alternatives to conventional methods of food analysis. However, few food analysts have the facilities to raise their own antisera, and most are therefore dependent on commercial suppliers of immunological reagents, either separately or in kit form, at reasonable cost. Only if such become available will the advantages of immunoassays in food analysis be realised.

ACKNOWLEDGEMENT

This work was partly funded by the Ministry of Agriculture, Fisheries and Food.

REFERENCES

JACKMAN, R. (1985) Determination of aflatoxins by ELISA with special reference to aflatoxin M_1 in milk. *Journal of the Science of Food and Agriculture*, **36**, 685–698.

MORGAN, M. R. A., MCNERNEY, R., MATTHEW, J. A., COXON, D. T. & CHAN, H. W.-S. (1983) An enzyme-linked immunosorbent assay for total glycoalkaloids in potato tubers. *Journal of the Science of Food and Agriculture*, **34**, 593–598.

MORGAN, M. R. A., COXON, D. T., BRAMHAM, S., CHAN, H. W.-S., VAN GELDER, W. M. J. & ALLISON, M. J. (1985) Determination of the glycoalkaloid content of potato tubers by three methods including enzyme-linked immunosorbent assay. *Journal of the Science of Food and Agriculture*, **36**, 282–288.

MORGAN, M. R. A., KANG, A. S. & CHAN, H. W.-S. (1986) Aflatoxin determination in peanut butter by enzyme-linked immunosorbent assay. *Journal of the Science of Food and Agriculture*, **37**, 908–914.

SANFORD, L. L. & SINDEN, S. L. (1972) Inheritance of potato glycoalkaloids. *American Potato Journal*, **49**, 209–217.

SHONE, C., WILTON-SMITH, P., APPLETON, N., HAMBLETON, P., MODI, N., GATELY, S. & MELLING, J. (1985) Monoclonal antibody-based immunoassay for Type A *Clostridium botulinum* toxin is comparable to the mouse bioassay. *Applied and Environmental Microbiology*, **50**, 63–67.

SESSION V

Novel Antibody-based Alternatives to Immunoassays

19

Immunosensors Based on Acoustic, Optical and Bioelectrochemical Devices and Techniques

E. KRESS-ROGERS
Leatherhead Food Research Association, Leatherhead, Surrey, UK

and

A. P. F. TURNER
Bioelectronics Division, Biotechnology Centre, Cranfield Institute of Technology, Bedford, UK

INTRODUCTION

With the increasing introduction of continuous processing, automated packaging and microprocessor-aided process and quality control, a need for more in-line and at-line instrumentation has arisen to provide up-to-date feedback information on the process stream as well as quality assurance. The requirements for this instrumentation are robustness, hygienic design, simple operation and rapid response. Such instruments are already available for the monitoring of pressure, temperature and the concentration of some food ingredients (McFarlane, 1983; Kress-Rogers, 1986), while for the assessment of the microbial status of food (Jarvis, 1982) or for the measurement of trace compounds or toxins (Hubbard & Wiseman, 1983) laboratory techniques are still without an at-line alternative.

One approach to the rapid assessment of the microbial state of food and to the prediction of product shelf-life is the electrochemical detection of a marker chemical consumed or produced by the microbes. This is the basis of an instrument under development by the Leatherhead Food Research Association, together with the Cranfield Institute of Technology, for meat shelf-life prediction based on the detection of glucose profiles in chilled meat joints (Kress-Rogers & D'Costa, 1986). (See Fig. 1.)

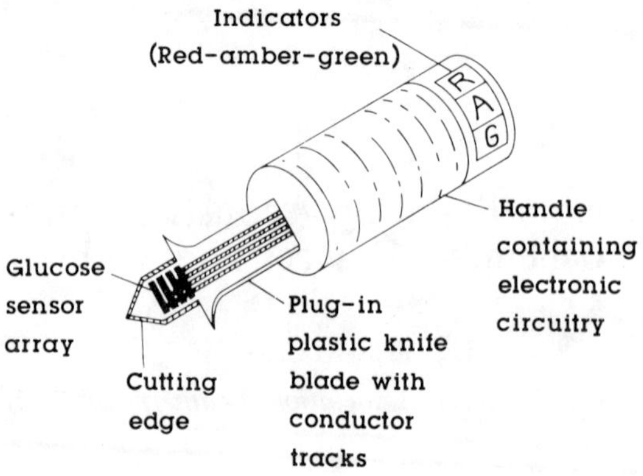

Fig. 1. The proposed instrument for the at-line shelf-life prediction of chilled meat joints by the measurement of the glucose profile from the surface to the bulk. The lead may transfer the output to, for example, a product labelling machine or to a product reject mechanism. A similar configuration could be used for at-line measurements with immunosensors.

It is now feasible to construct instruments suitable for at-line operation for the detection of analytes, such as microbial or fungal toxins, for the assay of vitamins or for the speciation of meat. Such instruments can be based on immunosensors which obviate the incubation phase and/or simplify the manipulation of the sample by eliminating the steps of reagent addition, volume measurement and/or separation of bound from free radio- or other labels which have to be carried out prior to measurement in a conventional immunoassay.

When antibodies are immobilised on a surface, the optical, acoustic and electrical properties of this surface change when the antigen binds. This change can be observed when the antibodies are immobilised on the surface of a sensor. Such an immunosensor, responding to changes in the layer thickness, density or elasticity, or to changes in a double layer potential, can operate in a kinetic mode where a time derivative of the response is measured. This signal is related to the concentration of the antigen in the sample and is obtained without prior incubation. Both direct and indirect immunosensors, relying on added labels or reporter groups, can be constructed. The separation of free from bound labels is unnecessary for a sensor responding to changes at the surface only.

For all direct immunosensors, whether optical, acoustic or potentiometric, it is important to ensure that non-specific binding of proteins to the sensing surface is avoided. The reduction of non-specific binding by the use of a 'blocking protein' has been demonstrated by Sutherland *et al.* (1984). (See also Place *et al.*, 1985, section 3.3.1.)

Instead of antibodies, other specific binding agents such as lectins, e.g. concanavalin A, may be immobilised on the sensors described below.

IMMUNOSENSORS BASED ON OPTICAL DEVICES

Devices Based on Surface Plasmon Resonance (SPR)

An example of a direct immunosensor is the surface plasmon resonance (SPR) device, modified with an antibody layer. The SPR device detects minute changes in the refractive index when the antigen binds (Liedberg *et al.*, 1983). This change in refractive index is related both to the size of the antigen and to the conformational change of the antibody–antigen complex on binding, which may involve solvent reorganisation and protein unfolding (Levison *et al.*, 1970; Place *et al.*, 1985, section 2.1). The refractive index change is detected as a shift in the angle of total absorption of light incident on a metal layer carrying the antibodies. The absorption of light occurs at an angle dependent on the refractive indices on either side of the metal film and is due to a collective excitement of electrons (the surface plasmons) in the metal film (Raether, 1977). The SPR device may consist of a prism on a glass slide carrying the thin metal layer (Fig. 2).

SPR devices have been used for the characterisation of the optical properties of dye monolayers (Pockrand *et al.*, 1978). They have also been configured as sensors for halothane gas by coating the device with a

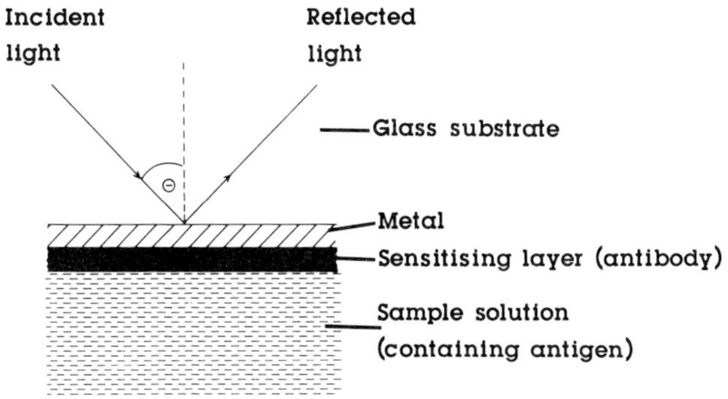

Fig. 2. The surface plasmon resonance (SPR) device for the measurement of minute changes in the refractive index. This device has been used by Liedberg *et al.* (1983) to measure IgG antibody concentrations in solution kinetically without prior incubation or separation steps.

specifically absorbing organic film (Nylander *et al.*, 1982; Liedberg *et al.*, 1983). The application of SPR devices to the measurement of antibody concentrations in liquids has been demonstrated by Liedberg *et al.* (1983). These workers immobilised γ-globulin (IgG) on the metal surface and observed the shift of the resonance angle when injecting a sample solution into the liquid contacting the sensor. The initial time derivative of the shift was proportional to the concentration of antibodies in the injected sample. The SPR immunoassay can thus yield a rapid concentration reading without prior incubation or separation steps. This first SPR immunoassay was carried out for the range 0·02–200 μg/ml. Flanagan & Pantell (1984) have immobilised human serum albumin (HSA) on a similar prism SPR device to observe the binding of anti-HSA. Alternatively, a metallised diffraction grating on a plastic support can form the basis of a more practical immunosensing device (Pettigrew, 1984) which can be manufactured inexpensively using holographic techniques already used in the production of compact discs. A fast diagnosis system for medical tests to be performed outside a centralised laboratory, based on such a grating SPR device, is being developed (Moffat, 1986). The devices carry antibodies specific to a virus, bacterium or other antigen and are to be used with a portable cassette-like instrument.

Devices Based on Total Internal Reflection (TIR)

Further optical immunosensors can be based on internal reflections in a light guide, with antibodies immobilised on the surface of the guide which is in contact with the analyte. These devices make use of the evanescent wave penetrating only a fraction of a wavelength into the optically rarer medium when light coming from an adjacent denser medium is incident on the interface (e.g. water on glass) with an angle above the critical angle (Fig. 3).

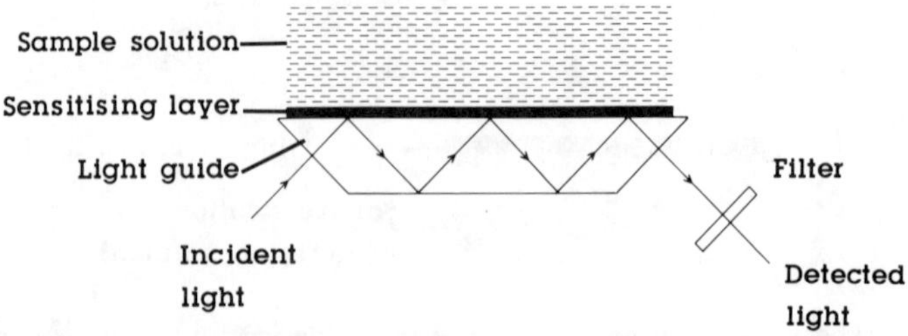

Fig. 3. Schematic design of immunosensors based on a total internal reflection (TIR) geometry, making use of the effect of antibody binding to the antigen immobilised on the surface, on the evanescent wave as announced in Biotech (1984).

When the refractive index or absorptivity at the surface changes, the transmission of light through the guide is reduced. Fluorescent techniques can be used to advantage with such a device since the fluorescent evanescent wave originating from fluorescent complexes at the surface is coupled back into the guide, yielding a high fluorescence intensity at the angle of total internal reflection. Separation of free labels in the sample solution is unnecessary and kinetic operation is possible (Lee *et al.*, 1979; Place *et al.*, 1985). An immunosensor based on the evanescent wave technique is being developed, for example by Biotech (1984). Optical devices of this type have been configured as disposable devices with automatic definition of sample volume by capillary tubes (Hirschfeld, 1984; Shanks, 1986).

The instrumentation for optical TIR immunosensors can be miniaturised for some applications by use of fibre-optic techniques and solid-state optical components. For other applications, a more versatile instrument

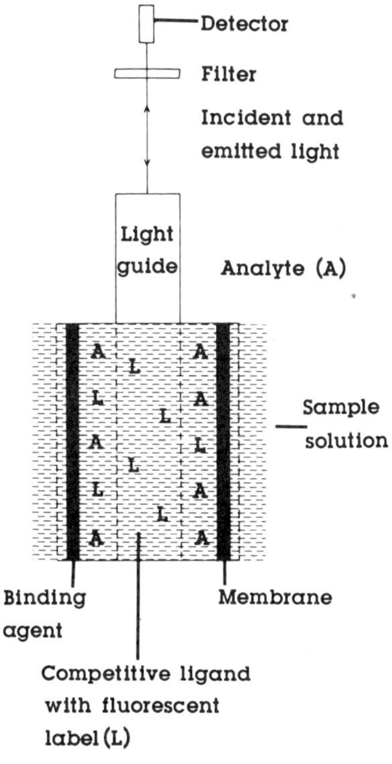

Fig. 4. Schematic design of fibre-optic sensing head for glucose as reported by Seitz (1984) using concanavalin A as the binding agent.

giving a choice of measuring and referencing wavelengths can be based on conventional components. Such an instrument could be used with a range of sensing heads, including not only immunosensors but also, for example, pH, dissolved oxygen or glucose probes based on, for instance, a fluorescence measurement (Lubbers & Opitz, 1983; Peterson *et al.*, 1984; Seitz, 1984). (See Fig. 4.)

Photon Correlation Spectroscopy

Photon correlation spectroscopy (PCS) is an optical technique for particle sizing in the submicron range. PCS is based on the measurement of the time constant of the Brownian motion of particles by dynamic light scattering. It yields information on particle size and asymmetry in the range from a few nanometres to a few micrometres (Chu & DiNapoli, 1984; Weiner, 1984). Where the formation of antibody–antigen complexes leads to agglomeration, the resultant change in particle size can be observed by PCS.

IMMUNOSENSORS BASED ON ACOUSTIC DEVICES

Devices Based on Surface Acoustic Waves (SAW)

Acoustic devices can also be turned into immunosensors. Devices sensitive to changes in the density, elasticity or electrical conductivity of a surface on which a surface acoustic wave propagates (SAW devices) can be configured as sensors. The SAW device consists of a piezoelectric crystal such as quartz or lithium niobate carrying thin-film interdigital electrode arrays. Radio frequency excitation of the electrode pair creates a synchronous mechanical surface wave, which is propagated on the surface of the piezoelectric substrate and received by another electrode pair (on a SAW delay line) or by the same pair after reflection (on a SAW resonator device). SAW devices are encountered as components in VHF circuits in, for example, televisions (Morgan, 1973; Lewis *et al.*, 1984), but SAW sensors for temperature and pressure (Reeder & Cullen, 1976; Risch, 1984) are already at the commercial stage and the usefulness of SAW sensors for specific gases and vapours has been demonstrated (Wohltjen & Dessy, 1979*a–c*; Bryant *et al.*, 1983; Wohltjen, 1984; Barendsz *et al.*, 1985). (See Fig. 5(a).)

A suitable choice of crystal cut and the use of a reference SAW device without the chemically sensitive layer ensure the insensitivity of the transducer to, for example, temperature in this latter application. It has also been shown that antigens can be detected with a SAW device carrying immobilised antibodies (Roederer & Bastiaans, 1983). This first SAW

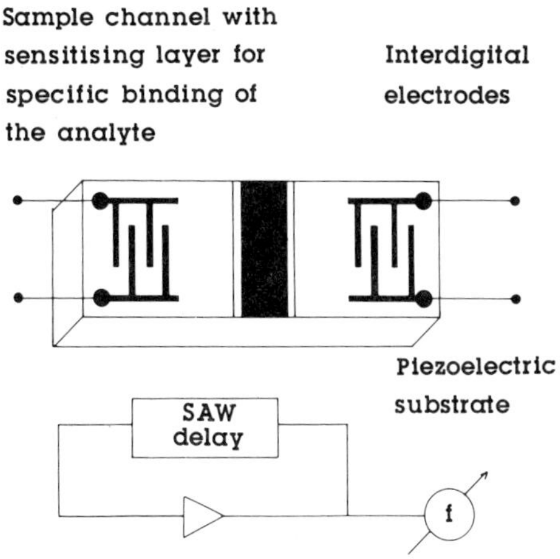

Fig. 5a. Schematic design of chemical sensor based on SAW delay line as used by Roederer & Bastiaans (1983) for the detection of IgG antigen. The basic circuit for the monitoring of the response of the SAW device is also shown.

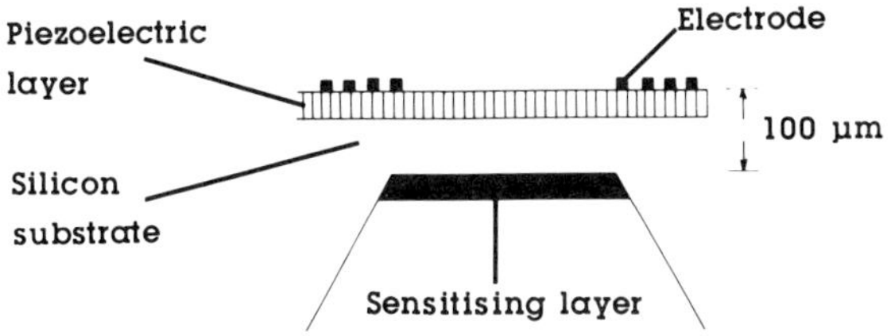

Fig. 5b. Schematic design of chemical sensor based on SAW membrane device as constructed by Chuang *et al.* (1982).

immunosensor carried a spring-loaded rubber O-ring sample cell and had a low sensitivity for the analyte. (In a recent review the detected quantity was quoted as nanograms, but in the cited source the figure is in fact 10 μg (Anon., 1984) of the analyte human IgG.)

A much higher sensitivity may be expected with a parallel sample channel, constructed on the device, similar to those used in SAW devices under development for viscosity measurements (Taylor, 1985, pers. comm.). Alternatively, a membrane SAW device as developed for vapour sensing (Chuang *et al.*, 1982) could be employed. The membrane device (Fig. 5(b)) provides spatial separation and thus protection of the SAW transducers from the sample solution. The sensitivity to be achieved with SAW immunosensors is yet to be established. An advantage of the SAW approach is the convenient output signal which is in the form of a frequency change and thus lends itself to digital signal processing and promotes low-noise signal transmission. Moreover, a simple instrument suitable for a range of SAW sensor heads for immunological, chemical, mechanical and thermal parameters can be envisaged.

Other Acoustic Devices

Another piezoelectric device employed as a sensor is the quartz microbalance or piezoelectric oscillator. This is based on the dependence of the resonance frequency of a vibrating quartz crystal on its mass. Such a crystal may be coated with a film specifically adsorbing an analyte gas or volatile component. The mass change on contact with the analyte is observed as a frequency shift. The estimated detection limit is 1 pg (10^{-12} g) (Hlavay & Guilbault, 1977; Guilbault, 1980). Devices of this type have, for instance, been configured as sensors for explosives in the ppb range (Tomita *et al.*, 1979). The crystal will also oscillate when immersed partially or completely in liquid (Nomura & Okuhara, 1982). If the solution properties such as density, viscosity and conductivity are kept constant, the weight change of the crystal can be detected and used to determine, for example, traces of 10^{-7}M iodide (Nomura & Mimatsu, 1982) or nanomolar concentrations of silver in solution (Nomura & Iijima, 1981). An immunosensor based on such a microbalance may be feasible. The commercialisation of an immunosensor based on the piezocrystal balance principle has been announced (Anon., 1985). The measurement of the bulk ultrasonic properties of a solution by the measurement of the velocity or attenuation of bulk ultrasonic waves transmitted through the liquid (Zacharias & Parnell, 1972; Wyn-Jones *et al.*, 1982; Asher, 1983), on the other hand, is too insensitive for immunoassays but may be used to monitor high yeast or bacteria cell concentrations in culture broths (Ishimori *et al.*, 1981).

IMMUNOSENSORS BASED ON SEMICONDUCTOR DEVICES

In addition to the acoustic and optical immunosensors, field effect transistor (FET) devices similar to the ion-sensitive FET (ISFET) (Janata & Huber, 1979; Bergveld, 1985) can be constructed for the detection of the minute potential changes associated with the formation of an antibody–antigen complex (Janata & Blackburn, 1984). These direct immunosensors have been termed IMFETs. ISFET devices and other microelectronic gas or ion sensors can also be used in indirect electrochemical immunoassays (using enzyme labels) in place of the traditional ion-selective electrodes or gas probes (Meyerhoff & Rechnitz, 1979). This approach has already been used for indirect biosensors based on enzyme-sensitised electrochemical devices such as the ENFET (Eddowes *et al.*, 1985). The advantages of the FET devices, namely fast response, good signal-to-noise ratio and small size, are particularly useful in flow injection analysis technqiues incorporating, for instance, an ammonia-sensitive CHEMFET and a urease column (Winquist *et al.*, 1985). Potentially, the FET devices can be constructed as inexpensive disposable devices, although their full potential has not yet been reached. The application of FET devices both as direct immunosensors and in indirect immunosensing applications are discussed in the section on electrochemical immunosensors.

There is also an indirect immunoassay based on another semiconductor device, namely the TELISA or thermistor ELISA, which has been shown to be highly sensitive. The thermistor, a heat-sensitive semiconductor device, can be chemically sensitised. The enzyme thermistor registers the heat evolved in an enzyme-catalysed reaction in a small well-insulated chamber. Ambient temperature changes can be compensated for by a split-flow system including a reference arm. Enzyme thermistors have been constructed, for example, for the determination of trace amounts of insecticides or heavy metal ions (Danielsson *et al.*, 1979; Mosbach & Danielsson, 1981). The thermometric enzyme-linked immunosorbent assay (TELISA) is based on the enzyme thermistor (Mattiasson *et al.*, 1977; Mosbach & Danielsson, 1981). The detection limits with the TELISA technique for the antigens albumin, gentamicin and insulin have been given as 10^{-13} mol/litre, 0·1 μg/ml and 0·1–1·0 U/ml respectively (Mosbach & Danielsson, 1981). The TELISA procedure has been automated for the monitoring of hormones and protcins produced by biotechnological methods (Birnbaum *et al.*, 1986; Danielsson & Mosbach, 1987).

IMMUNOSENSORS BASED ON ELECTROCHEMICAL TRANSDUCERS

Electrochemistry has dominated the field of biosensors and this has been reflected in the commercial availability of instruments relying on electrochemical detection (Scheller *et al.*, 1985). While there is little doubt that the newer acoustic and optical approaches will redress this monopoly, the wealth of experience gained with enzyme electrodes is immediately transferable to the area of immunoassay. The prevalence of electrochemical techniques is due to their unique blend of sensitivity with simplicity, resulting in a family of low-cost, rapid and portable chemical sensors capable of operation turbid solutions (Brooks & Turner, 1987; Owen & Turner, 1987; Turner *et al.*, 1987*c*).

Electrochemical measurements fall into two broad classes, both of which have been applied in chemical immunoassays (Green, 1987), although little work has been reported for either veterinary or food analysis. Potentiometric devices (e.g. the pH electrode) require the derived voltage to be determined with reference to a second electrode under conditions of essentially zero current flow. By contrast, amperometry involves measurement of the current flowing between two electrodes in response to the application of a defined voltage (e.g. the Clark oxygen electrode). The former produces a logarithmic response and is critically dependent on a precise reference electrode, but the response is largely independent of mass transport effects. Amperometric electrodes produce a linear response and are relatively insensitive to fluctuations in the reference voltage, but since the species being measured is consumed, they are affected by changes in the rate of diffusion of the analyte to the electrode. This problem is overcome either by precise hydrodynamic control or by the use of membranes to restrict the access of the species being measured (Wilson, 1986).

DIRECT POTENTIOMETRIC IMMUNOELECTRODES

Janata's (1975) proposal that the change in electrical charge when an antibody binds an antigen could be directly detected using a simple potentiometric system has caused considerable excitement in recent years. Proteins in aqueous solution possess an electrical charge which depends on their isoelectric point and the ionic strength of the solution. When two proteins complex, the net electrical charge differs from that of either of the individual components. Janata (1975) used the affinity of concanavalin A for yeast mannan as a model immunochemical system. Concanavalin A was covalently attached to a polyvinyl chloride membrane deposited on a platinum electrode. A change in the potential of the electrode in response to mannan could be detected when measured against a non-reacting protein reference electrode. Non-specific adsorption effects prohibited the use of a conventional reference electrode to measure relevant changes in potential. Janata (1975) also demonstrated a small potential difference (2 mV) when

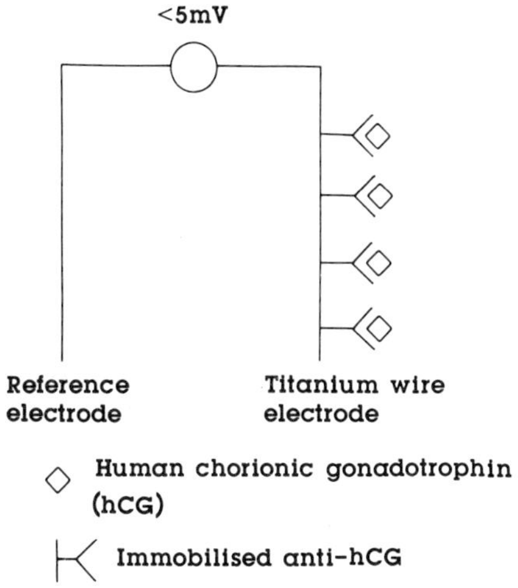

Fig. 6. Direct potentiometric immunosensor based on a titanium wire electrode as used by Yamamoto *et al.* (1978).

anti-ovalbumin was added to an ovalbumin immunoelectrode, but the effect could not be quantified.

Yamamoto *et al.* (1978) covalently immobilised anti-human chorionic gonadotrophin (anti-hCG) on a cyanogen bromide-activated titanium wire. The potential difference on addition of hCG ($5{\cdot}4 \times 10^{-9}$ g/litre) was measured against a titanium reference electrode (Fig. 6) and showed changes in the order of 5 mV with a response time of approximately 30 min. Yamamoto *et al.* (1978) considered that it would be feasible to measure voltage differences as low as 0·05 mV using their apparatus, but also drew attention to the problem of NSB which affected the observed potentials.

Aizawa *et al.* (1977) reported a thick polymer film immunoelectrode consisting of a complex of cardiolipin with cholesterol and phosphatidylcholine antigen immobilised in triacetyl cellulose. The cardiolipin membrane reacted with Wassermann antibody, which is used for non-treponemal serology tests for the detection of syphilis. Following the reaction the membrane was washed and mounted between two compartments of a cell, each containing various concentrations of sodium chloride. A transmembrane potential of up to −37·5 mV was measured compared with a negligible response from membrane contacted with antibody-free serum. Collins & Janata (1982), however, demonstrated that the membrane used by Aizawa *et al.* (1977) also responded to changes in the concentration of numerous inorganic ions, suggesting that the immunochemical response was a secondary effect on the ion-exchange properties of the membrane.

Field effect transistor (FET)-based biosensors have caught many people's imagination and the reader is referred to Bergveld (1985), Janata (1985) and Blackburn (1986) for comprehensive reviews of this area. One exciting possibility is to use the FET directly as a sensitive detector of the change in potential when an immobilised antibody binds an antigen (Janata & Huber, 1980; Collins & Janata, 1982; Janata & Blackburn, 1984). The so-called immunoFET or IMFET consists of an FET in which the metal gate is replaced by antibody or antigen immobilised on a membrane (Fig. 7). The conductivity of the n-channel region in the p-type silicon is controlled by the strength of the electric field at the gate and is measured by the application of a voltage between the source and drain electrodes. A prerequisite for such a device to function properly is that the solution/membrane interface should remain ideally polarised, i.e. be impermeable to the passage of charge. Failure to meet this requirement appears to be primarily responsible for the absence of realistic (high-sensitivity) immunoFETs, or indeed direct potentiometric sensors generally, despite intense research effort in this area (Blackburn, 1986).

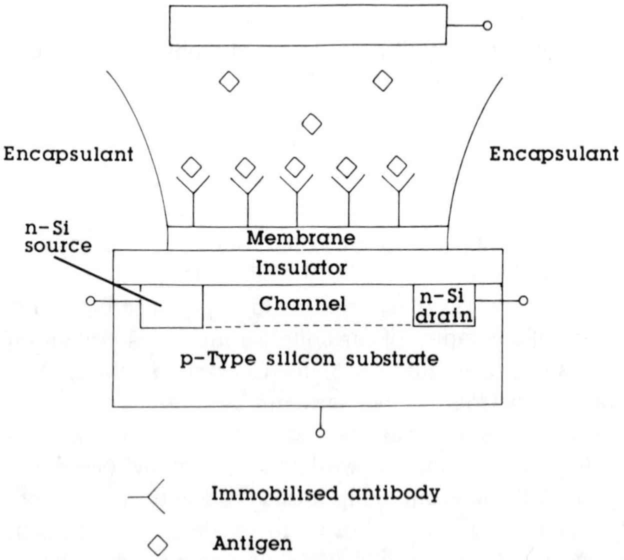

Fig. 7. Immuno field effect transistor (IMFET) device for the direct potentiometric monitoring of the antibody–antigen binding as constructed by Janata & Blackburn (1984) for the measurement of bovine serum albumin.

Indirect Potentiometric Immunosensors

Ion-selective electrodes (ISE) have been used relatively widely as alternative detectors in ELISAs (Boitieux *et al.*, 1979; Gebauer & Rechnitz, 1982; Brontman & Meyerhoff, 1984; Fonong & Rechnitz, 1984; Keating & Rechnitz, 1985) and, by inference, the ion-selective field effect transistor (ISFET) may also prove useful. It is now clear that the ISFET is a viable alternative to the ISE for many chemical sensing applications (Janata, 1985; Bergveld, 1986; Blackburn, 1986) and immunosensing principles elucidated with ISEs can be regarded as compatible with ISFETs.

Fonong & Rechnitz (1984) described an interesting homogeneous potentiometric immunosensor in which the product of the enzyme label was detected using an ISE (Fig. 8). A conjugate of chloroperoxidase and IgG was synthesised to provide labelled antigen for a competitive assay. The immobilised chloroperoxidase catalysed the bromination of β-ketoadipic acid in the presence of hydrogen peroxide and sodium bromide to form carbon dioxide, which could be detected. The enzymic activity of the conjugate was inhibited on binding anti-IgG and this effect was monitored by substrate addition following an initial incubation period of 30 min. The assay was sensitive in the mg/litre range.

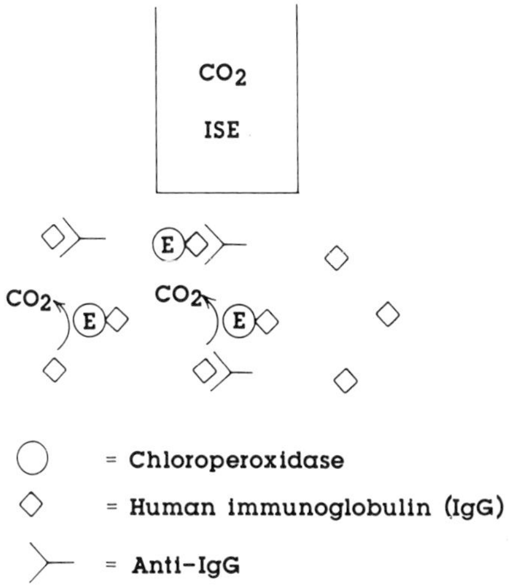

Fig. 8. Homogeneous potentiometric immunosensor in which the product of the enzyme label is detected using an ion-selective electrode (ISE) as described by Fonong & Rechnitz (1984).

A potentiometric complement electrode was described by D'Orazio & Rechnitz (1977) using sheep red blood cell ghosts loaded with the trimethylphenyl ammonium cation ($TMPA^+$). The blood cells bind haemolysins, which are activated by the complement system (nine serum protein compounds that react in a specific order to produce lysis of target cells), thus releasing the $TMPA^+$ marker, which can be detected using an ISE. The cascade effect made available by the complement system has also been applied to potentiometric immunoassay based on liposomes (D'Orazio & Rechnitz, 1977; Shiba *et al.*, 1980).

An ingenious immunosensor was recently detailed by Keating & Rechnitz (1984) and dubbed potentiometric ionophore-modulation immunoassay (PIMIA). The antigen, digoxin, was conjugated to two ionophores for potassium ions, benzo-15-crown-5 and *cis*-dibenzo-18-crown-6. One of the conjugates was then dissolved in a polyvinyl chloride support membrane, which was used as the ion-selective membrane in a conventional potentiometric configuration (Fig. 9). Digoxin antibodies were assayed against a constant activity of potassium ions in a background solution. When the antibody bound the conjugate the potential increased in

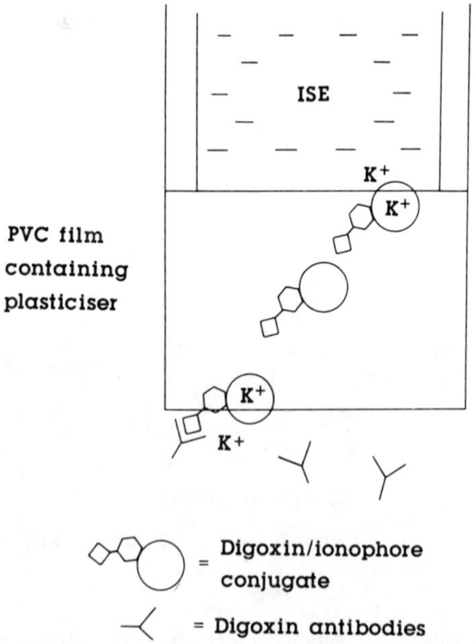

Fig. 9. Potentiometric ionophore modulation immunoassay (PIMIA) for digoxin as detailed by Keating & Rechnitz (1984).

proportion to the antibody concentration. Real samples required extensive dialysis against the background solution to eliminate any interfering ions prior to the assay. The electrodes responded to digoxin antibodies in buffer over the approximate range 1–20 mg/litre. Preliminary results using the electrodes in a competitive assay were also reported showing sensitivity to digoxin concentration in the range 1–1000 nM.

Indirect Amperometric Immunosensors

Amperometric electrodes have also been employed as the transducer in immunosensors. Aizawa *et al.* (1976) proposed an enzyme immunosensor for human immunoglobulin G (IgG) based on the Clark oxygen electrode (Fig. 10). Anti-IgG was immobilised on an acetylcellulose membrane, which was then placed over the active surface of an oxygen electrode. On exposure to a competitive mixture of labelled and unlabelled antigen, a proportion of the conjugated enzyme was bound to the electrode. Following a wash step the electrode was immersed in a dilute solution of hydrogen peroxide and the rate of increase in oxygen concentration monitored. IgG was determined in the range 0·1–2 g/litre in buffer. Aizawa and co-workers later expanded the applications of this principle to, for example, the assay of IgG in serum (Aizawa *et al.*, 1978), human chorionic gonadotrophin (Aizawa *et al.*, 1979) and biotin (Ikariyama *et al.*, 1983). Itagaki *et al.* (1983) showed that the method could be used for the assay of the drug theophylline.

Mattiasson & Nilsson (1977) described a similar enzyme immunoelectrode in which either catalase or glucose oxidase (GOD) was used as an enzyme label and the antibody was immobilised on a nylon net. Either oxygen consumption (GOD label) or oxygen production (catalase label) was monitored. Approximately 5–100 mg insulin/litre and 2·5–25 mg

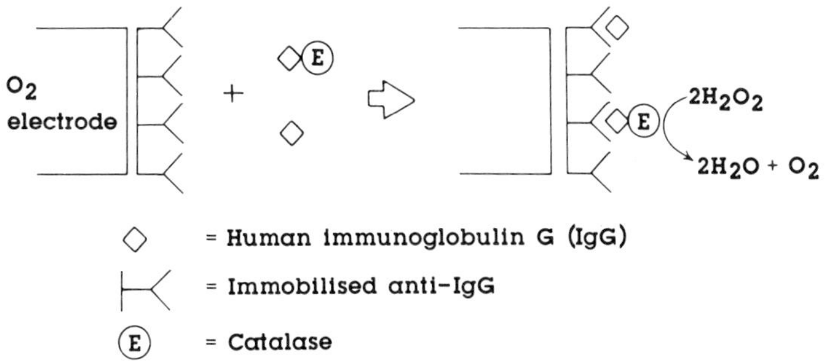

Fig. 10. Enzyme immunosensor for human immunoglobulin G based on the Clark oxygen electrode as proposed by Aizawa *et al.* (1976).

human serum albumin/litre were successfully assayed using the technique. Renneberg *et al.* (1983) also used the catalytic oxidation of glucose by GOD at an oxygen electrode as a detection mechanism. They, however, employed the classic antibody label alkaline phosphatase to convert glucose-6-phosphate to the substrate for GOD. An alternative approach to electrochemical detection of alkaline phosphatase labels is to use the enzyme to cleave the phosphate group off phenylphosphate, yielding electrochemically active phenol, which can be determined by direct amperometry (Doyle *et al.*, 1984).

Nicotinamide adenine dinucleotide (NAD^+)-dependent dehydrogenases have been used as enzyme labels for immunoassay and can be electrochemically coupled. Eggers *et al.* (1982) adapted a commercially available kit to assay phenytoin, using the electrochemical oxidation of NADH produced by a dehydrogenase in place of spectrophotometric detection. Good agreement was observed between the conventional and new method.

Chemically Mediated Amperometric Immunosensors

The electrochemistry of oxidoreductases has received considerable attention in relation to applications in enzyme electrodes. Many of the same considerations, however, apply to their use in immunoassay. In particular, highly efficient coupling of enzymic activity to the electrochemical detector is essential for sensitive and rapid assays. The realisation of electron transfer from biological systems to amperometric electrodes has been reviewed recently (Cardosi & Turner, 1987). A number of approaches have been described, but arguably the most effective is the use of low molecular weight mediators to shuttle electrons between the catalyst and an electrode. Of the mediators that have been reported for use in enzyme electrodes, ferricyanide (Racine & Mindt, 1971), tetracyano-*p*-quinodimethane (Kulys & Cenas, 1983), ferrocene (Aston *et al.*, 1984; Cass *et al.*, 1984; Turner *et al.*, 1984) and tetrathifulvalene (Turner *et al.*, 1987*b*) could also be useful in immunosensors (Fig. 11). They all exhibit rapid reactions with potential enzyme labels, have well-behaved electrochemistry and are unlikely to suffer from interference when used in real samples.

Mediated enzyme-linked immunoassay, in which a GOD label was monitored using a ferrocene derivative, was first reported by Robinson *et al.* (1985). They used an immunometric assay with a magnetic solid phase to facilitate separation of the bound from the free fractions and to promote localisation of the bound label at the surface of the electrode. Human choriogonadotrophin was detected over the range 0·1–2·5 IU/ml with a

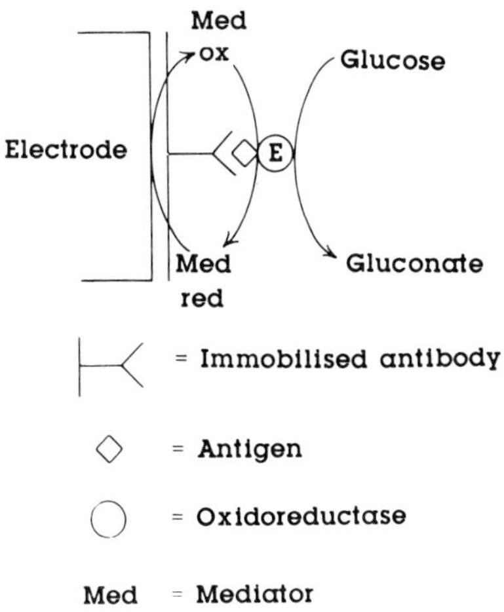

Fig. 11. Immunosensor for enzyme-labelled assay based on an electrode modified with a mediator such as ferrocene to shuttle electrons between the catalyst and the electrode.

sensitivity (2 × SD of determination of zero standard) of 0·15 IU/ml in a total assay time of 20 min.

A more elegant possibility is the use of the mediator molecule as a label. Weber & Purdy (1979) produced a conjugate of morphine and ferrocene carboxylic acid. They showed that the electrochemical oxidation of the ferrocene label was reduced when morphine antibody bound the conjugate and used this principle in a displacement assay for codeine (Fig. 12(a)). Since the key to practical oxidoreductase electrochemistry is the availability of a mediator such as ferrocene, it was apparent that this principle could be used to trigger an electrochemically coupled enzyme-catalysed reaction (Fig. 12(b)). The effective recycling of the ferrocene by GOD results in a further amplification of the signal over electrochemical noise due to electroactive substances present in the sample. Katalin *et al.* (1986) first applied this principle in a homogeneous competitive immunoassay for lidocaine. They detected antigen concentrations in the range 1·2–11·7 mg/litre with an SD of 3–6% and an assay time of 15 min.

Electrochemically-coupled enzyme reactions may also be activated by providing missing cofactors or coenzymes; see for example Ngo *et al.* (1985). It has been argued that quinoprotein dehydrogenases could prove particularly valuable in this respect (Turner *et al.*, 1987*a*). In one proposal D-amino acid oxidase was used as a label (Turner *et al.*, 1987*c*). The enzyme activity was monitored by its ability to liberate ammonium ions, thus

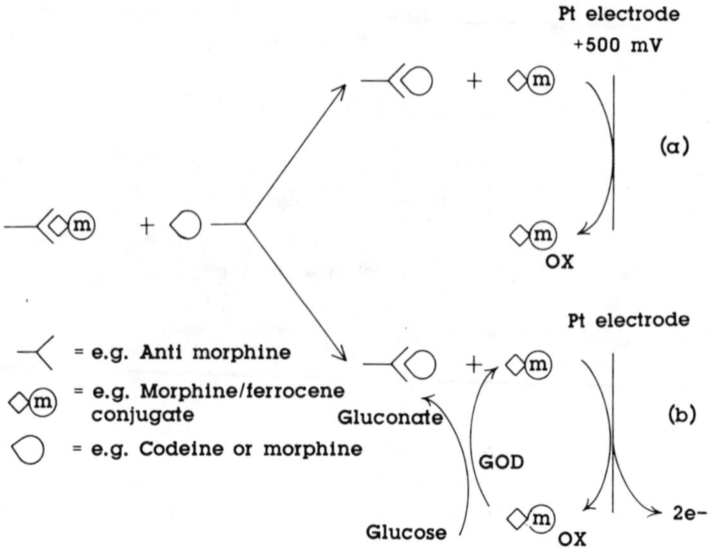

Fig. 12. Displacement assay for codeine using a mediator such as ferrocene as a label as proposed by Weber & Purdy (1979): (a) the signal due to the electrochemical oxidation of the label can be amplified by recycling of the mediator using glucose oxidase; (b) a principle applied by Katalin *et al.* (1986).

activating a second enzyme amplifier in the form of the quinoprotein methanol dehydrogenase (MDH), which has an absolute requirement for ammonium ions. The MDH reaction was carried out in the presence of excess substrate and was electrochemically coupled using ferrocene. The assay, however, requires care to avoid interference from ammonium ions in the sample. An alternative approach is the use of inactive derivatives of the quinoprotein coenzyme 2,7,9-tricarboxy-1H-pyrrolo (2,3-f) quinoline-4,5-dione (PQQ), which can be converted to an active form by an enzyme label (Turner *et al.*, 1987*a*). The apoenzyme of quinoprotein glucose dehydrogenase is preferred for use in this system (Fig. 13) since the holoenzyme has a high turnover number and can be efficiently coupled to an electrode (D'Costa *et al.*, 1986). Possible enzyme labels include aminoacylase to cleave, for example, L-methionine off the PQQ* molecule (Turner *et al.*, 1987*a*).

One particularly sensitive immunoassay which relies on enzyme amplification is marketed by IQ (Bio) Ltd, Cambridge (Stanley *et al.*, 1985) (See Chapters 3 and 5). The assay is shown schematically in Fig. 14. The catalytic activity of the enzyme label (alkaline phosphatase) used in a

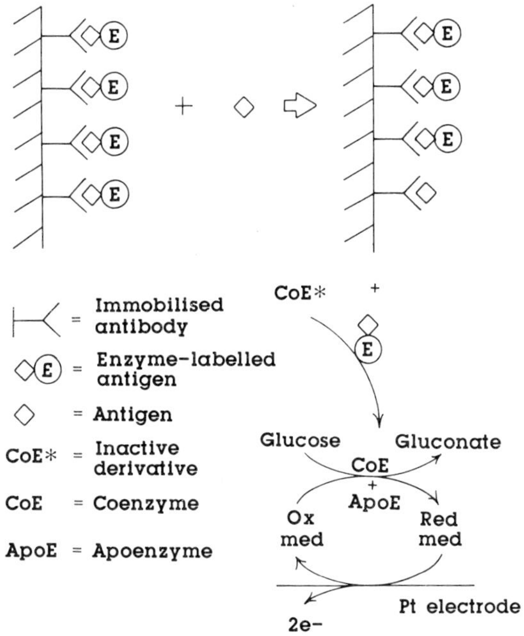

Fig. 13. Immunosensor based on the conversion of an inactive derivative of a coenzyme to the active form by an enzyme label (Turner *et al.*, 1986).

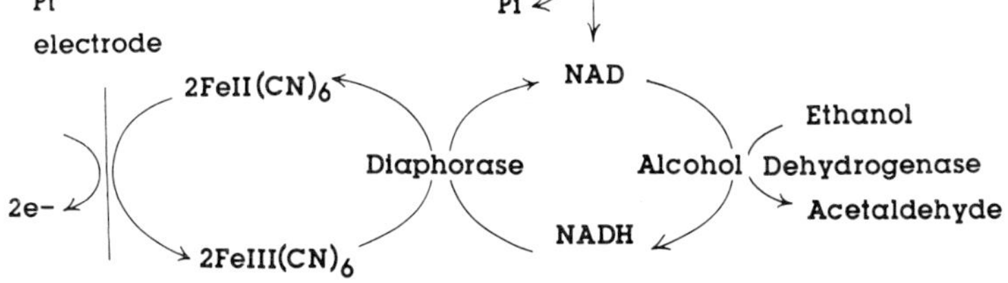

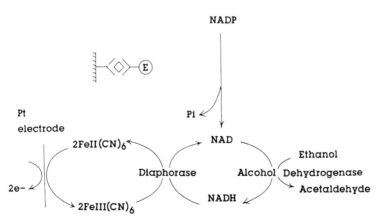

Fig. 14. Sensitive immunoassay relying on enzyme amplification; currently used with spectrophotometric detection (Stanley *et al.*, 1985).

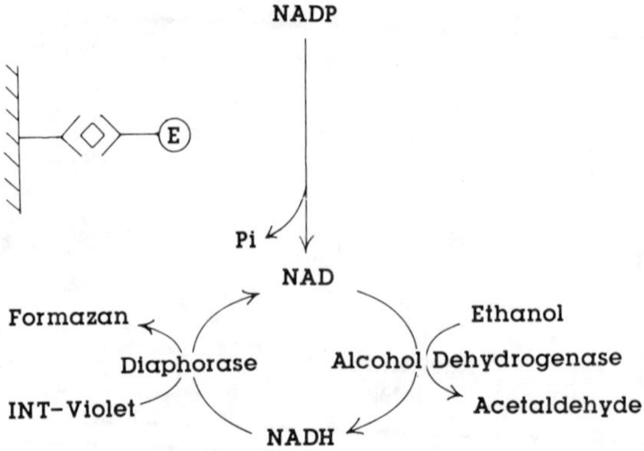

Fig. 15. Immunosensor relying on enzyme amplification with amperometric detection, yielding an improved dynamic range and reduced instrumentation costs (Cardosi & Turner, 1987).

sandwich assay is monitored by the addition of the substrate nicotinamide adenine dinucleotide phosphate (NADP), leading to the formation of the dephosphorylated product NAD. The NAD formed enters a redox cycle driven by the enzymes alcohol dehydrogenase and diaphorase (the enzyme amplifier), leading to the reduction of INT-violet to a coloured formazan dye. The dye is detected by measurement of the absorbance at 492 nm in a spectrophotometer in the form of a microtitration plate reader. An electrochemical version of this assay for prostatic acid phosphatase (PAP), a prostate tumour marker from human serum, has been reported recently (Stanley *et al.*, 1988). The procedure was essentially the same as that used in the commercial assay up to and including the formation of NAD from the substrate NADP by alkaline phosphatase. Then, however, an enzyme amplifier was added in which the INT-violet was replaced by ferricyanide (Fig. 15). Electrons from the NAD^+/NADH redox cycle passed via the diaphorase to the $Fe(III)(CN)_6$/$Fe(II)(CN)_6$ couple. The reduced species $Fe(II)(CN)_6$ was reoxidised at a platinum electrode at 450 mV versus a saturated calomel electrode producing an amperometric response. The optical and electrochemical detection techniques were compared using the PAP assay as an example. Both methods had similar detection limits in the order of 200 ng PAP/litre, but the electrochemical method had a greatly improved dynamic range (0–400 μg/litre compared with 0–7·5 μg/litre for the optical assay). This, coupled with greatly decreased instrumentation costs, suggests that amperometric detection of enzyme labels used in immunoassays could replace optical methods currently in use.

CONCLUSIONS

A range of direct immunosensors has been developed based on the immobilisation of antibodies or other specific binding agents on sensors detecting a change in the optical or acoustic properties of the sensor surface or an increase in the sensor mass when the antigen binds. The optical immunosensors based on surface plasmon resonance (SPR) or on total internal reflection (TIR) monitoring are already at the commercial development stage. They can be used in a kinetic mode, indicating the analyte concentration without prior incubation or separation steps. This is also possible for immunosensors based on the piezocrystal balance, which have also found commercial interest. Direct immunosensors based on surface acoustic wave (SAW) devices or on potentiometric devices have yet to prove that they can achieve the requirement of high sensitivity (detection limits of ng/ml or better).

Among the indirect immunosensors, the TELISA (thermistor enzyme-linked immunosorbent assay) is particularly sensitive, detecting less than picomolar analyte concentrations. Chemically mediated amperometric immunosensors offer detection limits similar to those provided by the indirect optical methods in current use, but with a greatly improved dynamic range.

The new immunosensors offer the possibility of instruments for immunoassays suitable for use by semi-skilled operators at a food processing or packaging line. Such instruments could be valuable in the detection of pathogens and also for meat speciation and vitamin assays.

ACKNOWLEDGEMENTS

The authors would like to acknowledge the support of the Ministry of Agriculture, Fisheries and Food for the development of sensors for process and quality control in the food industry.

REFERENCES

AIZAWA, M., MORIOKA, A., MATSUIKA, H., SUZUKI, S., NAGAMURA, Y., SHINOHARA, R. & ISHIGURO, I. (1976) An enzyme immunosensor for IgG. *Journal of Solid-phase Biochemistry*, **1**, 319–328.

AIZAWA, M., KATO, S. & SUZUKI, S. (1977) Immunoresponsive membrane. 1.

Membrane potential change associated with an immunochemical reaction between membrane-bound antigen and free antibody. *Journal of Membrane Science*, **2**, 125–132.

AIZAWA, M., MORIOKA, A. & SUZUKI, S. (1978) Enzyme immunosensor—II: Electrochemical determination of IgG with an antibody-bound membrane. *Journal of Membrane Science*, **4**, 221–228.

AIZAWA, M., MORIOKA, A., SUZUKI, S. & NAGAMURA, Y. (1979) Enzyme immunosensor—III: Amperometric determination of human chorionic gonadotropin by membrane-bound antibody. *Analytical Biochemistry*, **94**, 22–28.

ANON. (1984) Piezoelectric crystals detect proteins. *Chemical and Engineering News* (**April 23**), 18–19.

ANON. (1985) Microgravimetric assay to be marketed. *Chemical and Engineering News* (**Sept. 9**), 23.

ASHER, R. C. (1983) Ultrasonic sensors in the chemical and process industries. *Journal of Physics E: Scientific Instruments*, **16**, 959.

ASTON, W. J., ASHBY, R. E., HIGGINS, I. J., SCOTT, L. D. L. & TURNER, A. P. F. (1984) Enzyme-based methanol sensor. In: *Charge and Field Effects in Biosystems*, Allen, M. J. & Usherwood, P. N. R. (eds), Abacus Press, Tunbridge Wells, pp. 491–498.

BARENDSZ, A. W., VIS, J. C., NIEUWENHUIZEN, M. S., NIEUWKOOP, E., VELLEKOOP, M. J., GHIJSEN, W. J. & VENEMA, A. (1985) A SAW-chemosensor for NO_2 gas concentration measurement. IEEE Ultrasonics Symposium, San Francisco, 1985.

BERGVELD, P. (1985) The impact of MOSFET-based sensors. *Sensors and Actuators*, **8**, 109–127.

BERGVELD, P. (1986) The development and application of FET-based biosensors. *Biosensors*, **2**, 15–33.

BIOTECH 84 (1984) New Immunoassay Approach. Exhibitor Profiles. Batelle-Geneva. *Biotech 84 (Europe) News*, Online Conferences Ltd, Pinner, Middlesex.

BIRNBAUM, S., BULOW, L., HARDY, K., DANIELSSON, B. & MOSBACH, K. (1986) Automated thermometric enzyme immunoassay of human proinsulin produced by *Escherichia coli*. *Analytical Biochemistry*, **158**, 12–19.

BLACKBURN, G. F. (1986) Chemically sensitive field effect transistors. In: *Biosensors: Fundamentals and Applications*, Turner, A. P. F., Karube, I. & Wilson, G. S. (eds), Oxford University Press, Oxford, pp. 483–532.

BOITIEUX, J. L., DESMET, G. & THOMAS, D. (1979) An 'antibody electrode': preliminary report on a new approach in enzyme immunoassay. *Clinical Chemistry*, **25**, 318–321.

BRONTMAN, S. B. & MEYERHOFF, M. E. (1984) Homogeneous enzyme-linked assays mediated by enzyme antibodies: a new approach to electrode-based immunoassays. *Analytica Chimica Acta*, **162**, 363–367.

BROOKS, S. L. & TURNER, A. P. F. (1987) Biosensors for measurement and control. *Measurement and Control*, **20**, 37–43.

BRYANT, A., POIRIER, M., RILEY, G., LEE, D. L. & VETELINO, J. F. (1983) Gas detection using surface acoustic wave delay lines. *Sensors and Actuators*, **4**, 105–111.

CARDOSI, M. F. & TURNER, A. P. F. (1987) The realisation of electron transfer from biological molecules to electrodes. In: *Biosensors: Fundamentals and Applications*, Turner, A. P. F., Karube, I. & Wilson, G. S. (eds), Oxford University Press, Oxford, pp. 257–275.

CASS, A. E. G., DAVIS, G., FRANCIS, G. D., HILL, H. A. O., ASTON, W. J., HIGGINS, I. J., PLOTKIN, E. V., SCOTT, L. D. L. & TURNER, A. P. F. (1984) Ferrocene-mediated enzyme electrode for amperometric determination of glucose. *Analytical Chemistry*, **56**, 667–671.

CHU, B. & DINAPOLI, A. (1984) Application of photon correlation function profile analysis to molecular weight distributions of polymers in solution. In: *Particle Size Analysis*, Barth, H. G. (ed.), Wiley, New York, pp. 93–116.

CHUANG, C. T., WHITE, R. M. & BERNSTEIN, J. J. (1982) A thin-membrane surface acoustic wave vapour-sensing device. *IEEE Electron Device Letters EDL-3*, 145–148.

COLLINS, S. & JANATA, J. (1982) A critical evaluation of the mechanism of potential response of antigen polymer membranes to the corresponding antiserum. *Analytica Chimica Acta*, **136**, 93–99.

DANIELSSON, B. & MOSBACH, K. (1987) Theory and applications of calorimetric sensors. In: *Biosensors: Fundamentals and Applications*, Turner, A. P. F., Karube, I. & Wilson, G. S. (eds), Oxford University Press, Oxford, pp. 575–596.

DANIELSSON, B., MATTIASSON, B. & MOSBACH, K. (1979) Enzyme thermistor analysis in clinical chemistry and biotechnology. *Pure and Applied Chemistry*, **51**, 1443–1457.

D'COSTA, E. J., TURNER, A. P. F. & HIGGINS, I. J. (1986) Quinoprotein glucose dehydrogenase and its application in an amperometric glucose sensor. *Biosensors*, **2**, 71–87.

D'ORAZIO, P. & RECHNITZ, G. A. (1977) Ion electrode measurements of complement and antibody levels using marker-loaded sheep red blood cell ghosts. *Analytical Chemistry*, **49**, 2083–2091.

DOYLE, M. J., HALSALL, H. B. & HEINEMAN, W. R. (1984) Enzyme-linked immunoadsorbent assay with electrochemical detection for α_1-acid glycoprotein. *Analytical Chemistry*, **56**, 2355–2360.

EDDOWES, M. J., PEDLEY, D. G. & WEBB, B. C. (1985) Response of an enzyme-modified pH-sensitive ion-selective device: experimental study of a glucose oxidase-modified ion-sensitive field effect transistor in buffered and unbuffered aqueous solution. *Sensors and Actuators*, **7**, 233–244.

EGGERS, H. M., HALSALL, H. B. & HEINEMAN, W. R. (1982) Enzyme immunoassay with flow amperometric detection of NADH. *Clinical Chemistry*, **28**, 1848–1851.

FLANAGAN, M. T. & PANTELL, R. H. (1984) Surface plasmon resonance and immunosensors. *Electronics Letters*, **20**, 968–970.

FONONG, T. & RECHNITZ, G. A. (1984) Homogeneous potentiometric enzyme immunoassay for human immunoglobulin G. *Analytical Chemistry*, **56**, 2586–2590.

GEBAUER, C. R. & RECHNITZ, G. A. (1982) Deaminating enzyme labels for immunoassay. *Analytical Biochemistry*, **124**, 338–348.

GREEN, M. J. (1987) New approaches to immunoassays–immunosensors. In:

Biosensors: Fundamentals and Applications, Turner, A. P. F., Karube, I. & Wilson, G. S. (eds), Oxford University Press, Oxford, pp. 60–70.

GUILBAULT, G. G. (1980) Uses of the piezoelectric crystal detector in analytical chemistry. *Ion Selective Electrode Reviews*, **2**, 3–16.

HIRSCHFELD, T. E. (1984) US Patent No. 4 447 546.

HLAVAY, J. & GUILBAULT, G. G. (1977) Applications of the piezoelectric crystal detector in analytical chemistry. *Analytical Chemistry*, **49**, 1890–1894.

HUBBARD, R. & WISEMAN, A. (1983) Enzyme immunoassay and the use of monoclonal antibodies. *Trends in Analytical Chemistry*, **2**, VII–VIII.

IKARIYAMA, Y., FURUKI, M. & AIZAWA, M. (1983) Bioaffinity sensor with binding protein. *Analytical Chemistry Symposium Series*, **17**, 693–698.

ISHIMORI, Y., KARUBE, I. & SUZUKI, S. (1981) Determination of microbial populations with piezoelectric membranes. *Applied and Environmental Microbiology*, **42**, 632–637.

ITAGAKI, H., HAKODA, Y., SUZUKI, Y. & HAGA, M. (1983) Drug sensor: an enzyme immunoelectrode for theophylline. *Chemical and Pharmaceutical Bulletin*, **31**, 1283–1288.

JANATA, J. (1975) An immunoelectrode. *Journal of the American Chemical Society*, **97**, 2914–2916.

JANATA, J. (1985) Chemically sensitive field effect transistors: their application in analytical and physical chemistry. *Analytical Chemistry Symposium Series*, **22**, 129–154.

JANATA, J. & BLACKBURN, G. F. (1984) Immunochemical potentiometric sensors. *Annals of the New York Academy of Science*, **428**, 286–292.

JANATA, J. & HUBER, R. J. (1979) Ion-sensitive field effect transistors. *Ion Selective Electrode Review*, **1**, 31–79.

JANATA, J. & HUBER, R. J. (1980) Chemically sensitive field effect transistors. In: *Ion-selective Electrodes in Analytical Chemistry*, Freiser, H. (ed.), Plenum, New York, pp. 107–174.

JARVIS, B. (1982) Rapid methods in food microbiology. A practical approach. *Food Technology in Australia*, **34**, 518–523.

KATALIN, D. G., HILL, H. A. O. & MCNEIL, C. J. (1986) Homogeneous ferrocene-mediated amperometric immunoassay. *Analytical Chemistry*, **58**, 1203–1205.

KEATING, M. Y. & RECHNITZ, G. A. (1984) Potentiometric digoxin antibody measurements with antigen–ionophore based membrane electrode. *Analytical Chemistry*, **56**, 801–806.

KEATING, M. Y. & RECHNITZ, G. A. (1985) Potentiometric enzyme immunoassay for digoxin using polystyrene beads. *Analytical Letters*, **18**, 1–10.

KRESS-ROGERS, E. (1986) Instrumentation in the food industry: I. Chemical, biochemical and immunological determinands; II. Physical determinands in quality and process control. *Journal of Physics E: Scientific Instruments*, **19**, 13–21, 105–109.

KRESS-ROGERS, E. & D'COSTA, E. J. (1986) Biosensors for the food industry. *Analytical Proceedings*, **23**, 149–151.

KULYS, J. J. & CENAS, N. K. (1983) Oxidation of glucose oxidase from *Penicillium vitale* by one- and two-electron acceptors. *Biochimica Biophysica Acta*, **744**, 57–63.

LEE, E. H., BENNER, R. E., FENN, J. B. & CHANG, R. K. (1979) Angular distribution of fluorescence from liquids and monodispersed spheres by evanescent wave excitation. *Applied Optics*, **18**, 862–870.

LEVISON, S. A., KIERSZENBAUM, F. & DANDLIKER, W. B. (1970) Salt effects on antigen–antibody kinetics. *Biochemistry*, **9**, 322–331.

LEWIS, M. F., WEST, C. L., DEACON, J. M. & HUMPHREYES, R. F. (1984) Recent developments in SAW devices. *IEE Proceedings*, **A131**, 186–215.

LIEDBERG, B., NYLANDER, C. & LUNDSTROM, I. (1983) Surface plasmon resonance for gas detection and biosensing. *Sensors and Actuators*, **4**, 299.

LUBBERS, D. W. & OPITZ, N. (1983) Optical fluorescence sensors for continuous measurement of chemical concentrations in biological systems. *Sensors and Actuators*, **4**, 641.

MCFARLANE, I. (1983) *Automatic Control of Food Manufacturing Processes*, Elsevier Applied Science Publishers, London.

MATTIASSON, B. & NILSSON, H. (1977) An enzyme immunoelectrode—assay of human serum albumin and insulin. *FEBS Letters*, **78**, 251–254.

MATTIASSON, B., BORREBAECK, C., SANDFRIDSON, B. & MOSBACH, K. (1977) Thermometric enzyme linked immunosorbent assay: ELISA. *Biochimica Biophysica Acta*, **483**, 221–227.

MEYERHOFF, M. & RECHNITZ, G. A. (1979) Electrode-based enzyme immunoassay using urease conjugates. *Analytical Biochemistry*, **95**, 483–493.

MOFFAT, A. (1986) Making light work of detecting disease. *The Times*, **13 July**.

MORGAN, D. P. (1973) Surface acoustic wave devices and applications. I. Introductory review. *Ultrasonics*, **May 1973**. 121–131.

MOSBACH, K. & DANIELSSON, B. (1981) Thermal bioanalysers in flow streams: enzyme thermistor devices. *Analytical Chemistry*, **53**, 83A–94A.

NGO, T. T., BOVAIRD, J. H. & LENHOFF, H. M. (1985) Separation-free amperometric enzyme immunoassay. *Applied Biochemistry and Biotechnology*, **11**, 63–70.

NOMURA, T. & IIJIMA, M. (1981) Electrolytic determination of nanomolar concentrations of silver in solution with a piezoelectric quartz crystal. *Analytica Chimica Acta*, **131**, 97–102.

NOMURA, T. & MIMATSU, T. (1982) Electrolytic determination of traces of iodide in solution with a piezoelectric quartz crystal. *Analytica Chimica Acta*, **143**, 237–241.

NOMURA, T. & OKUHARA, M. (1982) Frequency shifts of piezoelectric quartz crystals immersed in organic liquids. *Analytica Chimica Acta*, **142**, 281–284.

NYLANDER, C., LIEDBERG, B. & LIND, T. (1982) Gas detection by means of surface plasmon resonance. *Sensors and Actuators*, **3**, 79–88.

OWEN, V. & TURNER, A. P. F. (1987) Biosensors: a revolution in clinical analysis? *Endeavour*, **11**, 100–104.

PETERSON, J. I., FITZGERALD, R. V. & BUCKHOLD, D. K. (1984) Fiber-optic probe for *in vivo* measurement of oxygen partial pressure. *Analytical Chemistry*, **56**, 62–67.

PETTIGREW, R. M. (1984) Assay Technique. International Patent Application. International Publication No. W084/02578.

PLACE, J. F., SUTHERLAND, R. M. & DAHNE, C. (1985) Opto-electronic immunosensors: a review of optical immunoassay at continuous surfaces. *Biosensors*, **1**, 321–353.

POCKRAND, I., SWALEN, J. D., SANTO, R., BRILLANTE, A. & PHILPOTT, M. R.

(1978) Optical properties of organic dye monolayers by surface plasmon spectroscopy. *Journal of Chemical Physics*, **69**, 4001–4011.

RACINE, P. & MINDT, W. (1971) On the role of substrate diffusion in enzyme electrodes. *Experientia*, **18**, 525–534.

RAETHER, H. (1977) Surface plasma oscillations and their applications. In: *Physics of Thin Films*, Volume 9, Academic Press, New York, pp. 145, 261.

REEDER, T. M. & CULLEN, D. E. (1976) Surface acoustic wave pressure and temperature sensors. *Proceedings IEEE*, **64**, 754–756.

RENNEBERG, R., SHLOSSLER, W. & SHELLER, F. (1983) Amperometric enzyme sensor-based enzyme immunoassay for Factor VIII related antigen. *Analytical Letters*, **16**, 1279–1289.

RISCH, M. R. (1984) Precision pressure sensor using quartz SAW resonators. *Sensors and Actuators*, **6**, 127–133.

ROBINSON, G. A., HILL, H. A. O., PHILO, R. D., GEAR, J. M., RATTLE, S. J. & FOREST, G. C. (1985) Bioelectrochemical enzyme immunoassay of human choriogonadotrophin with magnetic electrodes. *Clinical Chemistry*, **31**, 1449–1452.

ROEDERER, J. E. & BASTIAANS, G. I. (1983) Microgravimetric immunoassay with piezoelectric crystals. *Analytical Chemistry*, **55**, 2333–2336.

SCHELLER, F. W., SCHUBERT, F., RENNEBERG, R. & MULLER, H.-G. (1985) Biosensors: trends and commercialisation. *Biosensors*, **1**, 135–160.

SEITZ, W. R. (1984) Chemical sensors based on fiber optics. *Analytical Chemistry*, **56**, 16A–34A.

SHANKS, I. A. (1986) Optical biosensors for immunoassays. The Royal Society Discussion Meeting. *Biosensors*, London, 28 May 1986.

SHIBA, K., UMEZAWA, Y., WATANABE, T., OGAWA, W. & FUJIWARA, S. (1980) Thin-layer potentiometric analysis of lipid antigen–antibody reaction by tetrapentylammonium (TPA^+) ion loaded liposomes and TPA^+ ion selective electrode. *Analytical Chemistry*, **52**, 1610–1613.

STANLEY, C. J., PARIS, F., PLUMB, A., WEBB, A. & JOHANNSSON, A. (1985) Enzyme amplification: a new technique for enhancing the speed and sensitivity of enzyme immunoassays. *International Clinical Products Review*, **July/August**, 44–51.

STANLEY, C. J., COX, R. B., CARDOSI, M. F. & TURNER, A. P. F. (1988) Amperometric amplified immunoassay. *Journal of Immunological Methods*, in press.

SUTHERLAND, R. M., DAHNE, C., PLACE, J. F. & RINGROSE, A. R. (1984) Optical detection of antibody–antigen reactions at a glass–liquid interface. *Clinical Chemistry*, **30**, 1533–1538.

TOMITA, Y., HO, M. H. & GUILBAULT, G. G. (1979) Detection of explosives with a coated piezoelectric quartz crystal. *Analytical Chemistry*, **51**, 1475–1478.

TURNER, A. P. F., ASTON, W. F., BELL, J., COLBY, J., DAVIS, G., HIGGINS, I. J. & HILL, H. A. O. (1984) CO: Acceptor oxidoreductase from *Pseudomonas thermocarboxydovorans* strain C2 and its use in a carbon monoxide sensor. *Analytica Chimica Acta*, **163**, 161–174.

TURNER, A. P. F., MILLER, S. L. & D'COSTA, E. J. (1986) Specific binding assays. British Patent Application 8608435.

TURNER, A. P. F., D'COSTA, E. J. & HIGGINS, I. J. (1987*a*) Enzymatic analysis using quinoprotein dehydrogenases. In: *Enzyme Engineering*, Volume 541. *Annals of the New York Academy of Sciences*, Laskin, A. I., Mosbach, K., Thomas, D. & Winguard, L. B. (eds), Plenum, New York, pp. 283–287.

TURNER, A. P. F., HENDRY, S. P. & CARDOSI, M. (1987*b*) A new mediator for amperometric biosensors. *Instrumentation and Processing, World Biotechnology Report*, **1**, 125–137.

TURNER, A. P. F., HIGGINS, I. J. & FRANKLIN, A. (1987*c*) Biosensors for the food industry. In: *Food and Biotechnology*, De La Moue, Daulet, J. & Amiot, J. (eds), University of Quebec, Canada, pp. 51–68.

TURNER, A. P. F., MILLER, S. L., OWEN, V. M. & D'COSTA, E. J. (1987*d*) Quinoprotein-based enzyme amplifiers for use in immunosensors, *Diabetic Medicine*, in press.

WEBER, S. G. & PURDY, W. C. (1979) Homogeneous voltammetric immunoassay: a preliminary study. *Analytical Letters*, **12**, 1–9.

WEINER, B. B. (1984) Particle sizing using photon correlation spectroscopy. In: *Particle Size Analysis*, Barth, H. G. (ed.), Wiley, New York, pp. 117–134.

WILSON, G. S. (1986) Fundamentals of amperometric sensors. In: *Biosensors: Fundamentals and Applications*, Turner, A. P. F., Karube, I. & Wilson, G. S. (eds), Oxford University Press, Oxford, pp. 165–179.

WINQUIST, F., SPETZ, A., ARMGARTH, M. & LUNDSTROEM, I. (1985) Biosensors based on ammonia-sensitive metal–oxide–semiconductor structures. *Sensors and Actuators*, **8**, 91–100.

WOHLTJEN, H. (1984) Chemical microsensors and microinstrumentation. *Analytical Chemistry*, **56**, 87A–103A.

WOHLTJEN, H. & DESSY, R. (1979*a*) Surface acoustic wave probe for chemical analysis. I. Introduction and instrument description. *Analytical Chemistry*, **51**, 1458–1464.

WOHLTJEN, H. & DESSY, R. (1979*b*) Surface acoustic wave probe for chemical analysis. II. Gas chromatograph detector. *Analytical Chemistry*, **51**, 1465–1470.

WOHLTJEN, H. & DESSY, R. (1979*c*) Surface acoustic wave probe for chemical analysis. III. Thermo-chemical polymer analyser. *Analytical Chemistry*, **51**, 1470–1475.

WYN-JONES, E., PEREIRA, M. C. & MORRIS, E. R. (1982) Ultrasonic relaxation studies in sols and gels. *Progress in Food and Nutrition Science*, **6**, 21–31.

YAMAMOTO, N., NAGASAWA, Y., SAWAI, M., SUDO, T. & TSUBOMURA, H. (1978) Potentiometric investigations of antigen–antibody and enzyme–enzyme inhibitor reactions using chemically modified metal electrodes. *Journal of Immunological Methods*, **22**, 309–317.

ZACHARIAS, E. M. & PARNELL, R. A. (1972) Measuring the solids content of foods by sound velocimetry. *Food Technology*, **26**, 160–166.

20

The Uses of Flow Cytometry in Veterinary Diagnosis and the Food Processing Industry

N. M. MACKENZIE

Royal Veterinary College, University of London, UK

and

A. C. PINDER

AFRC Institute of Food Research, Norwich, UK

INTRODUCTION

Flow microfluorimetry is a new technology. However, the need to precisely identify and/or separate cells according to their specialised type is fundamental to virtually every biological process, both in the laboratory and in clinical and industrial applications. The flow cytometer (flow microfluorimeter or fluorescence activated cell sorter) is one of the most sophisticated machines dedicated to cell analysis and sorting available today. The applications of flow cytometric (FCM) techniques are ever widening and concomitantly the cost of the machines is falling. FCM has only recently made excursions into areas of interest to veterinarians and food analysts; therefore it is not possible to cite references covering the full range of uses from these fields. Comparisons will be made between FCM and ELISA, and the attributes and pitfalls of both techniques highlighted.

THE PRINCIPLE OF THE FLOW CYTOMETER

The power of a flow cytometer as an analytical tool is derived from its ability to measure simultaneously a number of properties of cells, on an individual basis, without the need to first isolate the cells of interest from the rest of the population, and to do this at high speed (up to 5000 cells per second). In principle, the cells (usually stained with fluorescent markers

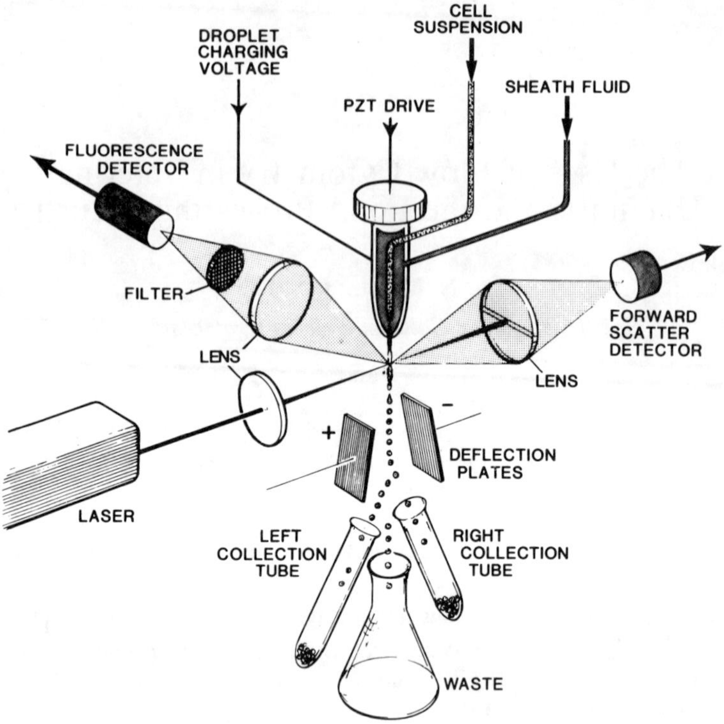

Fig. 1. Schematic diagram showing the principal components of a typical flow cytometer system (PZT drive: piezoelectric nozzle oscillating device).

indicative of biological properties) are made to pass one at a time through a focused laser beam. Strategically placed photo-sensors measure optical changes as each cell passes through the beam. These changes are characteristic of cell type, and the signals are fed to a computer for analysis. Cell sorting is accomplished by breaking up the fluid stream into droplets that are electrically charged according to the type of cell that each contains, and actual physical separation is achieved electrostatically (Herzenberg *et al.*, 1976; Melamed *et al.*, 1979; Parks *et al.*, 1986).

Figure 1 is a schematic diagram of a typical flow system. The cells need to be positioned very precisely on the optical axis of the cytometer, and this is accomplished by hydrodynamic focusing. A jet of biologically compatible fluid, called the 'sheath', is forced through a small orifice to form a very fine stream in air. The orifice is typically 50 to 100 μm in diameter, and the pressure on the sheath fluid is carefully adjusted so that the flow is laminar.

The cell suspension is then slowly introduced through a tube into the centre of the sheath, where the velocity gradient is such that the cells are accurately centred, causing them to pass one at a time through the orifice. A short distance below the orifice, the cell stream encounters the interrogating laser beam, focused to a spot. In the majority of machines this is an argon-ion laser. As each cell passes this spot a short (5 μs) pulse of light is emitted which is captured and imaged by lenses on to photo-sensors. One detector, co-linear with the interrogating beam, measures light scattered forward at shallow angles ($<15°$) as the cells pass in front of the laser; the intense laser beam itself is prevented from reaching the detector by an external obscurator or beam stop. This forward angle light scatter signal is related to the cross-sectional area and refractive index of the cell. A second detector, sited orthogonally to the laser beam, is generally used to detect emitted fluorescent light. Appropriate filters block stray light at the laser excitation wavelength and pass light only in the emission spectrum of interest.

Electrical pulses from the various optical detectors are shaped, amplified, digitised and then classified in a dedicated mini- or microcomputer. Statistical information can then be obtained on, for example, a sub-population of cells which is 'large' in size but 'weak' in fluorescence. Criteria based on logical combinations of cell parameters can be programmed into the computer, so that differences between two very similar sub-populations of cells can be identified.

All but the simplest flow cytometers incorporate facilities for cell sorting. Having identified the cell sub-population(s) of interest by computer, decision-making circuits are programmed to respond only to a particular combination of signals from the photo-detectors. These circuits cause the cell stream to be positively or negatively charged after a fixed time delay. The cell stream is broken up into droplets below the interrogation point by ultrasonically vibrating the nozzle assembly with a piezoelectric crystal (see Fig. 1). The time delay in the stream charging current is set equal to the cell transit time between the interrogation point and the droplet separation point. The result is a stream of individual droplets that are electrically charged according to the characteristics of the cell that each contains. The charged droplets are separated by passing the stream between a pair of electrostatic deflection plates (typically at ± 3 kV with respect to the earth). In this way, as shown in Fig. 1, positively charged droplets are deflected to the right, where they are collected in a sample tube, whilst negatively charged droplets are deflected to the left and similarly collected. Thus highly specific sub-populations of cells can be isolated to a high degree of purity and biological viability. The remainder of the droplets (which may contain debris or other unwanted cells) are uncharged, and are undeflected and discarded.

PARAMETERS MEASURABLE BY FLOW CYTOMETRY

Flow cytometry is without equal in its ability to measure quantitatively a diverse and ever-widening range of biological parameters. These are very briefly summarised in Table 1, which makes the distinction between 'intrinsic' measurements, those than can be measured without staining the cells, and 'extrinsic' ones that require highly specific fluorescent reagents (for reviews see Loken & Stall, 1982; Shapiro, 1983; Mackenzie & Pinder,

Table 1
Cellular Parameters Measurable by Flow Cytometry and Their Probes

Cellular parameters	*Probe*
Structural parameters	
Cell size	None required
Cell shape	None required
Cytoplasmic granularity	None required
Pigment content (e.g. haemoglobin)	None required
DNA content: Fixed cells	DAPI,[a] ethidium, propidium, mithramycin, etc.
Living cells	Hoechst 33342
RNA content	Acridine orange (+DNAase), pyronin
Chromatin structure	Fluorescently tagged specific antibody
Surface sugars	Fluorescently tagged specific lectin
Membrane-bound calcium	Chlorotetracycline
Functional parameters	
Enzyme activity	Non-fluorescent derivatives of coumarins, naphthols and fluorescein which yield coloured or fluorescent products
Endocytosis	Fluorescently tagged macromolecules
Hormone receptors	Fluorescently tagged hormones or anti-receptor antibodies
Membrane permeability	Hoechst 33342
Membrane integrity	Fluorescein diacetate
Intracellular pH	Fluorescein diacetate
DNA synthesis	Fluorescein-conjugated anti-bromodeoxyuridine antibody measuring BUdr[b] uptake during the cell cycle

[a] 4,6-Diamidino-2-phenyl-indole.
[b] Deuterated bromouridine.

1987). Using flow cytometry, both structural and functional measurements can be performed and, moreover, up to six parameters can be measured simultaneously on the same cell.

DIRECTLY MEASURABLE PARAMETERS

It is possible to derive a certain amount of information about cell structure through the use of the light scattering characteristics of the cells alone. It has already been mentioned that forward angle light scatter is a measure of cell size. Orthogonal or 90° light scatter, however, varies with cell size and, especially, intracellular granularity. Measuring both light scatter characteristics simultaneously provides a simple and elegant way to identify the

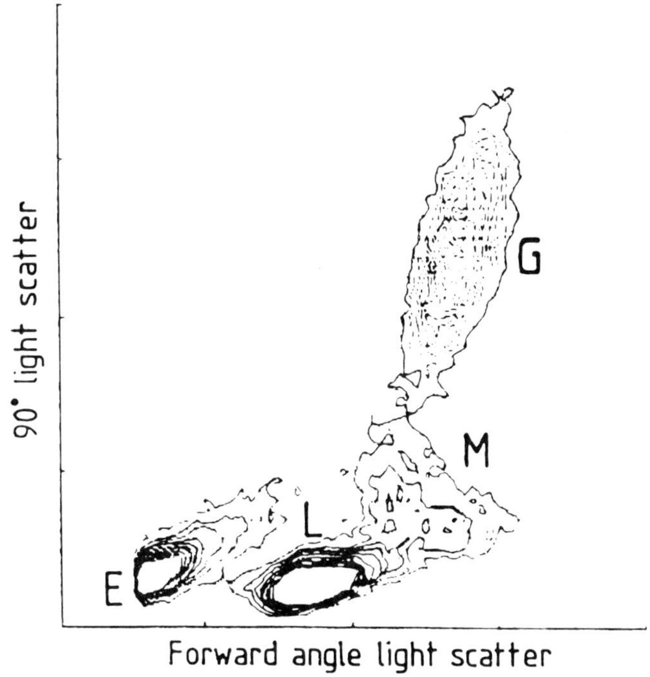

Fig. 2. Dual-parameter light scatter analysis of blood cells. Red cells (erythrocytes, E) and the major sub-population of white cells (lymphocytes, L; monocytes, M; granulocytes, G) can be clearly distinguished by their size (forward light scatter) and granularity (90° light scatter). Contours have been drawn through points on the diagram that occur with equal frequency.

mixed populations of cells in a whole blood sample, for instance (Mullaney *et al.*, 1969). Typical data are presented in Fig. 2 in the form of a contour plot of a correlated, two-parameter histogram. The horizontal axis represents the intensity of light scattered forward by each cell, and the vertical axis that scattered through 90°. Contours have been drawn through points on the diagram that occur with equal frequency. Thus it can be seen that most of the cells fall into one of four distinct types, which in this case can be shown to correspond to erythrocytes, lymphocytes, monocytes and granulocytes. Note that using forward scatter alone, it would not have been possible to resolve the latter two types, since both are of roughly the same cell size. With appropriately positioned electronic gates, each sub-population can be analysed further for other parameters, e.g. fluorescence, without having to isolate that sub-population first.

CELLULAR PARAMETERS MEASURABLE USING FLUORESCENT DYES

The full potential of flow cytometric analysis is realised only by the use of fluorescent dyes or probes. A range of dyes commonly used to determine cell structure is shown in Table 2, and can conveniently be categorised

Table 2
Fluorochromes Commonly Used in Flow Cytometry and the Probes Required

Fluorochrome	*Excitation spectrum*	*Emission spectrum*
For direct labelling of nucleic acids		
Ethidium bromide	blue/green	red
Acridine orange	blue/green	green (DNA), red (RNA)
Propridium iodide	blue/green	red
DAPI	ultraviolet	blue
Hoechst 33258, 33342	ultraviolet	blue
Chloromycin, mithramycin, oligomycin	blue	yellow
For conjugating to antibodies		
Fluorescein	blue/green	green
Rhodamine: RITC	green/yellow	green/yellow
XRITC	yellow	orange
Texas red	orange	red
Phycoerythrin	blue/green to yellow	yellow/orange
Phycocyanin	orange/red	red
Allophycocyanin	red	red

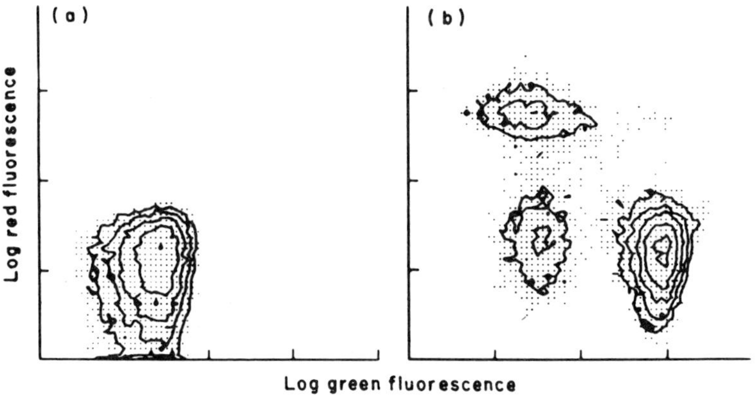

Fig. 3. Dual-parameter fluorescence analysis of sheep thymocytes showing the binding of a monoclonal anti-thymocyte antibody labelled with FITC (green fluorescence) and a monoclonal anti-MHC class I antibody labelled with phycoerythrin (red fluorescence) showing double negative cells with two other populations representing FITC positive and PE positive cells (no double positive cells were found) (b) versus unstained control (a). [Reproduced by permission of Blackwell Scientific from Mackay *et al.* (1985), *Immunology*, **55**, 729.]

according to whether they are used for staining nucleic acids or for linking to cell-specific antibodies or lectins.

An important use of flow cytometry is the study of cell surface markers using fluorescently labelled antibodies or lectins. This technique allows the rapid identification of sub-populations in heterogeneous populations of cells, without the need to isolate the cells of interest first. Antibodies, and monoclonal antibodies in particular, have revolutionised flow cytometry; any cell surface molecule can be used as a cell population marker, providing it can be made immunogenic. Two or more antibodies can be used together, provided they are conjugated to fluorescent dyes with non-overlapping emission spectra. The example in Fig. 3 is of cells that have been doubly stained with antibodies tagged with fluorescein isothiocyanate (FITC) and phycoerythrin (PE).

MICROBIOLOGICAL APPLICATIONS OF FLOW CYTOMETRY

The majority of the applications of flow cytometry relate at present to biomedical research. However, the technique is finding new fields in which to expand. Two of these fields are veterinary and food sciences. The use of flow cytometry in veterinary oncology, genetics, immunology, microbiology, cell biology and animal husbandry has been reviewed elsewhere (Mackenzie & Pinder, 1987).

Most bacteria and yeasts are large enough to generate a detectable scatter signal in flow (Hutter *et al.*, 1978; Van Dilla *et al.*, 1983). Staining bacteria with either DNA-binding stains (Steen *et al.*, 1982) or fluorescent antibodies (Cordery *et al.*, 1986) facilitates their detection in heterogeneous suspensions. The use of two or more antibodies (each conjugated to different coloured fluorochromes) would allow simultaneous detection of several bacteria in a sample, or, in combination with DNA stains, would enable the proportion of actively dividing cells to be determined.

FLOW CYTOMETRY IN IMMUNOASSAY

The ELISA is rapidly becoming the assay of choice for a wide range of applications. FCM overlaps with some of the areas where ELISA is used, particularly in bacteriology. Useful comparisons can be made between ELISA and FCM in this field. The fundamental difference between the use of FCM and ELISA is that FCM must be performed in the liquid phase whilst ELISA is a solid-phase assay. This does not pose problems for either assay in bacteriological applications as the sample would be in solution. However, in practice, most solid-phase immunoassays require at least one wash step to remove, for example, unbound conjugated antibody; this takes time. Washing is not a prerequisite for assays using FCM because unbound fluorochrome is not 'seen' by the machine. This means that very rapid assays can be performed using FCM; 15 min between application of antibody to readout of data is practicable using current methodology. This inherent rapidity is further enhanced because the binding of the fluorochromes used in FCM occurs immediately, whereas the chromogenic changes that form the basis of ELISA measurements take time to develop. Immunoassays using fluorochromes are also 10–20 times more sensitive than colorimetric assays; an approximately 50-fold greater dynamic range is obtainable from flow cytometers compared to microtitration plate readers.

These fundamental differences between the principles underlying the two techniques result in different trends for their development. In most cases it will not be too long before ELISAs are superseded by electronic immunosensors of some form (optical, acoustic or electrochemical). Developments in FCM, on the other hand, will be unlikely to affect profoundly the basic optical layout, but will involve miniaturisation and automation, or conversely increased sophistication of measurement or sorting capability.

FUTURE DEVELOPMENTS

There are two clearly discernible, and in some senses diametrically opposite, trends in the development of flow cytometry.

In the research laboratory, biologists are looking for increasingly subtle differences between cells, which require increasing sophistication in their measurements. Samples may be stained with a combination of fluorochromes, each of which may need to be excited at a different wavelength. The demand is now for instruments with multiple lasers and multi-parameter detection. Machine manufacturers are therefore offering krypton and dye laser options, in addition to the primary argon-ion source, with six or eight separate detection channels. More powerful computers are needed to handle the large amount of data that are generated, and increasing use is being made of 'list-mode' collection. In list-mode, the data are stored directly on disc or tape, as they are generated, and can then be replayed for more extensive analysis after the experiment.

At the other end of the scale, and of more immediate significance, are the flow cytometers that are being developed specifically for routine clinical or commercial applications. Research has demonstrated the usefulness of flow instruments in, for example, pathology and haematology, and created a demand for machines that are cheaper, simpler and easier to use. Machine control is being taken out of the hands of a skilled operator and placed directly under the influence of a central computer, paving the way towards eventual total process automation. There is intense research into new and more efficient dyes that may be excited at more convenient wavelengths. Therefore new cytometers could now be developed based on cheaper and more user-friendly lasers, rather than the expensive water-cooled ion lasers presently used.

There are also some exciting advances on the horizon that offer possibilities for the separation, purification or enrichment of high-value, low-yielding products on commercial scales. The cell-by-cell nature of the processing in a conventional flow cytometer, from which it derives its strength as an analytical tool, is also its greatest weakness in limiting the throughput to rates considerably less than those achievable using bulk separators. But new techniques offer potential increases in the sorting speed of one or two orders of magnitude. The advent of semi-preparative machines based upon these or other principles will then herald a new era in commercial bioseparation technology.

REFERENCES

Cordery, M. C., Mackenzie, N. M., Smith, I. M. & Parker, D. J. (1986) The quantification of flow microfluorimetry of specific binding of antibody to serotypes of *Haemophilus pleuropneumoniae*. *Research in Veterinary Science*, **41**, 277–278.

Herzenberg, L. A., Sweet, R. G. & Herzenberg, L. A. (1976) Fluorescence-activated cell sorting. *Scientific American*, **234**, 108–117.

Hutter, K. J., Punessen, U. & Eifel, H. (1978) Rapid determination of the purity of yeast cultures by immunofluorescence and flow cytometry. *Journal of the Institute of Brewing*, **85**, 21–22.

Loken, M. R. & Stall, A. M. (1982) Flow cytometry as a preparative and analytical tool in immunology. *Journal of Immunological Methods*, **50**, 85–112.

Mackenzie, N. M. & Pinder, A. C. (1987) Flow cytometry and its applications in veterinary medicine. *Research in Veterinary Science*, **42**, 131–139.

Melamed, M. R., Mullaney, P. F. & Mendelsen, M. L. (eds) (1979) *Flow Cytometry and Cell Sorting*, Wiley, New York.

Mullaney, P. F., Van Dilla, M. A., Coulter, J. R. & Dean, P. N. (1969) Cell sizing: light scattering photometer for rapid volume determination. *Review of Scientific Instruments*, **40**, 1029–1032.

Parks, D. R., Lanier, L. L. & Herzenberg, L. A. (1986) Flow cytometry and fluorescence-activated cell sorting (FACS). In: *Handbook of Experimental Immunology*, Weir, D. M. (ed.), Blackwell Scientific, Oxford.

Shapiro, H. M. (1983) Multistation multiparameter flow cytometry: a critical review and rationale *Cytometry*, **3**, 227–243.

Steen, H. B., Boye, E., Skastad, K., Bloom, B., Goodal, T. & Mustafa, S. (1982) Applications of flow cytometry on bacteria: cell cycle kinetics, drug effects and quantitation of antibody binding. *Cytometry*, **2**, 249–257.

Van Dila, M. A., Langois, R. G., Pinkel, O., Yajko, D. & Hadley, W. K. (1983) Bacterial characterization by flow cytometry. *Science*, **220**, 620–621.

21
Concluding Remarks

B. A. MORRIS
Department of Biochemistry, University of Surrey, Guildford, UK

The preceding chapters demonstrate without doubt that the application of immunoassay to veterinary and food analysis is now firmly established. The two years since the publication of *Immunoassays in Food Analysis* have seen an explosion in the application of the technique in these particular areas. The simplicity, sensitivity and specificity of the method, coupled with its capacity for large sample throughput, has now been fully appreciated and is being exploited. We are thus likely to see an even further increase in the number of analytes being measured and the number of laboratories performing immunoassay.

The readership of the present volume can no doubt be divided predominantly into three quite distinct categories. The first is those who are already using immunoassay and who are looking for ways of improving their existing assay performance, possibly to increase the sensitivity and hence the detection limit. They will no doubt have found much food for thought in the chapters by Barry Gould on the use of enzyme amplification systems to develop ultrasensitive immunoassays as well as in that by Chris Thorns and his colleagues from Weybridge on the use of monoclonal antibodies to impart greater specificity. Some of the alternative assay formats available have been very adequately described by Roy Jackman. However, I much regret that the literature is being flooded by a welter of acronyms. Perhaps we should try and keep the nomenclature as simple, rather than as complex, as possible.

Most of us have at some time had to overcome unacceptably high levels of non-specific binding in our assays and we will have to see how universally applicable Helena Windemann's solution is of including casein in the buffer. However, a considerable amount of interfering substances can be removed from the sample matrix by an adequate clean-up procedure and the experience of Richard Calverley and his colleagues, using solid-phase sample preparation columns, will no doubt be utilised by other workers.

The second category of reader is the new or potential recruit to the technique. He is forgiven if he now feels, having been lured into the arena with tales of how simple is the methodology, that it is too sophisticated and possibly too sensitive for his requirements. This would be entirely the wrong attitude to take. He must remember that each of the contributors to this volume gained his first experience of the technique with a simple assay system which was then modified and/or improved according to his particular requirements. The potential for increased sensitivity can either be exploited or it can be harnessed to reduce assay time or sample volume, with the latter option reducing any potential assay matrix interference. For many of you, this will be far more important than the sensitivity *per se*. To those readers who are contemplating immunoassay, but who are beginning to get cold feet, my advice is to jump in and get the feel of the technique with a fairly simple assay system. It may be all that is required for your particular problem.

For those readers who are looking for inspiration, there is no shortage of ideas for further application. Sheila Jones and Ron Patterson have shown how to produce more specific assays for the speciation of raw meats which exhibit reduced or negligible cross-reactivity between species. The next generation of assays in this area must be those applied to the speciation of cooked meats and those specific for individual offals, e.g. heart, liver, lung and intestine. Mike Harvey and his co-workers have shown the feasibility of using saliva in human epidemiological surveys for food contaminants and toxins, whilst Heather Kemp and her Norwich co-workers have demonstrated the use of immunoassay in controlling fermentation processes. There must be many more applications of these two strategies. Possibly one of the most convincing demonstrations of the superiority and convenience of immunological techniques over more tedious conventional methods of analysis is Alastair Robertson's method to replace the Howard mould count. Not only is it much simpler in that the number of filaments in the sample do not now have to be counted by eye, but the new method can also be used with homogenised samples, which previously was not possible.

On the other hand, one would be extremely naïve if one pretended that all was rosy in the garden of immunoassay development. John Allen's contribution outlining his first-hand experience in producing commercial immunoassay kits for food analysis has highlighted some of the problems involved. The chapter by Neil Griffiths has showed that public analysts who use ELISAs for food analytes in support of litigation should be aware of their limitations, though I feel that many of these would be overcome by the use of specific antibodies for more defined analytes. Anybody concerned about the cost effectiveness of these immunoassay methods compared with the more conventional alternatives will have found Mike Morgan's contribution a very fair assessment of the situation.

In any immunoassay, objective data reduction is of paramount importance if the care taken to perform an assay is not to be wasted. Barry Nix and Graham Groom, who have both had many years of experience of the subject in the clinical field, have highlighted some of the pitfalls which incorrect treatment of the data may produce. Nevertheless, Professor Mallinson has shown how useful computer-assisted data reduction and graphical presentation of the results can be in the Virginia-Maryland flock profiling system. Such a system need not be restricted to poultry, but could also be applied to any other intensively managed farm animal, for example pigs.

It would be both churlish and unreasonable to pretend that immunoassay is the perfect analytical method. Ask anybody who has to set up a classical immunoassay routinely whether he or she would prefer a method which did not require labelling each individual tube by hand, and the answer I am sure would be a resounding 'Yes'. The use of microtitration plates to a certain extent does eliminate some of the tedium. But how much simpler life would be if one could use an electrode incorporating all the specific characteristics of an antibody. In other words, an immunosensor. Although the main objective of this volume is to consider the application of immunoassay in these two areas, the editors felt very strongly that the readership should be aware of emerging analytical techniques using antibodies which were likely to compete with immunoassay in the future. Hence the reason for including chapters on immunosensors and flow cytometry in this volume. Although these methods may still be in their infancy, and currently lack the ease of application that immunoassay now has, I believe that in the years ahead they may prove to be realistic and attractive alternatives.

But, at present, immunoassays have no peer as far as practicality and reliability are concerned. Let us therefore use them imaginatively in tackling the many problems that confront us in veterinary and food analysis, and to replace more tedious and less sensitive methods. I hope that this volume will encourage all concerned to achieve those objectives.

Poster Presentations

Novel Hapten–Protein Conjugation Methods for the Synthesis of Immunogens and Coating Conjugates for Use in ELISA

A. S. KANG, H. W.-S. CHAN and M. R. A. MORGAN

AFRC Institute of Food Research, Norwich, UK

INTRODUCTION

This poster presentation demonstrates the well-known advantage of using a heterologous bridge when synthesising immunogens, coating conjugates and labelled antigens. The approach overcomes the problem of bridge recognition as encountered when the same site of attachment and condensation method are used in their preparation.

Conventional procedures for converting haptens with a hydroxyl group to immunogens most commonly use straight-chain aliphatic spacers (e.g. hemiglutarates, hemisuccinates). This poster presentation reports the preparation of heterologous conjugates using the bifunctional linking reagents sebacoyl dichloride and *trans*-1,4-cyclohexanedioic acid respectively for linking the hydroxyl groups on sterigmatocystin to a carrier protein.

METHODS

1. Synthesis of Immunogen

Heterologous conjugates were produced linking hapten hydroxyl groups to protein using the bifunctional linking reagent sebacoyl dichloride (Bailey & Butler, 1967) and *trans*-1,4-cyclohexanedioic acid respectively for preparing sterigmatocystin conjugates.

Antisera to sterigmatocystin hemiacetal were raised against a hapten–BSA conjugate synthesised using the bifunctional reagent sebacoyl dichloride.

2. Synthesis of Hapten–Protein Conjugates for ELISA Solid Phase

A conjugate of sterigmatocystin was synthesised with a homogeneous bridge using sebacoyl dichloride and KLH for the immunogen. A heterologous conjugate used a bridge containing a cyclohexane ring. *Trans*-1,4-cyclohexanedioic acid (0·5 g) was reacted with excess thionyl chloride (1·5 ml) by refluxing in tetrahydrofuran for 15 h. Excess thionyl chloride was removed under vacuum to leave a brown liquid containing the diacyl chloride derivative. An aliquot (0·2 ml) was added to sterigmatocystin (1 mg) in dioxan (1 ml) and pyridine (0·05 ml). The solution was refluxed for 1 h, concentrated under vacuum and then added to a solution of KLH (34 mg) in saline at room temperature to effect conjugation. Unbound hapten and reagents were removed by extensive dialysis.

3. Microtitration Plate ELISA

The indirect double antibody ELISA format used was that previously described by Morgan *et al.* (1986). The two coating conjugates were used for the ELISA solid phase, being passively adsorbed to the wells of the microtitration plates. Assay performance was then compared.

RESULTS AND DISCUSSION

Both conjugates allowed production of standard curves for the hapten. However, the use of the cyclohexyl bridge improved assay performance considerably compared with the straight-chain bridge. Background binding was reduced from 50% of the maximal binding to less than 5%. The limit of detection of the assay was also improved from 100 pg/well with the plates coated with homogeneous conjugate to 10 pg/well with the heterologous system.

Both the straight-chain and cyclic bifunctional coupling reagents can be prepared readily and may be applied to a wide range of functional groups such as hydroxyl, amino and thiol. It should be noted that the conventional route for sterigmatocystin conjugate synthesis (derivatisation with succinic anhydride) did not in this instance succeed due, it is thought, to intramolecular hydrogen bonding.

The tandem use of these two methods should find wide application in immunoassays for haptens. Conjugation of derivatised hapten to protein requires simple mixing of the two reagents and is not critically dependent on solvent composition. In this laboratory, several ELISAs have shown improved assay characteristics upon introduction of coating conjugates synthesised with the cyclohexyl spacer, including one for quinine (C. M. Ward & M. R. A. Morgan, unpublished results).

ACKNOWLEDGEMENTS

A.S.K. has an AFRC research studentship. The work was partly funded by the Ministry of Agriculture, Fisheries and Food.

REFERENCES

BAILEY, J. M. & BUTLER, J. (1967) Synthetic cholesterol–ester antigens in experimental atherosclerosis. In: *Reticulo–Endothelial System and Atherosclerosis*, De Luzio, N. R. & Paoletti, R. (eds), Plenum Press, New York, pp. 433–441.

MORGAN, M. R. A., KANG, A. S. & CHAN, H. W.-S. (1986) Production of antisera against sterigmatocystin hemiacetal and its potential for use in an enzyme-linked immunosorbent assay for sterigmatocystin in barley. *Journal of the Science of Food and Agriculture*, **37**, 873–880.

The Potential of Fluorescence Detection in ELISA

C. M. WARD, H. W.-S. CHAN and M. R. A. MORGAN
AFRC Institute of Food Research, Norwich, UK

INTRODUCTION

Since fluorescence can be detected with considerably greater sensitivity than can be achieved by other end-points (including optical density), it has often been suggested that assays relying on fluorimetry should show greater sensitivity. Unfortunately, this benefit has only occasionally been achieved in practice, mainly because the natural fluorescence of biological material gives rise to high background values. However, the use of microtitration plate ELISAs may be a more suitable vehicle in which to employ fluorescence detection because of the high efficiency of washing the immobilised phase and the large signal generated enzymically and specifically in the final assay stage.

In order to investigate this possibility, fluorogenic substrates have been substituted for chromogenic substrates in two assay procedures. Thus 4-methylumbelliferyl phosphate and 4-methylumbelliferyl-β-D-galactoside were used as the substrates in ELISAs with alkaline phosphatase and β-D-galactosidase labels respectively.

METHODS

Two-site Assay

Microtitration plates (Nunc), certified grade 1 (Gibco Europe Ltd), were coated with 1/5000 rabbit anti-rat IgG (Sigma). Following incubation with the sample containing the specific analyte they were visualised using 1/1000 alkaline phosphatase-labelled goat anti-rat IgG (Sigma) as the second antibody. Either 1 mg/ml 4-nitrophenyl phosphate or 100 μg/ml 4-methylumbelliferyl phosphate was used as substrate. The latter reaction was stopped after 30–60 min with 50 μl of 3M K_2HPO_4/KOH buffer (pH 10·4).

Hapten Assay

Measurement of quinidine was by an indirect competitive ELISA using quinidine–KLH-coated plates with alkaline phosphatase-labelled second antibody, as described by Morgan *et al.* (1985).

Fluorescence Determination

The enzyme-generated fluorescence in the microtitration wells was read on a conventional Perkin–Elmer LS-5 luminescence spectrometer. Excitation and emission wavelengths were 359 and 448 nm respectively. Samples were read by dilution to 3 ml in a quartz cell or by measuring the well contents directly using a microcell attachment. Both methods reduced the signal output by a factor of about 10. (A dedicated fluorescence plate reader could have been used.) Colorimetric reactions were read on a Kontron SLT210 plate reader at 405 nm.

RESULTS

Equivalent responses were obtained using 4-methylumbelliferyl phosphate or 4-methylumbelliferyl-β-D-galactoside as substrates. The former was used in the reported studies.

Two-site Assay

The standard curves for rat IgG measured by colorimetric and fluorescent end-points are compared in Fig. 1. The detection limit of the assay is improved by approximately 10-fold using a fluorescent substrate.

Hapten Assay

The measurement of quinidine by indirect ELISA produces a standard curve in which absorbance is inversely proportional to concentration. In this assay (data not shown) no significant improvement in sensitivity could be determined with a fluorescent end-point. However, the increased signal from the fluorogenic substrate enabled the reduction of reagent concentration. Thus the concentration of hapten–protein conjugate used for coating could be reduced from 1 μg/ml to 100 ng/ml and that of anti-quinidine antibody from 1/1000 to 1/10 000 dilution.

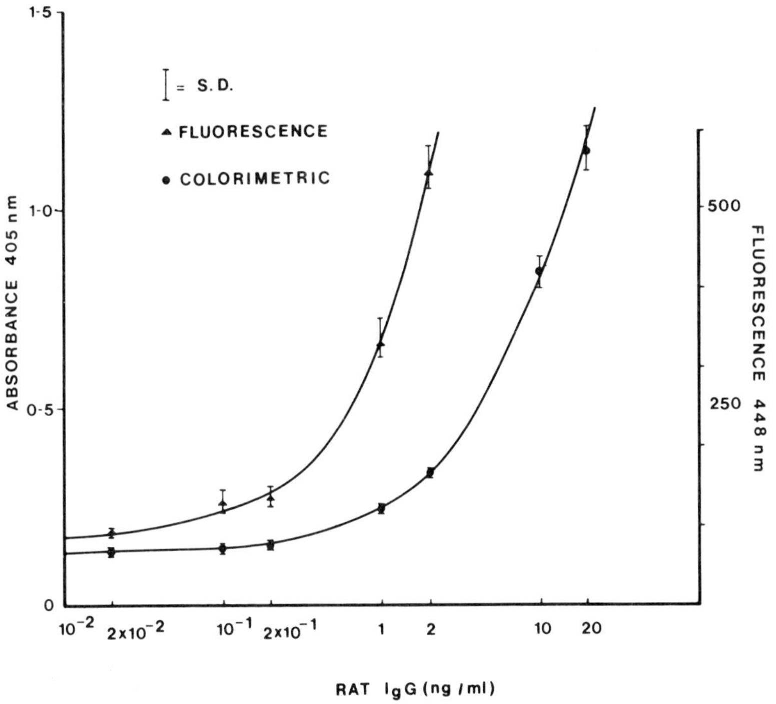

Fig. 1. Comparison of standard curves for rat IgG measured by fluorescent and colorimetric end-points.

The signal from the chromogenic substrate was less than that for the fluorescent substrate at low signal levels. However, the high background observed at these low levels of fluorescent product prevented any realisation of the potential for increase in assay sensitivity.

DISCUSSION

In a two-site assay, where the reading is directly proportional to analyte concentration, the use of fluorescence detection leads to greater assay sensitivity.

However, where there is an inverse relationship between the absorbance and analyte concentration, as in the competitive ELISA, no improvement in sensitivity was found.

The reaction products of the fluorescence assays were diluted 1 in 10 to give sufficient volume to read in a 3 ml fluorimetric cell. At a further 1 in 10 dilution, the fluorescence standard curve became indistinguishable from that of the colorimetric assay. Thus there is some loss of potential sensitivity.

Reduction of reagent concentrations, such as that of coating conjugate and second antibody, reduces the scale of the reaction. Although this can lead to improvements in other aspects of assay performance, there was no further improvement in assay sensitivity in the present study.

As the ratio of signal-to-noise generated in the assay is reduced, then the level of interference from the background fluorescence is proportionately increased. This is so, even with pure standards, and biological matrices were not tested in the present study. Thus high backgrounds have prevented exploitation of the full potential for increased sensitivity.

The use of fluorogenic substrates can therefore improve the limit of detection of certain assays, such as the two-site assay for rat IgG, but the advantage may not be universal in all assay formats.

REFERENCE

MORGAN, M. R. A., BRAMHAM, S., WEBB, A. J., ROBINS, R. J. & RHODES, M. J. C. (1985) Specific immunoassays for quinine and quinidine: comparison of radioimmunoassay and enzyme-linked immunosorbent assay procedures. *Planta Medica*, **51**, 237–241.

Development of Bovine and Ovine Monoclonal Antibodies to Testosterone

D. J. Groves, J. Clayton and B. A. Morris

AFRC Antibody Development Group, Division of Clinical Biochemistry, University of Surrey, Guildford, UK

INTRODUCTION

Investigations into the possibility of producing bovine and ovine monoclonal antibodies have been carried out as part of a programme of research into the immunomodulation of gonadal steroid feedback in domestic livestock to increase fecundity.

Since no myeloma line of either bovine or ovine origin was available, it was necessary to use the technique of inter-species fusion to produce a chimaeric hybridoma secreting the desired antibody. This approach has been adopted with varying success in the production of human (Teng *et al.*, 1983), ovine (Tucker *et al.*, 1981; Dicker *et al.*, 1985) and bovine (Srikumaran *et al.*, 1984; Tucker *et al.*, 1984) monoclonal antibodies.

This poster presentation reports the successful generation of ovine and bovine monoclonal antibodies to testosterone using inter-species fusion, and the characterisation and long-term production of these antibodies.

MATERIALS AND METHODS

Cell Lines

Lymphocytes

Sensitised lymphocytes were obtained from a Suffolk cross-bred wether and from a Friesian steer, both immunised against testosterone-3-carboxymethyloxime (CMO) ovalbumin. Blood was obtained from the sheep 10 days after boosting and from the steer three days after boosting. Blood was taken from the jugular vein and the lymphocytes separated by density gradient centrifugation on Lymphoprep (sheep) or Lymphopaque (steer) (Nyegaard, UK).

Mouse Myeloma

The mouse myeloma line used in the preparation of the ovine anti-testosterone hybridoma and the bovine/mouse heteromyeloma was the aminopterin-sensitive line NS1/1-Ag4-1. This line synthesises, but does not secrete, kappa light chains.

Heteromyeloma

A heteromyeloma cell line, sensitive to selective media, was made by fusing NS1/1-Ag4-1 mouse myeloma cells with bovine peripheral blood lymphocytes from an animal immunised against testosterone. Resulting hybridoma lines, which initially secreted antibodies to testosterone but which subsequently ceased to do so, were incubated with 8-azaguanine over 60 days to induce aminopterin sensitivity. The resulting cell line was used in place of the mouse myeloma line in the bovine fusions with a view to increasing the proportion of bovine chromosomes present in the resulting hybridomas, and therefore their potential stability (Tucker *et al.*, 1984).

SCREENING ASSAYS

Both bovine and ovine fusions were screened using an ELISA specific for the allogeneic anti-testosterone antibody. The ovine fusion was also screened with an ELISA for ovine IgG.

In the bovine (and ovine) anti-testosterone assay, PVC microtitration plates (Dynatech) were coated with a testosterone-3-CMO-chicken gammaglobulin conjugate before being incubated with cell supernatant samples and dilutions of a standard polyclonal bovine (or ovine) anti-testosterone antibody in cell culture medium. After washing, the plates were incubated with HRP-labelled rabbit anti-bovine IgG antibodies (Dakopatts) (or HRP-labelled donkey anti-ovine IgG, Guildhay Antisera) and then visualised with orthophenylenediamine (OPD).

The detection limit of the bovine assay was 15·6 pg/ml of specific IgG. The intra-assay coefficient of variation (CV%) was 8·1% and the inter-assay CV% was 8·9%. The corresponding values for the ovine assay were 1·18 pg/ml, 8·98% and 17·1%. In both systems mouse IgG (1 μg/ml) and allogeneic non-immune serum (1:5000) were both below the limit of detection.

For the ovine IgG assay, plates were coated with donkey anti-ovine IgG antibodies (Guildhay Antisera) and incubated with samples and standards. After washing, plates were incubated with HRP-labelled donkey anti-ovine IgG antibodies and visualised with OPD.

The detection limit of the assay was 4·5 ng/ml (due to high background from foetal calf serum (FCS) proteins), intra-assay CV% was 9·6% and inter-assay CV% was 26·5%. Mouse IgG (20 μg/ml) and chicken IgG (40 μg/ml) were both below the limit of detection.

FUSION AND MAINTENANCE

Exponentially dividing B/MF-2 heteromyeloma cells (or NS1/1-Ag4-1 mouse myeloma cells for the ovine fusion) were mixed with sensitised lymphocytes at a ratio of 4:1 (or 5:1) and a total cell number of 5×10^6 (or 6×10^6). Fusion was effected with 50% polyethylene glycol 1500 (BDH) added over 2 min and rapidly diluted out with Leibovitz serum-free medium according to the method of Galfre & Milstein (1981). The cells were transferred to hypoxanthine–aminopterin–thymidine (HAT) medium before being plated out over mouse thymocytes in multiwell plates (Gibco). Cultures were incubated at 37°C in an atmosphere of 5% CO_2 in air.

Following selection of hybridomas in aminopterin-containing medium over a period of seven days, the medium was replaced with Dulbecco's modified Eagle's medium (DMEM) containing 10% FCS supplemented with hypoxanthine and thymidine, and then by DMEM containing 10% FCS only. Colonies which were detected as secreting specific antibody were then cloned by limiting dilution and maintained in exponential growth by sequentially transferring cultures, subject to positive screening, from multidish wells to tissue culture flasks (Nunclon) of increasing size. Cell culture supernatants were collected by centrifugation, assayed and stored at −20°C.

RESULTS

Cell Culture

In the bovine fusion, colonies were first detected visually 11 days after fusion in 26% of the wells. Of these, 8% were secreting antibody to testosterone at 14 days. No further secreting colonies were detected over the following two months. Following two cloning stages and selection for the

Table 1
Results of Characterisation Studies

Antibody characteristics	
1. Bovine anti-testosterone:	
Cell line	B/MT.4A.17.H5.A5
Antibody class	IgG_1
Equilibrium dissociation constant (K_D)	$2{\cdot}50 \times 10^{-12}$M
Cross-reactivities	
Testosterone (4-androsten-17β-ol-3-one)	100%
Dihydrotestosterone (5α-androstan-17β-ol-3-one)	87·3%
Androstenedione (4-androsten-3,17-dione)	0·02%
Oestradiol (1,3,5(10)-estratrien-3,17α-diol)	<0·001%
Oestrone (1,3,5(10)-estratrien-3-ol-17-one)	<0·001%
Progesterone (4-pregnan-3,20-dione)	<0·001%
Optimal secretion rate	3·4 μg/10^6 cells/24 h
2. Ovine anti-testosterone:	
Cell line	O/M.4.22b.A24.17
Antibody class	IgG
Equilibrium dissociation constant (K_D)	$7{\cdot}63 \times 10^{-12}$M
Secretion rate at confluence	17 ng/ml

best line, hybridoma line B/MT.4A.17.H5.A5 was selected for expansion. This line is still growing and secreting after 30 months in culture.

In the ovine fusion, colonies were observed in 66% of the wells 14 days after fusion. The first positive assay results for testosterone antibodies were at 26 days and, like the bovine fusion, no positive lines were detected after this. Two of the positive lines were cloned and maintained in the culture for a period of four months before being frozen in liquid nitrogen.

Table 1 shows the results of characterisation studies on these cell lines and their respective antibodies.

DISCUSSION

This series of inter-species fusions has demonstrated the practicability of producing stable cell lines secreting monoclonal bovine or ovine antibodies, without the need for allogeneic myeloma fusion partners.

The fusion of a murine myeloma and ovine peripheral blood lymphocytes from an animal immunised against testosterone produced a hybridoma which secreted ovine antibody to testosterone. The antibody was an IgG of high affinity and was secreted at levels of up to 17 ng/ml by confluent cultures.

An aminopterin-sensitive murine–bovine heteromyeloma was developed. This line was fused with bovine peripheral blood lymphocytes from an animal immunised against testosterone to produce a hybridoma secreting a bovine antibody to testosterone. The antibody was an IgG_1 of high affinity secreted at a maximal rate comparable with that obtained in other inter-species fusions (e.g. Cote *et al.*, 1983; Butler *et al.*, 1983).

Simple and rapid ELISAs were developed to screen cell culture supernatants for specific ovine and bovine antibodies to testosterone. An assay was also developed for ovine IgG.

Repeated use of the bovine heteromyeloma will enable the production of further hybridomas secreting bovine monoclonal antibodies. The adaptation of this approach to the production of ovine monoclonal antibodies is also under investigation. This strategy has now been successfully applied to the production of ovine monoclonal antibodies to androstenedione and progesterone using an ovine–murine heteromyeloma fusion partner.

REFERENCES

Butler, J. L., Lane, H. C. & Fauci, A. S. (1983) Delineation of optimal conditions for producing mouse–human heterohybridomas from human peripheral blood B cells of immunised subjects. *Journal of Immunology*, **130**, 165–168.

Cote, R. J., Morrissey, D. M., Houghton, A. N., Beattie, E. J., Oettgen, H. F. & Old, L. J. (1983) Generation of human monoclonal antibodies reactive with cellular antigens. *Proceedings of the National Academy of Sciences, USA*, **80**, 2026–2030.

Dicker, P. D., Douglas, S., Jarman, D. J. & Brochas, A. J. (1985) Production of anti-luteinising hormone sheep monoclonal antibodies and their use in a luteinising hormone immunoassay. *The British Society for Immunology*, Autumn Meeting, London, 103 (Abstract).

Galfre, G. & Milstein, C. (1981) Preparation of monoclonal antibodics: strategy and procedure. *Methods in Enzymology*, **73**, 1–46.

Srikumaran, S., Guidry, A. J. & Goldsby, R. A. (1984) Production and characterization of monoclonal bovine immunoglobulins G_1, G_2 and M from bovine × murine hybridomas. *Veterinary Immunology and Immunopathology*, **5**, 323–342.

Teng, N. N. H., Lam, K. S., Riera, F. C. & Kaplan, H. S. (1983) Construction and testing of mouse–human heteromyelomas for human monoclonal antibody production. *Proceedings of the National Academy of Sciences, USA*, **80**, 7305–7312.

Tucker, E. M., Dain, A. R., Wright, L. J. & Clarke, S. W. (1981) Culture of sheep × mouse hybridoma cells *in vitro*. *Hybridoma*, **1**, 77–86.

Tucker, E. M., Dain, A. R., Clarke, S. W. & Donker, R. A. (1984) Specific bovine monoclonal antibody produced by a re-fused mouse/calf hybridoma. *Hybridoma*, **3**, 171–176.

Studies on the Specificity of some Commercially Available Antisera used in the Analysis of Meat Products

I. D. Lumley, I. Patel and C. J. Stanley

Laboratory of the Government Chemist, London, UK

INTRODUCTION

The majority of food analysts who use immunoassay techniques do not have access to animal house facilities and therefore rely on commercial organisations to supply consistently antisera of the required type and specificity. These are commonly anti-species or anti-vegetable protein antisera, but many of the commercial supplies from which the analyst can choose were prepared for use in immunodiffusion or immunoprecipitation procedures rather than for ELISAs. Using double diffusion and ELISA techniques, a wide range of commercially available antisera were examined for specificity, sensitivity and consistency, i.e. batch to batch variation. For most ELISA applications, an antiserum is required which is completely specific to its antigen.

ANTISERA SPECIFICITY USING ELISA

In this evaluation of commercially available antisera for meat speciation, the samples used were various cuts of the appropriate meat which had been finely minced. Offals, mechanically recovered meat and exudate from the meats have also been examined. Appropriate mixtures of the meats were prepared as required.

Table 1 indicates the intensity of some cross-reactions observed by ELISA for several types of antisera from several suppliers. The results indicate that antisera from four different suppliers are not species-specific, and in many instances are not suitable for use in ELISA. For example, the

Table 1
Specificity of some Antisera for Meat Speciation Investigated using ELISA

Supplier		*Intensity of signal*					
		Beef	*Pork*	*Chicken*	*Lamb*	*Bovine casein*	*Bovine whey proteins*
A	*Anti-porcine*[a]						
	Whole serum	++	+++	+	+	–	–
	IgG	++	+++	–	+	–	–
B	*Anti-porcine*[a]						
	Whole serum	++	+++	–	–	–	–
	IgG	++	+++	–	–	–	–
C	*Anti-porcine*[a]						
	Whole serum	–	+++	–	–	–	–
A	*Anti-bovine*[a]						
	Whole serum	+++	++	+	+	–	–
	IgG	+++	++	–	+	–	–
B	*Anti-bovine*[a]						
	Whole serum	+++	++	–	+	–	–
	IgG	+++	++	–	+	–	–
C	*Anti-bovine*[a]						
	Whole serum	+++	–	–	–	–	–
D	*Anti-bovine*[a]						
	Whole serum	+++	+	–	–	–	–
C	*Anti-bovine*						
	Casein	–	–	–	–	+++	–
C	*Anti-bovine*						
	Whey	–	–	–	–	–	+++

[a] *Note:* The antiserum is raised to either the whole serum or the IgG fraction of the whole serum from the species which it is intended to detect. These are *not* the whole antiserum or the IgG fraction of the antiserum.

+++ Strong signal typical of a specific antiserum; good discrimination between levels of desired antigen.

++ Medium strength signal, usually associated with non-specific antiserum, results in poor discrimination between levels of desired antigen and poor detection limits.

\+ Weak signal.

– No measurable signal.

anti-porcine protein antisera from suppliers A and B exhibited considerable cross-reaction with beef protein, and therefore high optical densities were recorded for 100% beef samples. Because of these cross-reactions, it was not possible to discriminate between the presence of 15 and 25% pork in admixture with beef. Various dilutions of antisera, enzyme conjugate and sample extract were used to optimise the assays, but these undesirable cross-reactions were still observed. From the pattern of results in Table 1 it is not surprising that the anti-porcine protein antiserum from supplier C gave the lowest detection limit for pork in admixture with beef (1% m/m). Some batches of antisera from supplier D were capable of detecting 1% pork in beef; however, the detection limit was variable due to batch to batch variation of the antisera.

Note that by stating a detection limit for pork in beef it is not implied that the analytical method used has been fully validated for the accurate determination of this amount of pork in samples alleged to be pure beef. Our results are based on the analysis of mixtures of meats of known composition.

Detection limits for bovine whey and casein, and for soya and gliadin, in admixture with meats are typically 0·5% (m/m) or less. The anti-soya and anti-gliadin antisera investigated to date show no cross-reactivity when tested against cereal rusks and soya flour, soya concentrate or soya isolate respectively, nor with the meat and milk proteins shown in Table 1.

REMOVAL OF CROSS-REACTING ANTIBODIES FROM ANTISERA

It is clear from our investigations that not all commercially available antisera are species-specific or suitable for use in ELISA. We have investigated several procedures for the removal of unwanted non-specific antibodies from commercial antisera. Two of the most promising have been a simple antibody–antigen precipitation method and affinity HPLC. (See Jones & Patterson, Chapter 10.) From the data shown, some anti-porcine antisera contain antibodies which cross-react with beef protein. The simplest way to remove these cross-reacting antibodies is to add BSA, allow the antibody–antigen complex to form, and then remove by centrifugation and filtration. Affinity HPLC requires the use of relatively sophisticated equipment, but the affinity columns can be simply produced in the laboratory, and can rapidly immunoadsorb antisera. The cross-reacting antibodies in a crude antiserum incapable in an ELISA of detecting less than 20% pork in beef were removed by both methods described above to produce an antiserum capable of detecting the presence of less than 2% pork.

SUMMARY

There is little doubt that immunoassay techniques will play an increasingly important role in food analysis, and consequently more analysts will need to become familiar with the methodology involved. This work has shown that care should be exercised when using commercially available antisera. Thorough tests for specificity should be performed and analysts must be prepared to change assay conditions in response to possible batch to batch variations in antisera (and enzyme conjugates). These precautions are necessary if sensitive, reliable and reproducible results are to be obtained.

Development of a Progesterone Field Test for Monitoring of Fertility in Large Domestic Animals

J. H. M. DAVINA, W. KOOPS and D. F. M. VAN DE WIEL
Research Institute for Animal Production, 'Schoonoord', Zeist, The Netherlands

Several commercial diagnostic test kits are currently available for the measurement of progesterone (Drew, 1986). All these tests are based on the EIA principle. Milk samples can now be tested on site without the need for expensive equipment or time-consuming postal services. These tests are suitable for use by veterinarians but they are less suitable for use by the farmer. It is difficult for the farmer to add very small quantities of each reagent and to prepare solutions for direct use, to carry out several subsequent incubations, and to wait for the test results after he has finished milking the cows. It was the aim of this research project to develop a field test for the measurement of progesterone for use by farmers. The test should have the following features: only one incubation; result to be rapidly available; easy to handle; reagents to be sufficiently stable; and usable by farmers in the tropics. Four models which may be suitable for application as progesterone field tests have been investigated. This study is not yet complete.

The first model is the dipstick EIA. This model has been derived from the progesterone EIA which has been developed in this laboratory (Wiel & Koops, 1986) and which is currently being applied in co-operation with the National Animal Health Service and the Federation of Societies for Artificial Insemination in The Netherlands. In the dipstick EIA model, a paper is used which is coated with a polyclonal anti-progesterone immunoglobulin. The paper has been attached to a dipstick. This stick is incubated for 15 min in a solution containing both the progesterone–peroxidase conjugate as well as the whole milk sample. After washing, the dipstick is incubated in a developer solution for 10 min. This method gives a result within 1 h and is relatively easy to handle, but this test consists of more than one incubation and the developer solution is not sufficiently stable.

The second model is based on the principle of the enzyme immunochromatographic test strip assay, as described by Zuk *et al.* (1985). This has been modified for use in the ng/ml range rather than the μg/ml range. This method is not critically dependent on the activity of the enzyme conjugate, because the height of the migration front is critical. For this reason this test is hardly influenced by environmental factors such as temperature, sample matrix effects or duration of assay. This model is suitable for measuring very low progesterone concentrations. However, the non-specific background staining is at present rather high. This can be reduced by purification of the enzyme conjugate and by an alternative method for the immobilisation of the antibody. As with the dipstick EIA, this chromatography EIA is not a one-step field test and still uses reagents which are insufficiently stable, especially for use in the tropics.

The third model for a field test is the 'litmus paper strip'. This is a one-incubation test that gives results within 1 h. It is also easy to handle by farmers in the tropics and the reagents are stable because all are kept in dry form. The paper strip consists of cellulose material as a support for the EIA reagents (Fig. 1). The sample is absorbed and comes into contact with the various reagents in the correct sequence. The second antibody is immobilised on a solid phase and acts as a filter for the anti-progesterone antibodies. So colour development will occur when a sample containing more than a critical amount of progesterone permits enzyme conjugate which is not bound by the anti-progesterone antibody to reach the enzyme indicator at the top of the strip.

One problem is the immunoreactivity of the progesterone–peroxidase conjugate. In addition to free peroxidase, conjugate which cannot be bound by the antiserum will produce a colour change, which is unrelated to a high sample progesterone content. An alternative conjugation method and the use of immunoaffinity chromatography are being investigated. Moreover, the separation of the conjugate from free peroxidase has been improved by hydrophobic interaction chromatography. Interference by milk lactoperoxidase is also a problem. It has been found that this can be excluded by pretreatment of the sample with the lectin concanavalin A. This can be included in the litmus paper strip by immobilising the lectin on the cellulose.

The fourth model is an agglutination SPIA (solid-phase immunoassay). It has been developed by Organon International for human pregnancy testing (Leuvering *et al.*, 1981). The advantages of this system are that this

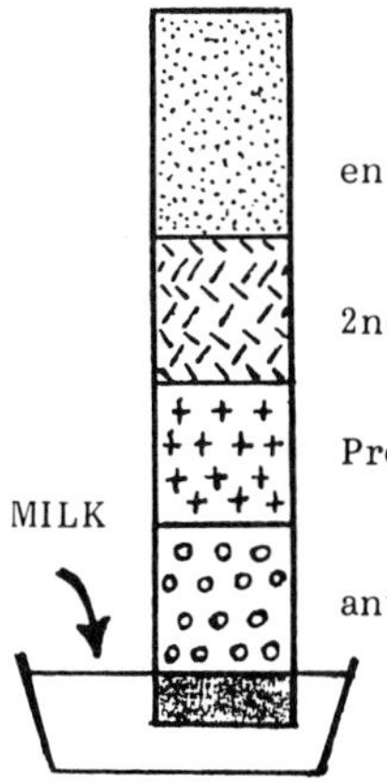

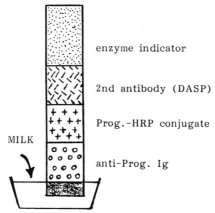

Fig. 1. Schematic representation of the 'litmus paper strip'. The milk sample is absorbed and migrates due to capillary action to reach the various reagents in turn which also migrate. However, the second antibody, which is immobilised on the cellulose, binds all the progesterone–anti-progesterone complexes. A high progesterone sample results in unbound enzyme conjugate which migrates further to reach the enzyme indicator at the top of the strip.

test is not based on an enzyme reaction, that only one incubation is needed, and that it is very easy to handle by the farmer. The system is based on the optical properties of properly dispersed antibody-coated gold particles and the optical phenomenon accompanying the agglutination of the particles in the presence of the antigen (colour change within 30 min: red → blue → grey → colourless). For the progesterone field test, an agglutination inhibition SPIA was used, because progesterone acts as a monovalent antigen. The principle of the test is as follows: colloidal gold sol particles of 50 nm are coated with anti-progesterone immunoglobulin. During incubation, milk progesterone and a protein which carries more than one progesterone molecule will compete for antibody binding sites. A low progesterone content causes agglutination because the conjugate can act as a bridge between individual gold sol particles. However, a high progesterone content in the sample will inhibit this agglutination process. Dose–response curves with a colour change in the range of 1 to 10 ng/ml progesterone have been determined for this analyte in buffer, in fat-free milk and in whole milk.

Evaluating the four models under investigation, the litmus paper strip and the gold agglutination assay are the most promising, because they only need one incubation step, employ dry reagents and are simple to use, not only by the veterinarian but also by the farmer, even in the tropics.

REFERENCES

DREW, B. (1986) Farm practice—milk progesterone testing as an aid to cow fertility management. In: *Practice, Veterinary Records*, supplement, **8**, 17–20.

LEUVERING, J. H. W., THAL, P. J. H. M., WAARDT, M. VAN DER & SCHUURS, A. H. W. M. (1981) A sol particle agglutination assay for human chorionic gonadotrophin. *Journal of Immunological Methods*, **45**, 183–192.

WIEL, D. F. M. VAN DE & KOOPS, W. (1986) Development and validation of an enzyme immunoassay for progesterone in bovine milk or blood plasma. *Animal Reproduction Science*, **10**, 201–214.

ZUK, R. F., GINSBERG, V. K., HOUTS, T., RABBIE, J., MERRICK, H., ULLMAN, E. F., FISCHER, M. M., SITZO, C. C., STISO, S. N. & LITMAN, D. J. (1985) Enzyme immunochromatography: a qualitative immunoassay requiring no instrumentation. *Clinical Chemistry*, **31**, 1144–1150.

Use of Serum Gastrin in the Diagnosis of Bovine Ostertagiasis

M. T. Fox, S. R. Pitt, D. Gerrelli and D. E. Jacobs
Department of Microbiology and Parasitology, The Royal Veterinary College, London, UK

INTRODUCTION

In Britain, the most important gastrointestinal parasite of cattle is the abomasal nematode, *Ostertagia ostertagi.* Infection with this parasite has been shown to impair the efficiency of digestion by lowering the production of hydrochloric acid resulting in a marked elevation in abomasal pH and an accumulation of pepsinogen. There is also an increase in permeability of the abomasal mucosa and of local capillary endothelial cells, thereby allowing pepsinogen to pass from the abomasal lumen into the circulation. Serum pepsinogen levels are significantly elevated by the time clinical signs appear, making this a useful diagnostic tool. However, methods for measuring pepsinogen are time-consuming and require considerable technical expertise.

Recent experimental work in sheep and cattle has demonstrated a marked increase in circulating levels of the gut hormone, gastrin, in association with *Ostertagia* infection. The aims of this investigation were (i) to monitor changes in pepsinogen and gastrin levels in calves exposed to *Ostertagia*, and (ii) to evaluate the use of serum gastrin for the diagnosis of bovine ostertagiasis.

MATERIALS AND METHODS

Experimental Infection

Changes in circulating pepsinogen and gastrin levels were monitored in two experimental *Ostertagia* infections. In each case, 20 three-month-old

Friesian bull calves were reared in individual pens under conditions designed to minimise the risk of parasitic infection. The calves were weight paired and then allocated to either pair-fed control or infected groups, the latter receiving (i) 100 000 *Ostertagia ostertagi* infective larvae on day 0 and (ii) the equivalent of 10 000 *O. ostertagi* larvae daily, given thrice weekly. The pattern of infection in each case was chosen to simulate the challenge to which calves are exposed at different times during the grazing season. All calves were treated with fenbendazole ('Panacur', Hoechst UK Ltd) at the manufacturer's recommended dose rate before and also towards the end of each investigation. Blood samples were collected three times per week.

Field Infection

Three trials were conducted on commercial farms in southern England to evaluate different prophylactic treatments in the control of bovine ostertagiasis. A total of 120 autumn-born calves were allocated to three matched groups on each farm. One group of calves acted as untreated controls, while the other two received alternative forms of prophylactic anthelmintic treatment. Blood samples were collected at approximately monthly intervals during the grazing season.

Serum Analysis

Serum pepsinogen levels were determined using the method of Mylrea & Hotson (1969). Serum gastrin assays were performed using a commercially available RIA kit for human gastrin (Serono Diagnostics Ltd, kit code 10994), validated for use in cattle using procedures outlined by Bolton (1982).

RESULTS AND DISCUSSION

Experimental Infection

Pronounced changes in digestive function, associated with the development and maturation of the worm burden, were recorded in both experimental studies. Infected calves exhibited an early rise in pepsinogen levels (from day 7) followed by a marked hypergastrinaemia (from day 16), when adult worms were present. The elevated gastrin levels were probably related to the concurrent increase in abomasal pH. This would stimulate hormone secretion by the gastrin cells in the pyloric antrum and, in turn, increase hydrochloric acid production by the parietal cells in the gastric glands. The marked elevation in gastrin levels demonstrated by the infected group

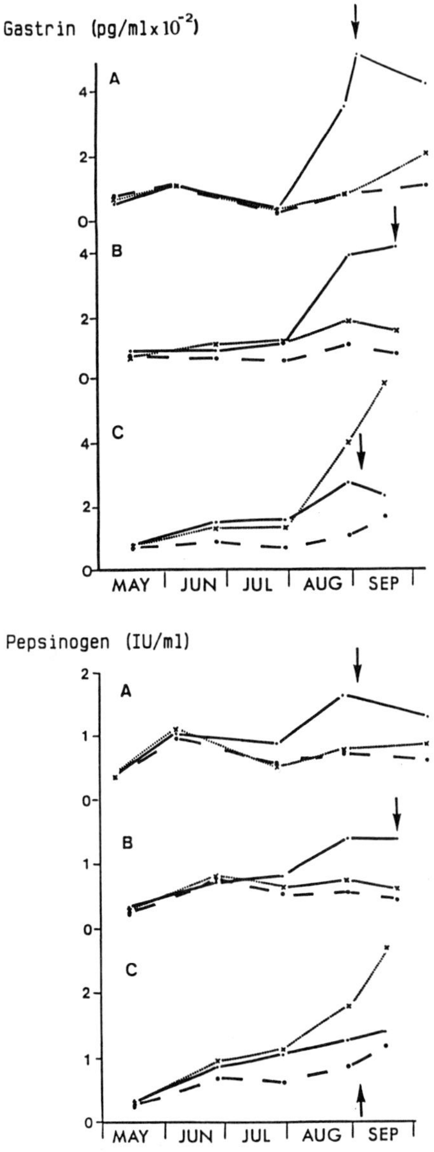

Fig. 1. Mean serum pepsinogen and gastrin values of calves in trials A, B and C. (Solid lines, untreated control groups; interrupted lines, alternative prophylactic anthelmintic treatment groups; arrows, therapeutic treatment of control groups.)

makes the hormone a potentially valuable tool in the diagnosis of ostertagiasis.

Field Infection

Worm eggs, deposited by first-season calves during spring and early summer, give rise to potentially dangerous levels of infective larvae on pasture during the latter half of the grazing season. This sequence of events was recorded on the control paddocks. In contrast, the prophylactic treatments reduced pasture contamination in all but one trial (farm C), with the result that the challenge to which calves were exposed later in the season was minimised. The degree of abomasal damage associated with *Ostertagia* infection in each group is reflected by the relative changes in pepsinogen and gastrin levels shown in Fig. 1.

In trials A and B the control group experienced the most severe abomasal damage. The correlation between mean pepsinogen and mean gastrin for the control group on each farm was highly significant ($r = 0{\cdot}85$ ($P < 0{\cdot}01$); $0{\cdot}93$ ($P < 0{\cdot}001$); and $0{\cdot}89$ ($P < 0{\cdot}001$) in trials A, B and C respectively), although gastrin levels rose later in the infection than pepsinogen levels. Furthermore, the difference in gastrin levels between control and treated groups was greater in each trial than the corresponding difference in pepsinogen values.

CONCLUSIONS

The magnitude of the gastrin response combined with its close correlation with changes in pepsinogen levels indicate that gastrin is of value in the diagnosis of bovine ostertagiasis in first-season animals. The fact that gastrin only appears to increase later during the course of *Ostertagia* infection, i.e. when adult worms are present, may also be an advantage in the diagnosis of infection in older immune cattle. Elevated pepsinogen levels in these animals may reflect increased larval intake which is not accompanied by a large adult-worm burden. Under these circumstances, gastrin levels might distinguish animals with elevated pepsinogen levels, associated merely with increased larval intake, from those harbouring a pathogenic worm burden.

ACKNOWLEDGEMENTS

Financial support was provided by the Agricultural and Food Research Council, Central Research Fund (University of London) and Coopers

Animal Health Ltd. The authors also wish to thank the Department of Parasitology, Glasgow Veterinary School, for providing the *Ostertagia* larvae.

REFERENCES

BOLTON, A. E. (1982) Validation of radioimmunoassays. *Irish Veterinary Journal*, **36**, 27–30.

MYLREA, P. J. & HOTSON, I. K. (1969) Serum pepsinogen activity and the diagnosis of bovine ostertagiasis. *British Veterinary Journal*, **125**, 379–388.

Quantitative Assay of 19-Nortestosterone in Meat by Chemiluminescence Immunoassay

C. Van Peteghem

Laboratory of Food Analysis, State University of Ghent, Belgium

The recently developed chemiluminescence immunoassay for 19-nortestosterone (Janssen *et al.*, 1984) was applied to the detection and quantitative assay of that compound in muscle tissue.

As in most other countries, 19-nortestosterone (19-NT) is prohibited in Belgium as an anabolic agent in cattle. Meat and organs intended for human consumption are considered harmful to human health if they contain residues of any anabolic or growth stimulating agent. Although muscle, except at implantation or injection sites, shows the lowest concentrations, it is generally the only matrix which is available for analysis.

Meat samples were digested enzymatically, extracted with diethyl ether, and purified by column chromatography on Lipidex and by reversed-phase HPLC. The final extract was then clean enough to permit quantitative measurements in the pg/g range.

The limit of quantification is 0·6 ng/g. This is calculated from the chemiluminescence signals from certified blank meat samples, which are significantly different ($p < 0{\cdot}001$) from the 125 pg standard of the standard curve but not from the 62·5 pg standard. The limit of detection, i.e. the minimum quantity of analyte which can be detected on the standard curve, is 12 ± 8 pg ($n = 8$). It depends on the slope of that curve and on the variance of the zero standard.

To check the reliability of the method, a certified negative sample and a spiked (1 ng/g) positive sample are run as quality controls in each assay. The within-day variation is 4·3% (concentration of 19-NT in muscle tissue is about 2 ng/g). Day-to-day variation has yet to be established.

REFERENCE

JANSSEN, E. H. J. M., ZOMER, G., VAN DEN BERG, R. H. & STEPHANY, R. W. (1984) Development of a chemiluminescent immunoassay for 19-nortestosterone (nandrolene). *Veterinary Quarterly*, **6**, 102–104.

Enzyme Immunoassay for the Feed Additive Monensin

M. E. MOUNT, D. L. FAILLA

Department of Clinical Pathology, School of Veterinary Medicine, University of California, Davis, California, USA

and

S. WIE

Environmental Diagnostics Inc., Burlington, North Carolina, USA

Monensin (Fig. 1) is an important representative of the polyether ionophore antibiotics which are finding numerous applications in the field of livestock production and veterinary medicine (Goodrich *et al.*, 1984). However, poisoning has occurred as a result of extensive usage (Beck & Harries, 1979). Various analytical methods to detect monensin are available but, in general, these assays are restricted to specialised laboratories. The advantages which immunoassay offers could potentially overcome many of the current difficulties. Immunoassays give flexibility in analyte determination (Ngo, 1985), and a modified indirect enzyme immunoassay (miEIA) has been developed, as has a research prototype which is a spot test using competitive enzyme immunoassay (cEIA) principles (Voller *et al.*, 1979). Although monensin is a carboxylic acid ionophore, this functional group was not chosen as the coupling site since this serves as an important site biologically. The primary 26-hydroxyl group of monensin was chosen as an alternative site to derivatise for coupling; it was believed to have reacted with bromoacetyl bromide which introduced a leaving group, allowing for protein coupling with lysyl residues. The reaction of bromoacetyl bromide and laidlomycin, which is also a carboxylic acid ionophore and closely resembles monensin structurally, has served as a model, since selective acylation of the 26 position has been demonstrated (Clark *et al.*, 1982). The resulting monensin bromoacetate then alkylated protein primary amines by displacement of bromide (Sweet *et al.*, 1972).

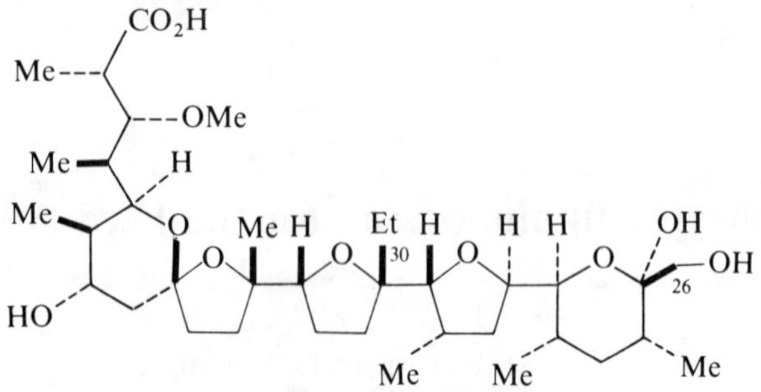

Fig. 1. Structure of monensin.

Monensin sodium (639 mg, 1 mmol) was dissolved in 10 ml of dichloromethane with 20 μl pyridine and stirred on ice. Bromoacetyl bromide (200 μl) was added dropwise over 30 s. The residue containing monensin bromoacetate following clean-up was dissolved in 25 ml tetrahydrofuran (THF) and added to 25 ml of 0·5 M lithium borate buffer (LBB, pH 9·35) containing 250 mg of BSA. The mixture was then dialysed exhaustively to remove uncoupled monensin derivative. KLH and HRP conjugates of monensin were both prepared in similar fashion. New Zealand white rabbits were immunised (Vaitukaitis *et al.*, 1971) with a 1 mg/ml antigen mixed 50:50 with Freund's complete adjuvant initially, followed by Freund's incomplete adjuvant thereafter. Antisera were collected and purified by equivalence zone adsorption (Garvey *et al.*, 1977) and ammonium sulphate precipitation (Herbert *et al.*, 1973), and stored at −60°C. A solid-phase miEIA was established using ABTS/H_2O_2 as the substrate.

A research prototype of a rapid card test (Environmental Diagnostics) was made incorporating a zone treated with monensin-specific antibodies. A standard or sample was then added to the zone, followed by the enzyme–monensin conjugate and then the substrate. The addition of three drops of substrate allowed for removal of unbound enzyme conjugate via the absorbent design. Inhibition of colour development indicated the presence of monensin.

Spiked horse sera and horse urine were diluted serially in PBST and analysed directly. Faecal samples (1 g) were extracted with dichloromethane (5 ml). Following evaporation, 1 ml of PBST was added followed by analysis. The miEIA had a detection limit of 10 ng/ml sodium monensin. Direct analysis of serum or urine spiked with 10 ng/ml sodium monensin or a dichloromethane extract of faeces spiked with 100 ng/ml sodium monensin resulted in recovery of monensin ranging from 53 to 130%.

Cross-reactivity studies were performed with other polyether ionophores such as narasin, lasalocid and laidlomycin. The antibody had a 52% cross-reactivity with laidlomycin, a striking result since this ionophore differs from monensin only in a propionyl substituent in place of a methyl group at carbon number 30 (Fig. 1). No cross-reactivity was observed with the other ionophores.

This assay provides an excellent screening technique to detect monensin in biological samples. This will greatly aid diagnostic laboratories in evaluating the potential for monensin intoxication of poultry or livestock. The rapid card test kit when available for field application will need further testing with biological samples. It is anticipated that veterinary practitioners would be able to use this in the field with minimal effort and that this would provide them with an excellent diagnostic tool.

REFERENCES

Beck, B. E. & Harries, W. N. (1979) The diagnosis of monensin toxicosis: a report on outbreaks in horses, cattle, and chickens. *Proceedings of the 22nd Annual Meeting of the American Association of Veterinary Laboratory Diagnosticians*, **22**, 269–282.

Clark, R. D., Hedden, G. L., Kluge, A. F. & Modox, M. L. (1982) Enhancement of the activity of the antibiotic laidlomycin by acylation and the ^{13}C-NMR spectra of laidlomycin and its esters. *Journal of Antibiotics*, **35**, 1527–1537.

Garvey, J. S., Cremer, N. E. & Sussdorf, D. H. (1977) In: *Methods in Immunology*, 3rd edn, The Benjamin/Cummings Publishing Company, Massachusetts, pp. 273–299.

Goodrich, R. D., Garrett, J. E., Gast, D. R., Kirick, M. A., Larson, D. A. & Meiske, J. C. (1984) Influence of monensin on the performance of cattle. *Journal of Animal Science*, **58**, 1484–1498.

Herbert, G. A., Pelham, P. L. & Pittman, B. (1973) Determination of the optimal ammonium sulfate concentration for the fractionation of rabbit, sheep, horse, and goat antisera. *Applied Microbiology*, **25**, 26–36.

Ngo, T. T. (1985) Enzyme-mediated immunoassay: an overview. In: *Enzyme-mediated Immunoassay*, Ngo, T. T. & Lenhoff, H. M. (eds), Plenum Press, New York, pp. 3–6.

Sweet, F., Arias, F. & Warren, J. C. (1972) Affinity labeling of steroid binding sites. *Journal of Biological Chemistry*, **247**, 3414–3433.

Vaitukaitis, J., Robbins, J. B., Nieschlag, E. & Ross, G. T. (1971) A method for producing specific antisera with small doses of immunogen. *Journal of Clinical Endocrinology*, **33**, 988.

Voller, A., Bidwell, D. E. & Bartlett, A. (1979) The enzyme-linked immunosorbent assay (ELISA). Dynatech Laboratories Inc., Alexandria, Virginia, pp. 7–21.

The Analysis of Chloramphenicol Residues in Animal Tissue by RIA

K. W. Freebairn, N. T. Crosby
Laboratory of the Government Chemist, London, UK

and

J. Landon
Department of Chemical Pathology, St Bartholomew's Hospital, London, UK

INTRODUCTION

The antibiotic chloramphenicol (CAP) is now only used clinically in humans as a last resort. This is because the drug has in some cases been found to cause bone marrow damage. Since CAP is a very effective and therefore widely used drug for the treatment of a number of infections in cattle, poultry and swine, concern has been voiced over the possibility of residues finding their way into food for human consumption. A RIA procedure has been developed for monitoring CAP levels in the low part per billion range with a view eventually to adapting the technique to an ELISA.

EXPERIMENTAL DETAILS

Production of Anti-Chloramphenicol Antiserum

A polyclonal anti-CAP antiserum was prepared by the Department of Chemical Pathology, St Bartholomew's Hospital, London. CAP was rendered immunogenic by conjugating it, or various derivatives, to keyhole limpet haemocyanin (KLH) as listed below (see Fig. 1).

Immunogen 1 was prepared from CAP hemisuccinate using a carbodiimide reaction. Immunogen 2: after preparation of the amine derivative

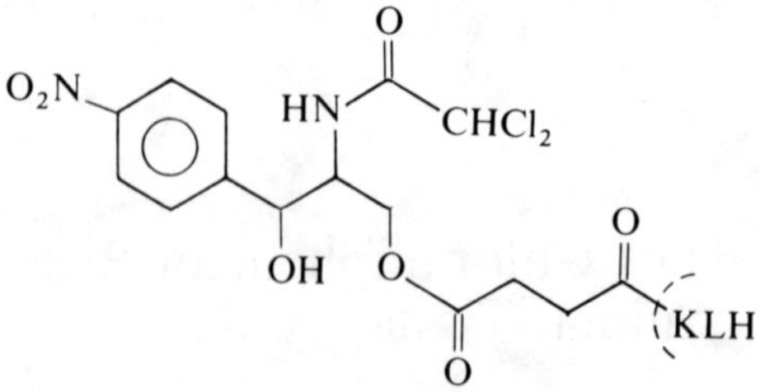

Immunogen 1

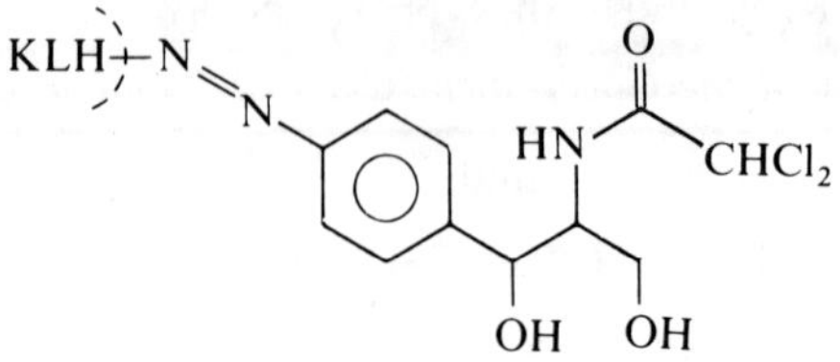

Immunogen 2

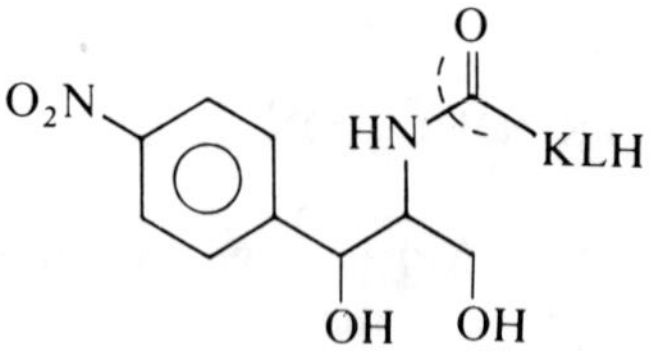

Immunogen 3

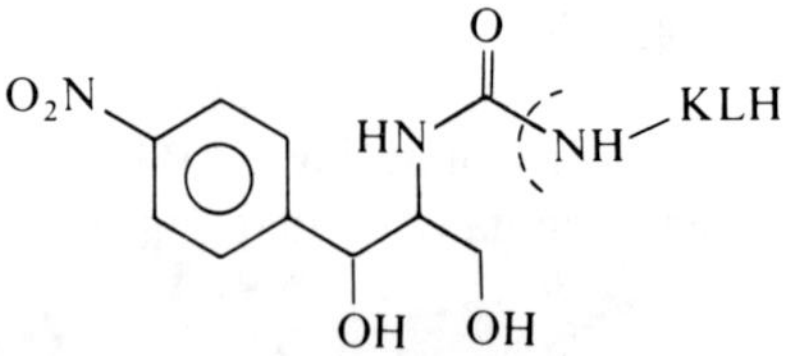

Immunogen 4

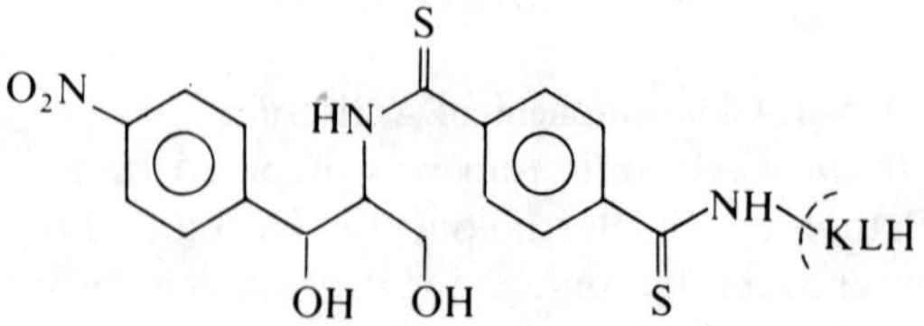

Immunogen 5

Fig. 1. Immunogens used for antisera production.

of CAP by reducing the nitro group (high-pressure hydrogenation), the reduced CAP product was diazotised and coupled to KLH. Immunogen 3 was prepared from CAP base using 1-ethyl-3-(dimethylaminopropyl)-carbodiimide HCl and KLH. Immunogen 4 was prepared by reacting the bifunctional reagent *N,N*-disuccinimidyl carbonate with CAP base, the resulting products being reacted with KLH under alkaline conditions. Immunogen 5 was prepared by reacting the bifunctional reagent phenylenediisothiocyanate with CAP base and reacting the products with KLH under alkaline conditions.

Only the antisera raised against immunogen 1 recognised ^{14}C-labelled CAP (Amersham International plc, Amersham, Bucks).

Chloramphenicol in Tissue—Extraction and Clean-up

Samples of unheated tissue were freeze-dried and defatted before homogenising with PBS. The homogenate was then, if necessary, incubated with glucuronidase/aryl sulphatase to hydrolyse conjugates arising from CAP metabolism.

After centrifugation at high speed, C_{18} solid-phase extraction cartridges were used to clean up methanolic aliquots of the supernatant, CAP being eluted directly into RIA tubes.

RIA Protocol

^{14}C-CAP (100 pCi, equivalent to ~2 pM) was incubated with CAP standards or sample extracts and a 1:4200 dilution of antiserum. Separation of the antibody-bound fraction was achieved with high molecular weight (200 000 to 275 000) dextran-coated charcoal.

RESULTS

To estimate the efficiency of the extraction and clean-up technique, a number of spiked beef samples of high fat content were analysed, together with unspiked samples. The spiked samples, equivalent to 950 pg CAP per tube, corresponded roughly to 2 ng CAP/g of raw meat.

No CAP was detected in any of the unspiked samples, while variable recoveries (ranging from 15 to 90%) were obtained for the spiked samples. The limit of detection of the RIA is in the region of 100 pg/tube, which with the extraction procedure described roughly corresponds to 0·2 ng CAP/g of raw meat.

DISCUSSION

Sensitivity is limited by the low specific activity of the ^{14}C-CAP. A tritium-labelled CAP tracer would allow a far greater specific activity to be obtained. Amersham International produces such a product (propionylated CAP base) but unfortunately this compound is not recognised by this anti-CAP antiserum.

The recovery problem is being investigated. It has already been shown, using radiotracer experiments, that losses are not occurring at the clean-up stage. It is thought that the problem may be due to the high fat content of the samples. A more efficient defatting procedure is now being investigated, and a competitive ELISA using an in-house-produced CAP–BSA coating conjugate and a phosphatase-labelled donkey anti-sheep (Serotec) second antibody is being developed based upon the work of Campbell *et al.* (1984).

REFERENCE

Campbell, G. S., Mageau, R. P., Schwab, B. & Johnston, R. W. (1984) Detection and quantitation of chloramphenicol by competitive enzyme-linked immunoassay. *Antimicrobial Agents and Chemotherapy*, **25**, 205–211.

Development of an ELISA for the Detection of Antibodies to *Pasteurella anatipestifer*

R. M. Hatfield, B. A. Morris and R. R. Henry

Division of Clinical Biochemistry, Department of Biochemistry, University of Surrey, Guildford, UK

INTRODUCTION

Pasteurella anatipestifer (PA), species incertae sedis, is responsible for an economically important disease of commercially raised ducks (*Anas platyrhynchos*). Ducks of all ages are susceptible to infection, but the disease is usually associated with birds aged between three and six weeks. Unacceptable losses as a result of high mortality and the necessity for increased culling and condemnation at slaughter usually follow. The poultry industry currently uses rapid slide agglutination (RSA) and agar gel precipitin (AGP) methods to detect antibodies to this organism; however, these procedures are insensitive and only detect agglutinating and/or precipitating antibodies. There is a need for a rapid, sensitive and reproducible method capable of screening large numbers of sera for anti-PA antibodies. This poster presentation describes the first development and validation of an ELISA for the detection of anti-PA antibodies in duck sera.

MATERIALS AND METHODS

Antigen

A freeze–thawed extract of PA type 2 containing 50 mg protein/100 ml was diluted 1:8 in carbonate–bicarbonate buffer (pH 9·6) and 100 μl volumes of this preparation used to coat the assay wells of the microtitration plate.

Positive and Negative Reference Sera

Four birds were inoculated with an alhydrogel-adsorbed formalised PA vaccine given at 23 and 48 days after hatching. These birds were bled

10 days following the booster injection and the harvested sera combined to form the positive control pool.

Non-vaccinated birds, reared in special isolation units, were bled at 27 days of age and these samples used to provide the negative control pool.

Effect of Sodium Chloride Concentration in PBS/Tween 80 Wash Buffer on Non-specific Binding (NSB)

Positive and negative reference sera were diluted to 1:100 in each of a series of PBS/Tween 80 buffers containing NaCl concentrations ranging from 0·15 to 2·0M (Case *et al.*, 1982) and the ELISA performed. NSB was evaluated as the amount of colour developed in the absence of antigen.

ELISA protocol

100 μl volumes of the test sera diluted to 1:100 in PBS/Tween 80 were pipetted into the antigen-coated wells of a microtitration plate and incubated for 1 h at 37°C. The plate was then washed and 100 μl of a 1:600 dilution of rabbit anti-duck immunoglobulin antiserum were added. After incubation for 1 h, the plate was again washed and 100 μl of a horseradish peroxidase (HRP)-labelled donkey anti-rabbit IgG antiserum diluted to 1:4000 were added, followed by a further incubation for 1 h. Unbound conjugate was removed by washing and the substrate hydrogen peroxide with *o*-phenylenediamine, prepared in phosphate–citrate buffer (pH 5·0), added. The reaction was stopped after 45 min at 22°C by the addition of 100 μl of 2·5M H_2SO_4.

Prediction Curve

Nineteen sera were assayed at a 1:100 dilution in the ELISA and the measured absorbance obtained for each of these samples plotted against the serum end-point titre. The line of best fit was obtained using the method of least squares regression analysis.

Precision

Three duck serum QC pools, representing varying levels of anti-PA antibodies, were added randomly to ten antigen-coated wells of the assay plate and the ELISA performed. From the standard deviation of the absorbance measurements, the within-assay CV was derived for the serum QC pools. The between-assay CV ($n = 60$) was derived by assaying the same QC pools in the ELISA over six consecutive assays.

Specificity
Antisera were raised against PA types 1 and 2, *Salmonella typhimurium*, *Salmonella anatum*, *Pasteurella multocida*, *Escherichia coli* and *Acinetobacter calcoaceticus*, and samples shown by RSA to contain agglutinating antibodies to the homologous antigen. These sera were then assayed in the ELISA.

Comparison of ELISA, RSA and AGP Tests for Detecting Anti-PA Antibodies
Ducks were injected 27 days after hatching with a PA vaccine and bled at intervals thereafter. Serum samples were stored at −20°C until required.

RESULTS

Preparation of PA Antigen
This organism was found to grow very readily on blood agar, and the stock antigen preparation used for the duration of these investigations demonstrated no loss of immunoreactivity in the ELISA.

Reduction of NSB in the ELISA
It was found that by increasing the NaCl concentration in the PBS/Tween 80 diluent progressively from 0·15 to 1·0M the NSB value was reduced from 0·25 to 0·04 absorbance units. NaCl was added to the PBS/Tween 80 wash buffer to give a final concentration of 1·0M in all further work.

Prediction Curve
Significant correlation ($r = 0{\cdot}99$) was demonstrated between the absorbance measurements obtained for a 1:100 dilution of sample in the ELISA and its end-point titre (Fig. 1). This enabled serum antibody levels to be expressed as a titre value.

Precision
Within-assay CVs of 3·2, 4·9 and 6·3% respectively were found for the three duck serum QC pools representing high, mid-range and low levels of anti-PA antibodies. Similarly, between-assay CVs of 6·8, 8·3 and 8·6% respectively were obtained.

Specificity
Samples known to contain agglutinating antibodies to the potentially interfering bacterial antigens gave no significant reactions. There were no

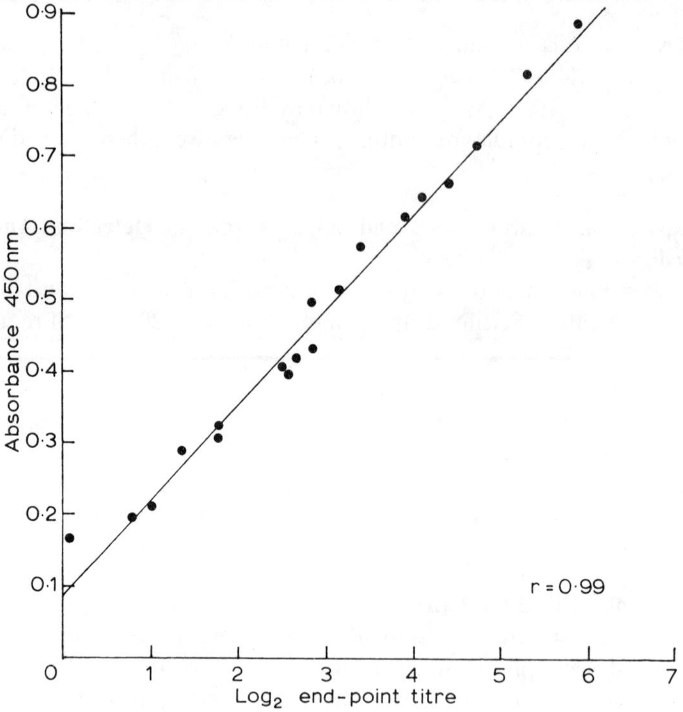

Fig. 1. Correlation between end-point titre and A_{450} of a 1:100 dilution of 19 duck sera as determined by ELISA.

false positives, the ELISA detecting antibodies to PA only in serum samples from birds inoculated with that organism.

Comparison of ELISA, RSA and AGP

Four days after vaccination, anti-PA antibodies were just detectable in two of the five birds. Three days later, antibodies were detected by ELISA in all five birds, but not by RSA or AGP. Ten days after vaccination, agglutinating antibodies were detected in two of the experimental birds by RSA. Not until four days later were precipitating antibodies shown to be present in one of these birds by AGP.

CONCLUSIONS

A reproducible and specific ELISA has been developed for the detection of anti-*P. anatipestifer* antibodies. High NSBs initially encountered were reduced by the use of 1·0M NaCl in the sample diluent.

It was established that $\log_2$ end-point titre exhibited a significant correlation with A_{450} of a 1:100 dilution of serum in the ELISA and enabled a prediction curve to be constructed.

This assay is able to detect anti-*P. anatipestifer* antibodies earlier than either RSA or AGP and therefore provides a much earlier warning of onset of infection.

REFERENCE

Case, J. T., Ardans, A. A., Bolton, D. C. & Reynolds, B. J. (1982) Optimisation of parameters for detecting antibodies against infectious bronchitis virus using an enzyme-linked immunosorbent assay: temporal response to vaccination and challenge with live virus. *Avian Diseases*, **27**, 196–210.

Development of a Practical ELISA for the Detection of Trichina in Pork

P. SINGH, D. G. OLIVER, M. ABAD, N. VAIL, L. JANG, T. BROCK and D. ALLISON

Idetek Inc., San Bruno, California, USA

INTRODUCTION

Ninety million hogs are slaughtered each year in the US, of which 0·1% are infected with the worm *Trichinella spiralis* (Woods *et al.*, 1985; National Pork Producers' Council, 1984). This translates into over 13 million pounds weight of pork that is contaminated with the trichina worms. Responsibility for trichinosis control in the US is centred on the processing of pork by commercial producers or the consumer. The processing methods used for trichina control involve curing, freezing or cooking to destroy encysted trichina larvae. The US pork industry is convinced that the domestic demand and export of pork would substantially increase if certified trichina-safe pork were available. To ensure this, it is critical to identify and eliminate trichina-infected hogs at the time of slaughter.

METHOD

The system that has been developed for routine use in a slaughterhouse is based on a standard ELISA technique. This ELISA detects the presence of antibodies to *T. spiralis* in hogs by utilising an excretory–secretory (ES) antigen produced by the trichina worm (Gamble *et al.*, 1983). The ES antigen is coated on to the wells of a standard microtitration plate. The absorbance measurement for the sample, when compared to the negative and positive reference standards, is calculated as a per cent EIA. Results greater than 15% EIA are considered positive.

Table 1
Intra-assay Variability of Control Samples ($n = 30$)

	Run 1	*Run 2*	*Run 3*
Negative			
Mean optical density	0·178	0·243	0·219
Standard deviation	0·012	0·038	0·012
%CV	6·7	15·6	5·3
Positive			
Mean optical density	0·925	1·103	1·074
Standard deviation	0·044	0·042	0·033
%CV	4·7	3·8	3·0

RESULTS

Intra-assay variability for negative and positive samples exhibits a CV of less than 16% ($n = 30$) (see Table 1). Day-to-day precision of less than 10% CV was also found for high and low positive control samples tested over a three-week period. (High positive: $\bar{x}$ (%EIA), 66·06; SD, 5·62; CV, 8·52; *n*, 83. Medium positive: $\bar{x}$, 49·42; SD, 4·5; CV, 9·0; *n*, 83.) Inter-operator variability of three trichina antibody test kits, which contained different sets of reagents and plates coated with ES antigen, was determined by three different workers. The reproducibility of results for negative and positive reference standards, and negative and positive control samples, between operators was less than 5%.

In a study carried out in a slaughterhouse* (Oliver *et al.*, 1986), blood samples and corresponding diaphragm muscle sections were collected from 3005 hogs at the time of slaughter. The diaphragm muscle sections were tested for trichina larvae using a standard pooled digestion technique. Of the 3005 samples tested by ELISA, one sample appeared to be a false negative and 2·6% of the samples were considered to be false positives when compared to the digestion technique. The false negative sample had less than one-tenth larvae per gram of diaphragm. The false positive samples occurred in a single group of hogs, indicating a common origin, and are therefore assumed to be real positives.

* Field trial studies were carried out at Lundy Packing Company in Clinton, North Carolina, USA. The studies were funded by the North Carolina Pork Producers and the National Pork Producers' Council, USA.

Samples were collected from 26 trichina-infected hogs (22 positive, 4 negative) in which larvae concentrations were known. No false negative or false positive results were obtained for these samples when tested by ELISA for anti-trichina antibodies. There was no correlation between the larvae count and the observed ELISA values.

DISCUSSION

The ELISA is capable of detecting trichina-infected hogs even when the level of infection is quite low. Differences in antigenic response, the level and duration of infection can account for the lack of correlation between %EIA for samples and corresponding larvae counts. Hogs with very light infection can be detected provided that there has been time to develop anti-trichina antibodies. Such lack of time may be the reason for the false negative sample found in the slaughterhouse group. The manufacturing of antigen and reagents for this assay has shown that they can be reproduced and results for different reagents are repeatable with various operators.

Automation is necessary if the operator is to keep up with the high kill rate at slaughterhouses and test each hog. This is possible with the use of a robotic sample handler. The analysis time for the assay with the automated system is less than 90 min. This allows for sufficient time to identify a trichina-infected hog before it reaches the cutting and processing areas. A bar-code identification system has been developed in order to track and identify infected hogs. Trichina-positive animals can also be traced to the farm of origin so that the source of infection can be identified and eliminated.

CONCLUSION

The ELISA for trichina antibody in swine could allow the US pork industry to provide the consumer with certified trichina-safe pork, allowing domestic demand and US export of pork to increase. Combining this assay with high-speed automated instrumentation and a bar-code identification system, slaughterhouses would be able to track, identify and eliminate trichina-infected hogs. Use of this system by slaughterhouses could eventually lead to the eradication of human trichinosis caused by infected pork.

REFERENCES

GAMBLE, H. R., ANDERSON, W. R., GRAHAM, C. E. & MURRELL, K. D. (1983) Diagnosis of swine trichinosis by enzyme-linked immunosorbent assay (ELISA) using an excretory–secretory antigen. *Veterinary Parasitology*, **13**, 349–361.

NATIONAL PORK PRODUCERS' COUNCIL (1984) *Trichina safe pork*, Des Moines, Iowa 50306, USA.

OLIVER, D. G., SINGH, P., ABAD, M. & VAIL, N. (1986) Development of high volume testing systems for certifying trichina free pork. *Proceedings IVth International Symposium of Veterinary Laboratory Diagnostics*, 296–299.

WOODS, G. T., BIEHL, L. G., HANKENS, R. & MURRELL, K. D. (1985) Trichinosis. In: *Pork Industry Handbook*, Cooperative Extension Service, Purdue University, Indiana, USA.

Application of ELISA in Sheep Lungworm (*Dictyocaulus filaria*) Infection

S. M. Thamsborg

Institute of Internal Medicine, Royal Veterinary and Agricultural University, Copenhagen, Denmark

INTRODUCTION

Dictyocaulus filaria is a bronchial parasite which may spread to the gastrointestinal tract and cause varying degrees of coughing and weight loss. In Denmark, the epidemiology and the prevalence of *D. filaria* infection is not fully understood. Traditionally, the infection is diagnosed by the demonstration of larvae in faeces. However, *Dictyocaulus* infections are known to produce circulating antibodies and a variety of serological tests have been developed for their detection (Cornwell, 1963; Movsesijan & Lalić, 1971; Bokhout *et al.*, 1979; Boon *et al.*, 1982; Joshi *et al.*, 1984).

The aim of this work was to develop an ELISA capable of detecting antibodies to *D. filaria* and to investigate the assay as a diagnostic tool.

MATERIALS AND METHODS

ELISA

The assay was performed as a non-competitive indirect ELISA, measuring antibody binding to *D. filaria* antigen. The antigen was a crude aqueous extract of adult worms, diluted in carbonate buffer to approximately 5 μg protein per ml. Polystyrene plates (Nunc, DK) were coated for 18 h at 20°C, followed by saturation with 4% horse serum in PBS. All washings were done with tap water containing 0·5% Tween 20. Sera were added to the plate in two-fold serial dilutions ranging from 1/20 to 1/2560. HRP-conjugated rabbit anti-sheep Ig (Dakopatt, DK) was used for antibody detection. The colour reaction with the substrate 2,2′-azinobis(3-ethylbenzothiazoline-6-sulphonic acid) (ABTS) was stopped with 96% ethanol after 30 min at 20°C and the absorbance read at 405 nm using an EIA plate reader (Bio-Tek).

A titration of a positive standard serum was included on every plate, together with controls. The titre of a serum was defined as the highest dilution which gave a positive reaction (end-point titre) (Voller *et al.*, 1979). A titre of 1 corresponded to a dilution of 1/20, a titre of 2 to 1/40, and so forth. A serum negative at any dilution was assigned the titre of 0. The threshold value of absorbance for positive reaction was calculated as the mean of absorbance in dilutions 1/640 and 1/1280 of the standard positive serum on the same plate. Consequently the standard positive serum was always assigned the titre of 6. The precision of the assay was evaluated by the coefficient of variation (CV) for the threshold value. Intra-assay CV was 5·1%.

Faecal Method

10 g of faeces obtained from the rectum were examined for larvae by a modified Baermann technique (Nevenić *et al.*, 1962).

EXPERIMENTAL DESIGN

Experiment 1

Six four-month-old lambs raised indoors were infected with *D. filaria* and slaughtered 35 days later. Serum samples were also obtained from 14 lambs and ewes infected with gastrointestinal worms, but no lungworms.

Experiment 2

Twenty-six ewes with 18 lambs were allocated to two groups and put on worm-free pasture in two adjacent pens from late May to mid-October 1984. Some ewes were naturally infected with *D. filaria.* In one group, lambs and ewes were treated intensively with anthelmintics until August. The other group was untreated. This experimental design was repeated in 1985.

Experiment 3

Sera and faeces were collected in 18 flocks of grazing sheep in late August. Five lambs from each flock were sampled.

RESULTS AND DISCUSSION

Experiment 1

At necropsy, *D. filaria* were recovered from all infected lambs. Mean group titres were below 1·0 for 11 weeks before infection. The lambs showed a marked rise in titres, beginning two weeks after infection. All had a titre of 4 or above (mean 5·0) at the time of patency four weeks after infection.

Animals infected with gastrointestinal worms only had titres between 0 and 2, with the exclusion of a lamb and a ewe with titres of 3. A titre of 4 or above seemed indicative of *D. filaria* infection.

Experiment 2

In October, 80% of untreated lambs were found to be excreting *D. filaria* larvae. A rise in mean titres during the season from 0·0 to 5·0 was noticed for the same lambs (Fig. 1).

Some lambs had titres below 4 in early patency. Untreated ewes had a 66% incidence rate for the season as a whole, with a rise in mean titre from 3·3 to 7·0.

The eight lambs treated with anthelmintics did not excrete larvae at any time and had a mean titre rising from 0·0 to 1·8 in October.

Comparison of the faecal method and the ELISA for examination of the samples from lambs at the end of seasons 1984 and 1985 yielded an 83% sensitivity (22/26) and an 80% specificity (20/25). The low specificity is probably due to low sensitivity of the faecal technique used for comparison

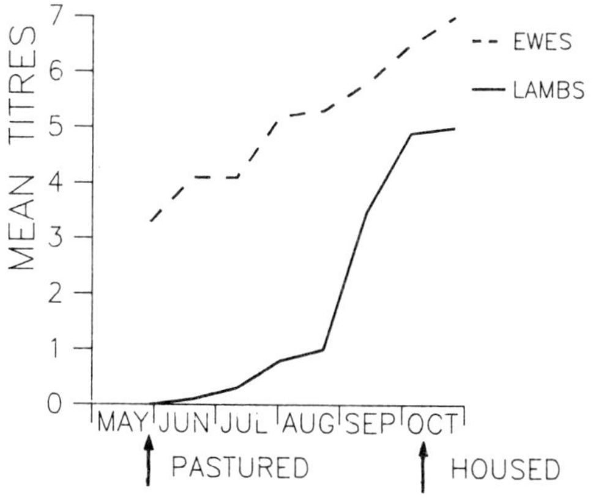

Fig. 1. Mean titres of lambs and ewes in the untreated flock during the 1984 grazing season.

(Thomas *et al.*, 1970), but cross-reactions with gastrointestinal worms may also play a part (Boon *et al.*, 1982).

A highly positive correlation was found between numbers of lambs excreting larvae and average antibody titre, but the assay did not seem so sensitive in early patency as found in experiment 1.

In both groups, some ewes had persistently high titres, apparently without excreting larvae, and it was therefore impossible to determine a cut-off level for ewes. Infection earlier in life or a higher degree of cross-reaction with gastrointestinal worms in older animals cannot be excluded.

Experiment 3

In the survey, no larvae were demonstrated in faeces of any animal on the day of sampling. The assay revealed mean titres above 4 in two flocks. The finding is suggestive of previous *D. filaria* exposure.

CONCLUSIONS

This preliminary work shows that ELISA is a practical technique capable of detecting antibodies against the sheep lungworm, *D. filaria*. The assay is sensitive in lambs, showing a marked rise in titre at the time of patency or in some cases 2–3 weeks later. Use of larval antigen instead of that of adult worms for coating the plates may, however, detect antibodies produced at an earlier stage of the infection (Bos *et al.*, 1986). The specificity is rather low, which results in a low predictive value in areas of low prevalence. The application of the ELISA in ewes is more complex, due to the low and intermittent excretion of larvae and therefore sometimes inexplicable high titres.

Field application of this assay, found suitable under controlled experimental conditions, appears to require further investigation.

REFERENCES

Bokhout, B. A., Boon, J. H. & Hendriks, J. (1979) Operational diagnostics of lungworm infections in cattle: preliminary investigation into the usefulness of IHA. *The Veterinary Quarterly*, **1**, 195–203.

Boon, J. H., Kloosterman, A. & Brink, R. van den (1982) The incidence of *D. viviparus* in cattle in The Netherlands. I. The ELISA as a diagnostic tool. *The Veterinary Quarterly*, **4**, 155–160.

BOS, J. H., BEEKMAN-BONESCHANSCHER, J. & BOON, J. H. (1986) Use of ELISA to assess lungworm infection in calves. *Veterinary Record*, **118**, 153–156.

CORNWELL, R. L. (1963) Complement fixing antibody response of calves to *D. viviparus*. *Journal of Comparative Pathology*, **73**, 297–308.

JOSHI, P., SINGH, B. P. & TEWARI, H. C. (1984) Use of the ELISA in the diagnosis of *D. filaria* infection. *Research in Veterinary Science*, **37**, 258–259.

MOVSESIJAN, M. & LALIĆ, R. (1971) Radioactive antibody studies on *D. filaria* infection. *Research in Veterinary Science*, **12**, 282–284.

NEVENIĆ, V., JOVANIĆ, M., SOKOLIĆ, A., CUPERLOVIĆ, K. & MOVSESIJAN, M. (1962) Jednostavan postupak za ustanovljenje larvica *D. filaria* (English abstract). *Veterinarski Glasnik*, **16**, 203–209.

THOMAS, R. J., NUNNS, V. J. & BOAG, B. (1970) The incidence of lungworm infection in sheep in north-east England. *Veterinary Record*, **87**, 70–75.

VOLLER, A., BIDWELL, D. E. & BARTLETT, A. (1979) *The Enzyme-linked Immunosorbent Assay*, Dynatech-Europe, Guernsey.

Amplification Systems in ELISA: Use of NAD Recycling System in the Immunoassay of *Clostridium botulinum* Toxins Types A and B in Food

N. K. Modi
Porton International Ltd, London, UK

C. C. Shone, P. Hambleton and J. Melling
PHLS, Centre for Applied Microbiology and Research, Porton Down, Salisbury, UK

INTRODUCTION

Clostridium botulinum produces eight serologically distinct toxins (Hobbs, 1976). These when ingested cause botulism, a disease with a relatively rare occurrence but high fatality. Detecting and serotyping these toxins therefore form important steps in identification of the organism responsible.

The mouse lethality test, being simple and sensitive (one mouse LD_{50} is approximately 5 pg pure neurotoxin (Shone *et al.*, 1985)), is at present widely used for detecting botulinum toxins. However, for the test to be specific, neutralisation tests have to be performed in parallel and in consequence large numbers of mice are needed, increasing the cost of the assay. Furthermore, the assay is slow, taking up to four days.

Although various *in vitro* assays for toxin have been reported, few are as sensitive and reliable as the mouse lethality test (Kazaki *et al.*, 1973; Notermans & Kazaki, 1981; Hobbs *et al.*, 1982; Neaves & Gibbs, 1983; Shone *et al.*, 1985). This poster presentation describes: (a) amplified ELISAs for botulinum neurotoxin types A and B, using a commercially available NAD recycling system; (b) the ability of these ELISAs to detect the toxins present in food extracts; and (c) the specificity of various monoclonal antibodies (Mabs) used in these assays.

METHODS

Production of Monoclonal Antibodies

Purified neurotoxin type A (from NCTC 2916) and type B (from Danish strain) were used to immunise BALB/c mice (Hambleton *et al.*, 1981; Shone *et al.*, 1985; Evans *et al.*, 1986) and hybridoma cell lines obtained as described earlier (Irons *et al.*, 1983; Shone *et al.*, 1985). Mabs were purified from ascites fluid using protein A–Sepharose 4B (Ely *et al.*, 1978). The four Mabs, BA11 and BA56 obtained using toxin A and BB68 and BB75 obtained using toxin B, belonged to the subclass IgG_1 (Modi *et al.*, 1986).

ELISA for Anti-Neurotoxin Antibody

Sixty inner wells of a 96-well microtitration plate (Dynatech 129A or Nunc Immuno plate I) were coated overnight at 4°C with neurotoxin A or B (100 μl/well, 20 μg/ml). The toxin solutions were prepared using PBS (8·1 mM Na_2HPO_4, 1·5 mM KH_2PO_4, 140 mM NaCl and 2·7 mM KCl). The wells were emptied, shaken and blocked with GPB (0·7 M Na_2HPO_4, 0·2% (w/v) gelatin and adjusted to pH 6·5 with HCl) containing 1% (w/v) BSA (GPBSAB). Alternatively RPMI cell culture medium (Imperial Laboratories, Salisbury) containing 10% (v/v) FCS (RPMI-S10) at 150 μl/well, was used, and incubated at 37°C for 2 h. The wells were emptied, dried and serial dilutions of antibody samples added at 100μl/well. The plate was incubated at room temperature with shaking for 2 h, emptied, washed three times with PBST (containing 0·1% (v/v) Tween 20) and dried by shaking. Rabbit anti-mouse IgG–HRP conjugate (Dako Products), diluted 1:200 with GPBSAB or RPMI-S10, was added at 100 μl/well and incubated at room temperature with shaking for a further 2 h. The wells were emptied, washed three times with PBST, dried and the peroxidase substrate (see below) added at 100 μl/well. The plate was then incubated at room temperature with shaking for 30 min.

Ten milligrams of 3,3′,5,5′-tetramethylbenzidine were dissolved in 1 ml of dimethylsulphoxide. An aliquot (100 μl) of this solution was added to 10 ml of 0·1 M sodium acetate–citric acid buffer of pH 6·0. 8 μl of 6% (w/v) H_2O_2 were then added to the above solution. After substrate incubation, the reaction was stopped by adding 2 M H_2SO_4 at 50 μl/well and the absorbances read at 450 nm using a Dynatech MR580 plate reader.

ELISAs for Neurotoxins

These were performed similarly, except that the order of addition of reagents to the plate was immobilised monoclonal or polyclonal antibody, neurotoxin (serially diluted in GPB) and appropriate anti-neurotoxin–HRP conjugate. The sensitivity of an ELISA was defined as the concentration of neurotoxin (mouse LD_{50}/ml) which gave an absorbance of 0·1 units above the neurotoxin negative control.

Amplified ELISAs

These were performed as described earlier (Shone *et al.*, 1985) and as diagrammatically depicted in Fig. 1. The sensitivity of an amplified ELISA was defined as the concentration of neurotoxin (mouse LD_{50}/ml) which gave an absorbance of 0·3 units above the neurotoxin negative control.

The absence of a matrix effect was demonstrated by establishing that assay performance was not affected when neurotoxin standards were diluted in an extract from 'uncontaminated' salmon.

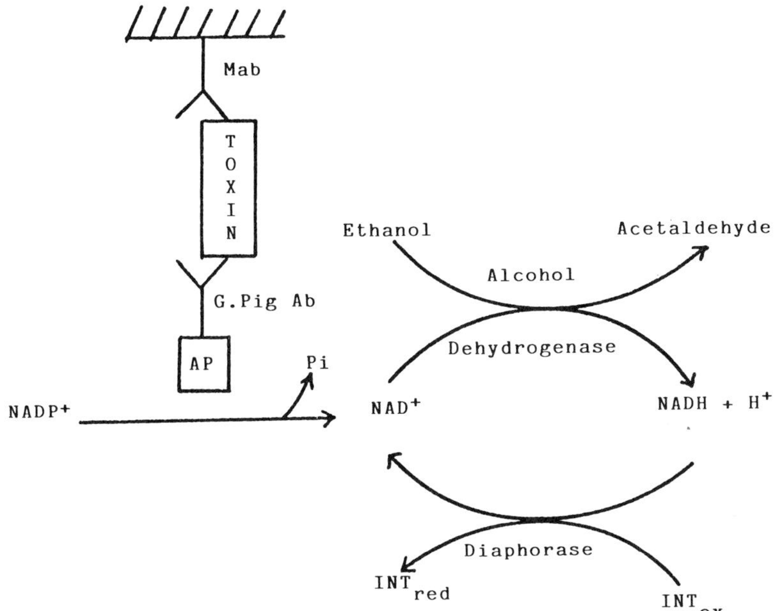

Fig. 1. The amplified ELISA. Mab, monoclonal antibody; G.Pig Ab, guinea pig polyclonal antibody; AP, alkaline phosphatase; INT_{red}, reduced iodonitrotetrazolium; INT_{ox}, oxidised iodonitrotetrazolium.

Preparation of Antibody–Enzyme Conjugates

Guinea pig antibodies against neurotoxin types A and B were raised and purified as described earlier (Shone *et al.*, 1985). These antibodies were conjugated to alkaline phosphatase using succinimidyl-4-(*N*-maleimidomethyl)cyclohexane-1-carboxylate by IQ Bio Ltd, Cambridge. HRP was conjugated to appropriate antibodies as previously described (O'Sullivan & Marks, 1981).

Preparation of Food Extracts

A total of approximately 5×10^4 mouse LD_{50} units (approximately 0·5 ml of a culture supernatant) was mixed with 100 g of food material and 100 ml of TGS (100 mM Tris-HCl buffer of pH 7·5 containing 0·2% (w/v) gelatin and 150 mM NaCl) added. The mixture was processed for about 5 min in a stomacher and centrifuged at 10 000*g* for 30 min at 4°C. An aliquot of the supernatant was subjected to amplified ELISA. Parallel mouse-bioassays in duplicate were performed to estimate the neurotoxin in the food extract. The recovery of added neurotoxin averaged $78 \pm 13\%$ ($n = 8$).

Neurotoxin Neutralisation Test

This was performed as previously described (Shone *et al.*, 1985).

Table 1
Comparison of Amplified and Unamplified ELISAs for Purified Neurotoxin Types A and B (in buffer)

ELISA format	*Limit of detection, mouse LD_{50} units/ml*
BA11–NTA–G.Pig.HRPO	530, SD = 448 (7)
BA56–NTA–G.Pig.HRPO	820, SD = 278 (6)
G.Pig–NTA–G.Pig.HRPO	990, SD = 425 (6)
BA11–NTA–G.Pig.AP–Amplifier	12, SD = 6·5 (9)
BB68–NTB–G.Pig.HRPO	790, SD = 480 (3)
G.Pig–NTB–G.Pig.HRPO	750, SD = 290 (6)
BB68–NTB–G.Pig.AP–Amplifier	19, SD = 3·6 (7)

NTA, neurotoxin type A.
NTB, neurotoxin type B.
G.Pig.HRP, guinea pig polyclonal anti-mouse γ-G antibodies conjugated to HRP.
G.Pig.AP, guinea pig polyclonal antibodies conjugated to alkaline phosphatase.
BA11, BA56 and BB68 are Mabs.

RESULTS AND DISCUSSION

The amplified ELISA for neurotoxin types A and B were more than forty times more sensitive than the corresponding unamplified ELISA.

The sensitivities of these amplified ELISAs were approximately the same even in the presence of various food materials (Table 2). The specificity of the Mabs towards various bacterial toxins was examined in the ELISA, in which the toxin was immobilised on the solid phase, followed by serial dilution of Mab preparation and rabbit anti-mouse IgG–HRP conjugate. All four Mabs (BA11, BA56, BB68 and BB75) are specific for their toxin

Table 2
Detection of Neurotoxin Types A and B in Food Materials using Amplified ELISAs

Food material	*Minimum mouse LD_{50} units/ml detected*	
	Neurotoxin type A	*Neurotoxin type B*
Salmon (canned)	6	18
	7	21
	10	18
	14	26
	10*	
	4*	
	6*	
Corned beef	8·5	21
	12	29
Liver paté	ND	13
	ND	16
Processed peas	14	7
	13	12
Canned carrots	7·5	11
	8	8

Neurotoxin was added as culture supernatants except (*) where *C. botulinum* was grown in food containers.
Amplified ELISAs were as follows:
BA11–NTA–G.Pig.Alkaline phosphatase conjugate–Amplifier;
BB68–NTB–G.Pig.Alkaline phosphatase conjugate–Amplifier.
NTA, neurotoxin A; NTB, neurotoxin B; ND, not determined.

Table 3
Specificity of the Four Monoclonal Antibodies Towards Various Antigens

Antigen	*Monoclonal antibody*			
	BA11	*BA56*	*BB68*	*BB75*
Clostridium botulinum				
Neurotoxin type A	$1{\cdot}7 \times 10^6$	$4{\cdot}2 \times 10^6$	<100	<100
SDS neurotoxin type A	<100	<100	<100	<100
Neurotoxin type B	<100	540	$1{\cdot}1 \times 10^6$	$1{\cdot}2 \times 10^6$
SDS neurotoxin type B	<100	<100	<100	$4{\cdot}4 \times 10^3$
Neurotoxin type E	<100	ND	<100	ND
Clostridium perfringens				
Enterotoxin A	<100	<100	<100	<100
Clostridium difficile				
Toxin A	<100	ND	ND	ND
Toxin B	<100	<100	<100	<100
Clostridium tetani				
Neurotoxin	<100	ND	ND	ND
Corynebacterium diphtheriae				
Toxoid	<100	<100	<100	<100
Staphylococcus aureus				
Enterotoxin A	<100	ND	ND	ND
Enterotoxin B	<100	ND	ND	ND
Vibrio cholerae				
Toxin	<100	ND	ND	ND

The numbers represent antibody titre (dilution at which absorbance = 0·1 units above negative control in ELISA); ND = not determined.

type (Table 3). Although BB75 shows binding activity with the SDS-treated neurotoxin type B, this is about 270-fold less than with the native neurotoxin B.

Mabs BA56, BB68 and BB75 could not neutralise the toxicity of their respective neurotoxins as assayed by the mouse lethality test. Even when combined BB68 and BB75 could not neutralise the toxicity of neurotoxin B. BA11 has only weak neurotoxin neutralising activity for type A neurotoxin (Shone *et al.*, 1985), and the neutralising ability was not enhanced even in the presence of the second Mab, BA56.

Both these amplified ELISAs have detection limits approaching that of the mouse assay (4–5 mouse LD_{50} units/ml). Since the detection limits are unaltered by food matrices, these ELISAs have considerable potential for replacing the conventional mouse lethality test. Since the capture Mabs (BA11 and BB68) used in the amplified ELISAs are specific for the respective botulinum neurotoxins, the need to perform parallel neutralisations for serotyping may be eliminated in some instances.

REFERENCES

ELY, P. L., PROWSE, S. J. & JENKIN, C. R. (1978) Isolation of pure IgG_1, IgG_{2a} and IgG_{2b} immunoglobulins from mouse serum using protein A–sepharose. *Immunochemistry*, **15**, 429–436.

EVANS, D., WILLIAMS, R. S., SHONE, C. C., HAMBLETON, P., MELLING, J. & DOLLY, J. O. (1986) Botulinum neurotoxin type B: its purification, radioiodination and interaction with rat-brain synaptosomal membranes. *European Journal of Biochemistry*, **154**, 409–416.

HAMBLETON, P., CAPEL, B., BAILEY, N., HERON, N., CROOKS, A., MELLING, J., TSE, C. & DOLLY, J. O. (1981) Production, purification and toxoiding of *Clostridium botulinum* type A toxin. In: *Biomedical Aspects of Botulism*, Lewis, G. E. (ed.), Academic Press, London, pp. 247–260.

HOBBS, G. (1976) *Clostridium botulinum* and its importance in fishery products. *Advances in Food Research*, **22**, 135–185.

HOBBS, G., CROWTHER, J. S., NEAVES, P., GIBBS, P. A. & JARVIS, B. (1982) Detection and isolation of *Clostridium botulinum*. In: *Isolation and Identification Methods for Food Poisoning Organisms*. The Society for Applied Bacteriology's Technical Series No. 17, Corry, J. E. L., Roberts, D. & Skinner, F. A. (eds), Academic Press, London, pp. 151–164.

IRONS, L. I., ASHWORTH, L. A. E. & WILTON-SMITH, P. (1983) Heterogeneity of the filamentous haemagglutinin of *Bordetella pertussis* studied with monoclonal antibodies. *Journal of General Microbiology*, **129**, 2769–2778.

KAZAKI, S., DUFRENNE, J., HAGENAARS, A. M. & NOTERMANS, S. (1973) Enzyme-linked immunosorbent assay (ELISA) for detection of *Clostridium botulinum* type B toxin. *Japanese Journal of Medical Science and Biology*, **32**, 199–205.

MODI, N. K., SHONE, C. C., HAMBLETON, P. & MELLING, J. (1986) Monoclonal antibody-based amplified enzyme-linked immunosorbent assays for *Clostridium botulinum* toxin types A and B. In: *Proceedings of 2nd World Congress Foodborne Infections and Intoxications*, Institute of Veterinary Medicine, Robert von Ostertag-Institute, Berlin (West), **2**, 1184–1188.

NEAVES, P. & GIBBS, P. A. (1983) Alternatives to the mouse toxicity test for detection of *Clostridium botulinum* and its toxins. In: *Scientific & Technical Surveys No. 138*, Leatherhead Food Research Association, Leatherhead, UK.

NOTERMANS, S. & KAZAKI, S. (1981) Isolation and identification of botulinum toxins using the ELISA. In: *Biomedical Aspects of Botulism*, Lewis, G. E. (ed.), Academic Press, London, pp. 181–189.

O'SULLIVAN, M. J. & MARKS, V. (1981) Methods for the preparation of enzyme–antibody conjugates for use in enzyme immunoassays. *Methods in Enzymology*, **73**, 147–166.

SHONE, C., WILTON-SMITH, P., APPLETON, N., HAMBLETON, P., MODI, N., GATLEY, S. & MELLING, J. (1985) Monoclonal antibody-based immunoassay for type A *Clostridium botulinum* toxin is comparable to the mouse bioassay. *Applied and Environmental Microbiology*, **50**, 63–67.

The Prevention of Protein A Interference in Immunoassays for *Staphylococcus aureus* Enterotoxins

P. D. PATEL* and P. A. GIBBS†

**Biopolymers Section and †Applied Microbiology Section, Leatherhead Food Research Association, Leatherhead, Surrey, UK*

Some strains of *Staphylococcus aureus* produce potent enterotoxins that cause food poisoning when present at levels of about 1 μg/100 g food. Because of their inherent sensitivity and specificity, immunoassay techniques, especially ELISAs, are well suited to the detection and quantification of such enterotoxins in foods.

However, foods contaminated with *S. aureus* may also contain non-toxic extracellular proteins, including protein A (PA) (Notermans, 1985). PA binds to the F_c portion of IgC of many species, leaving the $F_{(ab')_2}$ portions free to interact with specific antigens (Goding, 1978). It has thus been pointed out that when PA is present it may interfere in some ELISAs by causing non-specific binding (whatever the analyte), as illustrated in Fig. 1. The risk of such interference is smaller in the competitive ELISA (Fig. 1(d)),

Table 1
Elimination of Protein A Interference in the Direct MEIA for Staphylococcal Enterotoxin B

Cheese extract/Added components	*Enzyme activity* (A_{490})
Extract only (control)	≤0·05
Extract + enterotoxin B[1]	0·1
Extract + enterotoxin B[1] + protein A[2]	0·75
Extract + enterotoxin B[1] + protein A[2] + Spicer–Edwards serum	0·08

[1] 1 μg/100 g cheese.
[2] 1 mg/100 g cheese.

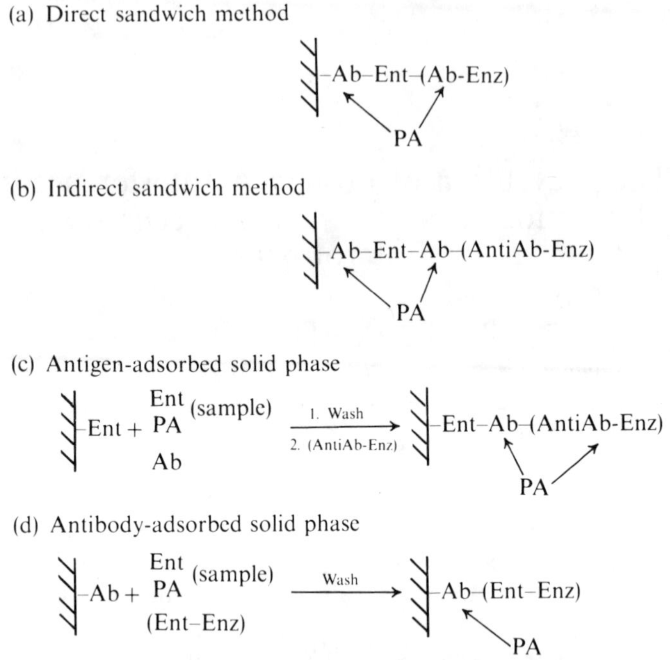

Fig. 1. Interference of protein A in ELISA techniques: Ent, toxin; PA, protein A; Ab, antibody to toxin; Ab-Enz, enzyme-labelled antibody; AntiAb-Enz, enzyme-labelled second antibody, Ent–Enz, enzyme-labelled toxin.

where the primary antibody from a species other than sheep or goat is adsorbed to a solid phase and there is no second primary antibody or antibody–enzyme conjugate.

A direct magnetic enzyme immunoassay (MEIA) has been developed (Patel *et al.*, 1985) for *S. aureus* enterotoxin B in which antibodies against the enterotoxins were covalently coupled to magnetic beads. It has been observed that PA at levels ≥ 50 ng/ml may interfere in the assay. Interference was demonstrated by treating the beads with PA, or with extracts of food containing PA, followed by HRP-labelled anti-enterotoxin B antibodies.

Such interference by PA, even at levels up to 100 μg/ml, was completely and conveniently eliminated by pre-reacting the PA, or extracts of cheese containing the PA, with non-specific rabbit antibodies (in this case Spicer–Edwards anti-*Salmonella* antiserum). The results are presented in Table 1.

Alternatively, antibodies produced in sheep and goats may be used since

PA has a lower affinity for the F_c fragments of the IgGs of these species compared with that of rabbit (Van der Ouderaa & Haas, 1981). However, as yet there is no commercial source of sheep antibodies to the staphylococcal enterotoxins.

PA has been regarded as a universal antibody binding reagent because of its affinity for the F_c fragments of a number of different species and hence, ironically, it finds many useful applications in both immunochemical assays and histocytochemical studies. For example, Fey *et al.* (1982) have used a PA–alkaline phosphatase conjugate instead of an enzyme-labelled second antibody in an ELISA, while staphylococcal cells containing cell-wall PA have been used to precipitate the antigen–antibody complexes in a RIA for staphylococcal enterotoxins (Reiser & Bergdoll, 1980).

ACKNOWLEDGEMENT

This work was supported by the Ministry of Agriculture, Fisheries and Food and is Crown copyright.

REFERENCES

FEY, H., STIFFLER-ROSENBERG, G., WARTENWEILER-BURKHARD, G., MÜLLER, CHR. & RÜEGG, O. (1982) Der Nachweis von Staphylokokken-Enterotoxinen (SET). *Schweizer Archiv für Tierheilkunde*, **124**, 297–306.

GODING, J. W. (1978) Use of staphylococcal protein A as an immunological reagent. *Journal of Immunological Methods*, **20**, 241–253.

NOTERMANS, S. (1985) Enzyme-linked immunosorbent assay of staphylococcal enterotoxins in foods. In: *Rapid Methods and Automation in Microbiology and Immunology*, Habermehl, K. O. (ed.), Springer-Verlag, Berlin, pp. 649–655.

PATEL, P. D., HAINES, S. D. & GIBBS, P. A. (1985) Development of a direct magnetic enzyme immunoassay (MEIA) technique for the rapid determination of staphylococcal enterotoxin B in foods. *Leatherhead Food RA Research Report*, No. 534.

REISER, R. F. & BERGDOLL, M. S. (1980) Application of radioimmunoassay for detection of staphylococcal enterotoxins in foods. *Journal of Food Protection*, **43**, 68–72.

VAN DER OUDERAA, F. & HAAS, H. (1981) Use of immunoassays to detect enterotoxin B of *Staphylococcus aureus* in foods. *Antonie van Leeuwenhoek*, **47**, 186–187.

EIAs with Chromogenic and Fluorogenic Substrates for the Quantitative Analysis of Heat-resistant Hydrolases from Psychrotrophic Pseudomonads

G. VAGIAS, S.-E. BIRKELAND, L. STEPANIAK and T. SØRHAUG

Department of Dairy and Food Industries, Agricultural University of Norway, Ås, Norway

INTRODUCTION

Cold storage of raw milk is a common practice in the modern dairy industry. Hydrolases produced by psychrotrophic bacteria have the potential to impair both the processing properties of raw milk and the shelf-life of milk products (Cousin, 1982; Birkeland *et al.*, 1985). The microflora of refrigerated raw milk is dominated by the genus *Pseudomonas* with *P. fluorescens* as the most common species (Cousin, 1982). The intention of the present work was to increase the sensitivity of a previously developed ELISA (Birkeland *et al.*, 1985) for quantitation of the heat-stable proteinase P1 from *P. fluorescens*. Other aims were to apply ELISA for the detection of lipase and phospholipase C produced by the same bacterium, and to study by ELISA the production by *Pseudomonas* sp. of proteinases related or unrelated to proteinase P1.

MATERIALS AND METHODS

Proteinase P1, lipase P1 and phospholipase C P1 from *P. fluorescens* P1 and proteinase AFT 21-III from *Pseudomonas* sp. AFT 21 were produced in shaken skimmed milk cultures at 7°C and purified by ion exchange and gel filtration chromatography. The enzymes, used as immunogens, were homogeneous, as shown by SDS gel electrophoresis. Proteinase P1 (Birkeland *et al.*, 1985) and proteinase AFT 21-III (Stepaniak & Fox, 1985) have been characterised earlier. Lipase P1 and phospholipase C P1 are heat stable (unpublished work). The immunisation protocol was as previously

Table 1

Conjugation method Enzyme[a]	Substrates	Detection limits (ng/ml)			Minimum CFU/ml for detection of enzymes in milk, 4°C		Comments
		Enzymes[b]	PBST	Milk	P. fluorescens P1	Pseudomonas sp. AFT 21	
2 step glutaraldehyde							
Peroxidase	Chromogenic	PP1	0·25	0·25	10^7	—	Suitable
(Voller *et al.*, 1979)	*o*-phenylenediamine	LP1	100	100	10^6	—	Low NSB
		P AFT 21-III	2·5	2·5	—	10^8	
1 step glutaraldehyde							
(a) Alkaline	Chromogenic	PP1	0·25	0·25	10^7	—	Suitable
phosphatase	*p*-nitrophenyl phosphate	LP1	—	—	—	—	High NSB
(Birkeland *et al.*, 1985)		P AFT 21-III					
(b) *β*-galactosidase	Chromogenic	PP1	—	—	—	—	High NSB
(Neurath &	O-nitrophenyl-*β*-D-galactopyranoside	LP1	—	—	—	—	
Strick, 1981)	and Fluorogenic	PLCP1	—	—	—	—	
	4-methylumbelliferyl-*β*-D-galactopyranoside						
N-*succinimidyl-3-(2-pyridyldithio)-propionate*							
β-galactosidase	Chromogenic	PP1	100	100	—	—	High NSB
(Neurath &	O-nitrophenyl-*β*-D-galactopyranoside	LP1	—	—	—	—	
Strick, 1981)		PLCP1	—	—	—	—	
	Fluorogenic	PP1	0·01	0·08	10^6	—	Suitable
	4-methylumbelliferyl-*β*-D-galactopyranoside	LP1	20	40	10^6	—	Low NSB
		PLCP1	40	85	—	—	Cross reactivity with PP1

[a] References for methods of conjugation are mentioned in parentheses.
[b] Proteinase P1, PP1; lipase P1, LP1; proteinase AFT 21-III, P AFT 21-III; phospholipase C P1, PLCP1.

described (Birkeland *et al.*, 1985). Rabbit IgG was purified on protein A–Sepharose CL-4B (Pharmacia, Uppsala).

Four different types of enzyme conjugates were prepared (Table 1) and the sandwich ELISA procedure (Birkeland *et al.*, 1985) was followed except that the incubation time was 30 min with the chromogenic substrates and 15 min with the fluorogenic substrate. The performance of conjugates was compared and detection limits with purified enzymes were evaluated for the different types of conjugates. A number of *Pseudomonas* strains (*Pseudomonas* sp., *P. fluorescens*) were grown at 7°C in shaken skimmed milk cultures, and cell-free liquors were analysed for the presence of proteinase P1, lipase P1 and proteinase AFT 21-III after various periods of cultivation. Immunoreactivity of supernatants showing strong positive hydrolytic activity was checked by agar diffusion methods with casein and tributyrin as substrates.

RESULTS

The detection limits of the ELISAs for the four hydrolases, with different conjugates and substrates, are summarised in Table 1. The lowest number of cells/ml (in cultures), with detectable amounts of the enzymes, are also given. Purification of conjugates with Sepharose 6B, or introduction of BSA, did not reduce the NSB significantly. Proteinase P1 and proteinase AFT 21-III were immunologically unrelated. No cross-reaction was observed with the lipase P1 preparations against anti-proteinase antibodies. Phospholipase C P1 cross-reacted with antibodies raised against proteinase P1.

Fourteen out of 16 pseudomonad isolates produced proteinases serologically related to proteinase P1. Culture supernatants from six of these strains also showed a limited cross-reactivity with antibodies against proteinase AFT 21-III. *Pseudomonas* sp. AFT 21 and AFT 7 both produced proteinase AFT 21-III, whereas proteinase P1 was not detectable by ELISA with these strains.

DISCUSSION

The results show that the type of enzyme conjugate and conjugation method greatly influence the sensitivity of the ELISA for the detection of heat-stable hydrolases. Conjugates of β-galactosidase used in conjunction with a fluorogenic substrate gave the highest sensitivity in the ELISA. Proteinase P1 was detected at equal sensitivity with peroxidase or alkaline phosphatase labels. However, with these only HRP-labelled conjugates were suitable for the detection of lipase P1 and proteinase AFT 21-III. Some differences were observed in the performance of HRP conjugates produced with two different batches of antiserum, but detection limits were not affected.

Pseudomonads possess complex proteolytic enzyme systems and immunologically unrelated proteinases can be found within and among strains of these micro-organisms (unpublished work). However, production of proteinases immunologically identical with or related to proteinase P1 is rather common among pseudomonads and the enzyme was also detected in samples of raw milk stored at 4°C (Birkeland *et al.*, 1985).

Milk processed in modern dairies rarely contains more than 10^6 psychrotrophs/ml (Cousin, 1982). Thus methods even more sensitive than those described here are desirable for the detection of heat-resistant hydrolases in raw milk. Some methods have been explored for increasing the sensitivity of the ELISA (Ishikawa & Kato, 1978; Vaag, 1985).

CONCLUSION

The present work shows that highly specific and sensitive ELISAs, especially with fluorogenic substrates, can be used for the detection of heat-resistant hydrolases from psychrotrophs in milk.

REFERENCES

Birkeland, S. E., Stepaniak, L. & Sørhaug, T. (1985) Quantitative studies of heat-stable proteinase from *Pseudomonas fluorescens* P1 by the enzyme-linked immunosorbent assay. *Applied and Environmental Microbiology*, **49**, 382–387.

Cousin, M. A. (1982) Presence and activity of psychrotrophic microorganisms in milk and dairy products: a review. *Journal of Food Protection*, **45**, 172–207.

Ishikawa, E. & Kato, K. (1978) Ultrasensitive enzyme immunoassay. *Scandinavian Journal of Immunology*, **8**, Suppl. 7, 43–55.

Neurath, A. R. & Strick, N. (1981) Enzyme-linked immunoassays using β-galactosidase and antibodies covalently bound to polystyrene plates. *Journal of Virological Methods*, **3**, 155–165.

Stepaniak, L. & Fox, P. F. (1985) Isolation and characterization of heat-stable proteinases from *Pseudomonas* isolate AFT 21. *Journal of Dairy Research*, **52**, 77–89.

VAAG, P. (1985) Enzyme-linked immunosorbent assay (ELISA) for quality control in beer. *Proceedings of the European Brewery Convention, 20th Congress*, 2–7 June 1985, Helsinki, IRL Press, Oxford, pp. 547–554.

VOLLER, A., BIDWELL, D. E. & BARTLETT, A. (1979) *The Enzyme-linked Immunosorbent Assay (ELISA)*, Dynatech-Europe, Borough House, Rue du Pre, Guernsey, Channel Islands.

ELISA of Aflatoxins

A. P. WILKINSON, A. S. KANG, H. W.-S. CHAN and M. R. A. MORGAN
AFRC Institute of Food Research, Norwich, UK

INTRODUCTION

As part of our programme of improving analytical methods for use by the food industry, we have produced both monoclonal and polyclonal antibodies for various mycotoxins and used them in microtitration plate ELISAs, usually of the indirect format (for example, see Morgan *et al.*, 1985, 1986*a* and see Mills *et al.*, p. 347, this volume). This report is concerned with two of our assays for aflatoxins which are a group (see Fig. 1) of secondary metabolites produced by *Aspergillus flavus* and *A. parasiticus*. One such, aflatoxin B_1, has LD_{50} values in the range 0·3 to 10·2 mg/kg (Smith & Moss, 1985), making it in some animal species the most carcinogenic compound known. Aflatoxins are present in a wide range of important agricultural produce, particularly nuts and cereals (Jarvis, 1982), and thus there is a need for rapid, specific and sensitive yet simple and cost-effective analytical methods such as described below.

DETERMINATION OF AFLATOXINS B_1 AND G_1 IN PEANUT BUTTER

One of the range of antibodies that have been produced recognised aflatoxins B_1 and G_1 equally well but B_2 and G_2 poorly. Since B_1 and G_1 are the carcinogenic members of this group, this is a particularly useful property. The ELISA involving this antibody has been applied to peanut butter samples (Morgan *et al.*, 1986*b*). The validated extraction procedure was a simple solubilisation of toxins by homogenisation of the sample with

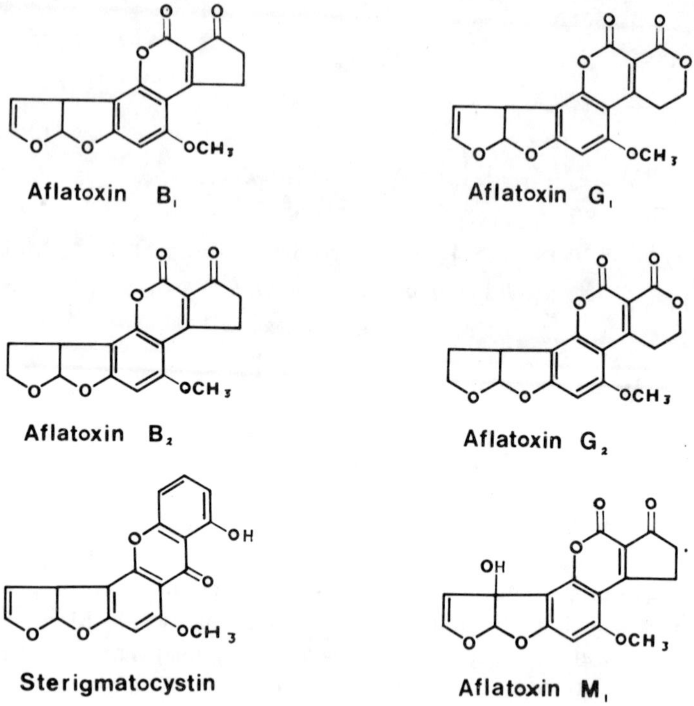

Fig. 1. Structures of aflatoxins B_1, B_2, G_1, G_2 and M_1, and sterigmatocystin.

an acetonitrile–water mixture. After filtering, the filtrate can then be diluted in assay buffer and put through the ELISA procedure. Under these conditions, there was no matrix interference and recovery was quantitative. The limit of detection of the assay was 1 pg per well. Trials with other laboratories have shown the efficacy of the method, which should find wide application in the future because of the rapidity and simplicity with which large numbers of samples can be analysed.

DETERMINATION OF STERIGMATOCYSTIN IN BARLEY

The same indirect ELISA protocol has been employed. In order to avoid potential solubility problems, the ready conversion of toxin to the hemiacetal derivative has been exploited to increase aqueous solubility. Hence the antibody preparation has been raised against the hemiacetal form of the toxin (Morgan *et al.*, 1986*c*). The antibody was of high specificity, cross-reacting with aflatoxins B_1, B_2, G_1 and G_2 by less than 0·01%. The extraction procedure validated for barley was simple: extraction with chloroform, removal of solvent, acid-catalysed conversion of toxin to hemiacetal derivative, neutralisation and immunoassay. Assay limit of detection was 10 pg per well.

CONCLUSIONS

The ELISAs for aflatoxin determination that have been developed are highly sensitive, rapid and simple, permitting quantitative aflatoxin analysis of large numbers of samples at low cost. They should find wide application in the future.

ACKNOWLEDGEMENTS

A.S.K. has an AFRC studentship. The work was funded in part by the Ministry of Agriculture, Fisheries and Food.

REFERENCES

JARVIS, B. (1982) The occurrence of mycotoxins in UK foods. *Food Technology in Australia*, **34**, 508–514.

MORGAN, M. R. A., MCNERNEY, R. & CHAN, H. W.-S. (1985) An ELISA for the analysis of the mycotoxin ochratoxin A in food. In: *Immunoassays in Food Analysis*, Morris, B. A. & Clifford, M. N. (eds), Elsevier Applied Science Publishers, London, pp. 159–168.

MORGAN, M. R. A., MCNERNEY, R., CHAN, H. W.-S. & ANDERSON, P. H. (1986*a*) Ochratoxin A in a pig kidney determined by enzyme-linked immunosorbent assay (ELISA). *Journal of the Science of Food and Agriculture*, **37**, 475–480.

MORGAN, M. R. A., KANG, A. S. & CHAN, H. W.-S. (1986*b*) Aflatoxin determination in peanut butter by enzyme-linked immunosorbent assay. *Journal of the Science of Food and Agriculture*, **37**, 908–914.

MORGAN, M. R. A., KANG, A. S. & CHAN, H. W.-S. (1986*c*) Production of antisera against sterigmatocystin hemiacetal and its potential for use in an enzyme-linked immunosorbent assay for sterigmatocystin in barley. *Journal of the Science of Food and Agriculture*, **37**, 873–880.

SMITH, J. E. & MOSS, M. O. (1985) In: *Mycotoxins, Formation, Analysis and Significance*, Smith, J. E. & Moss, M. O. (eds), Wiley & Sons, Chichester, p. 7.

Production of Anti-Trichothecene Antibodies and Their Use in the Analysis of Food

E. N. C. MILLS, H. A. KEMP,
H. W.-S. CHAN and M. R. A. MORGAN

AFRC Institute of Food Research, Norwich, UK

INTRODUCTION

Trichothecenes are a class of metabolites possessing a characteristic ring structure containing a double bond and an epoxy group at positions 9,10 and 12,13 respectively (Fig. 1). These are produced by various genera of fungi such as *Fusarium* and *Trichoderma*, and infestations of such fungi, especially in cereal crops, have been associated with outbreaks of conditions such as alimentary toxic aleukia in both humans and livestock. The trichothecenes have been implicated as the causative agents, and thus their analysis in feedstuffs is of considerable importance. Physico-chemical analytical techniques such as TLC or LC have been hampered by the weak or non-existent UV absorbance or fluorescence of these compounds. Although immunoassay does not itself require the analyte to have such spectral properties, their absence can hinder the development of such assays by causing difficulties in assessing the quality of conjugates synthesised. Antisera raised to trichothecenes reported in the literature have been of poor quality.

METHODS

Trichothecene–Protein Conjugate Synthesis

Hemisuccinate or hemiglutarate derivatives of the trichothecenes were prepared using the methods of Lau *et al.* (1981) or Chu *et al.* (1979), and were purified on a silica gel (SG60) column using either chloroform: propan-2-ol:acetone (81:1, v:v:v) or chloroform:methanol (95:5, v:v) as eluting solvents. The purity of products was first analysed by TLC using the methods of Trucksess *et al.* (1984) or Takitani *et al.* (1979), and their

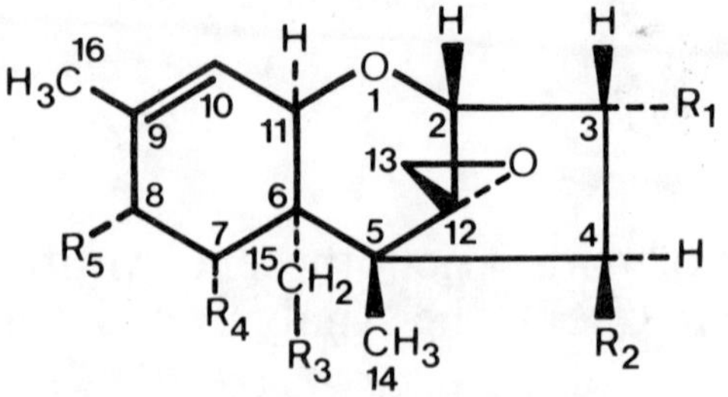

Fig. 1. Structures of some trichothecenes.

Trichothecene	R_1	R_2	R_3	R_4	R_5
3-Acetyldeoxynivalenol	OAc	H	OH	OH	=O
Deoxynivalenol	OH	H	OH	OH	=O
Nivalenol	OH	OH	OH	OH	=O
Diacetoxyscirpenol	OH	OAc	OAc	H	H
T-2 toxin	OH	OAc	OAc	H	$-OCOCH_2-CH(CH_3)_2$

structure was later confirmed by mass spectrometry and NMR. These derivatives were then coupled to protein using the mixed anhydride procedure, as described by Kemp *et al.* (1986). In some instances the protein was first derivatised with 6-aminohexanoic acid to introduce a spacer-arm. The degree of conjugation was monitored using a microtitration plate format of the trinitrobenzenesulphonic acid (TNBS) method for measuring free amino groups (Habeeb, 1966).

Antisera Production and ELISA Protocol

Antisera were raised in New Zealand white rabbits (Kemp *et al.*, 1986) and used in an indirect ELISA performed on microtitration plates. An anti-rabbit Ig-alkaline phosphatase-labelled second antibody was used. Samples of ground wheat or rice were spiked with trichothecenes in methanol and the solvent allowed to evaporate. The samples were then extracted with 10 volumes of the appropriate solvent by shaking for 60 min. The debris was removed by filtration and the extract diluted into assay buffer.

RESULTS AND DISCUSSION

Assessment of Conjugate Quality

In order to ensure that effective conjugates were produced, the trichothecene hemiglutarate or hemisuccinate derivatives to be used for conjugate synthesis were first rigorously characterised, using mass spectrometry and

NMR. Secondly, the degree of hapten–protein coupling was monitored by following the loss of free amino groups in the protein.

A TNBS standard curve was constructed using unconjugated protein. When assaying 6-aminohexanoic acid derivatives of a protein, about 30% loss of free amino groups was observed, probably resulting from cross-link formation during derivatisation. From such curves, the loss of free amino groups during conjugation was ascertained. Typically, losses ranged from 65–90%. These results suggested that the coupling procedure was more than adequate for generating conjugates for use as immunogens or as the solid phase in ELISA.

ELISA for 3-Acetyldeoxynivalenol (3-ADON)

A highly specific antiserum was raised against 3-ADON, which exhibited a cross-reactivity of 0·007% with deoxynivalenol, indicating that the antibodies were highly specific for the C_3 acetyl group. The specificity was further emphasised by the fact that T-2 toxin and diacetoxyscirpenol would not depress antibody binding to 50% at any level tested. A typical standard curve gave an assay limit of detection of 1 pg/well (equivalent of 1 ng 3-ADON/g rice). The assay has been validated for the analysis of rice samples. Recoveries from spiked samples, extracted in 60% (v:v) methanol:water diluted and added directly to the assay, were quantitative.

ELISA for Diacetoxyscirpenol (DAS)

A high titre anti-DAS antiserum was produced and was used at a dilution of 1:20 000 in the ELISA. As for the 3-ADON ELISA, the anti-DAS antibodies exhibited a high degree of specificity. The highest cross-reaction obtained was 1%, against the related compound neosolaniol. This differs from DAS by possessing a hydroxyl group at the C_8 position. Cross-reactivity against T-2 toxin was low (0·2%), and against the 'B'-type trichothecenes, such as deoxynivalenol, it was virtually non-existent since they were unable to depress antibody binding to 50% of the zero. The assay limit of detection is 2 pg DAS/well ($\pm$two standard deviations from the zero point). This ELISA has been applied to the analysis of wheat samples. A simple methanol extraction procedure has been employed which allows samples to be diluted and added directly to the assay. Recoveries of 80–90% for spiked samples have been achieved.

CONCLUSIONS

One of the key areas in the development of hapten ELISAs is that of synthesising the hapten–protein conjugates which are effective as either immunogens or the adsorbed phase of ELISA. The trichothecenes present a particular problem in that their lack of spectral properties makes it difficult to assess the quality of such conjugates.

By careful characterisation of the conjugates specific ELISAs for 3-ADON and DAS have been developed. Assays for T-2 toxin, deoxynivalenol and nivalenol are in the course of development. The ELISAs for 3-ADON and DAS have been applied to the analysis of cereals. Simple extraction into water miscible solvents avoids the need for lengthy clean-up procedures prior to analysis.

ACKNOWLEDGEMENT

This work was funded by the Ministry of Agriculture, Fisheries and Food.

REFERENCES

CHU, F. S., GROSSMAN, S., WEI, R. D. & MIROCHA, C. J. (1979) Production of antibody against T-2 toxin. *Applied and Environmental Microbiology*, **31**, 104–108.

HABEEB, A. F. S. A. (1966) Determination of free amino groups in proteins by trinitrobenzenesulphonic acid. *Analytical Biochemistry*, **14**, 328–336.

KEMP, H. A., MILLS, E. N. C. & MORGAN, M. R. A. (1986) Enzyme-linked immunosorbent assay of 3-acetyldeoxynivalenol applied to rice. *Journal of the Science of Food and Agriculture*, **37**, 888–894.

LAU, P. H., GAUR, P. K. & CHU, F. S. (1981) Preparation and characterization of aflatoxin B-2a hemiglutarate and its use for the production of antibody against aflatoxin B_1. *Journal of Food and Safety*, **3**, 1–13.

TAKITANI, S., YOSHIHIRO, A., KATO, T., SUZUKI, M. & UENO, Y. (1979) Spectrodensitometric determination of trichothecene mycotoxins with 4-(*p*-nitrobenzyl)pyridine on silica gel thin-layer chromatography. *Journal of Chromatography*, **172**, 335–342.

TRUCKSESS, M. W., NESHEIM, S. & EPPLEY, R. M. (1984) Thin-layer chromatographic determination of deoxynivalenol in wheat and corn. *Journal of the Association of Official Analytical Chemists*, **67**, 40–43.

Determination of Ochratoxin A by a Monoclonal Antibody-based Immunoassay

A. A. G. Candlish, W. H. Stimson and J. E. Smith
Department of Bioscience and Biotechnology, University of Strathclyde, Glasgow, UK

INTRODUCTION

Ochratoxin A (OA) is a low molecular weight, toxic, non-immunogenic secondary metabolite produced by a number of fungal species in the *Aspergillus* and *Penicillium* genera. The toxin is widely detected as a contaminant of food and feed products, especially cereals, in many European and North American countries (Shotwell *et al.*, 1969; Krogh *et al.*, 1977; Steyn, 1984). OA may induce an acute toxic response at high concentrations and is a potent nephrotoxin and hepatotoxin in a number of animals. Furthermore, OA is thought to cause porcine nephropathy (Krogh *et al.*, 1973) and has been implicated in human endemic Balkan nephropathy (Krogh *et al.*, 1977).

The present methods of analysis to determine OA most commonly involve TLC or HPLC (Howell & Taylor, 1981). Such techniques are protracted, involving solvent extraction of toxin, clean-up, separation, fluorescence detection and confirmation by chemical derivatisation. Immunoassays have recently been shown to possess many advantages, including reduced sample preparation, less expense, increased sensitivity and specificity, greater throughput of samples and potential for large-scale screening of samples. Polyclonal antisera to OA have been used in RIA (Chu *et al.*, 1976; Rousseau *et al*, 1985) and ELISA (Morgan *et al.*, 1983). This poster presentation reports the development of a highly sensitive monoclonal antibody to OA and its application in an ELISA system to detect OA.

METHODS AND RESULTS

Due to its low molecular weight, OA was conjugated directly to BSA and KLH by the water-soluble carbodiimide method (Chu *et al.*, 1976), and the molar ratio of OA/protein determined by A_{333}/A_{280}. This was found to be 20:1 for the OA–BSA conjugate and 1240:1 for the OA–KLH conjugate. Female NZB/BALB/c F_1 hybrid mice were injected intraperitoneally with 50 μg OA–KLH conjugate per injection. The sensitised spleen cells from such mice were fused with myeloma cells in a ratio of 4:1 in the presence of 46% polyethylene glycol 1500. Hybridomas were produced at a rate of $1/10^6$ spleen cells used, and hybridomas secreting specific antibody were selected by indirect ELISA with OA–BSA-coated plates. From a total of 204 hybridoma cultures 27 proved positive for anti-OA antibodies. However, only one hybridoma (10E2) was further selected on the basis of growth characteristics, both *in vitro* and *in vivo*, and ability to detect OA in an indirect competitive ELISA. The hybridoma cell line was cloned twice by limiting dilution, grown in tissue culture on a large scale and as ascites. The monoclonal antibodies so produced were safely stored in liquid nitrogen with dimethylsulphoxide as a cryoprotective agent.

An indirect competitive ELISA was performed by coating microtitration plates with OA–BSA (5 μg/ml OA) overnight at 37°C in 0·02M Tris/HCl buffer (pH 9·0). The following morning the plates were washed and 100 μl of standard OA solution in 0·1M Tris/HCl buffer (pH 8·5) were added, together with 100 μl of MAb (1:40 000 dilution of ascites fluid in 0·1M Tris/HCl buffer (pH 8·5)). After incubation for 1 h at 37°C, the plates were washed and 200 μl of HRP-labelled sheep anti-mouse IgG conjugate (1:2000 dilution prepared in 0·15M NaCl containing 25% normal sheep serum) were added and incubated for a further hour at 37°C. After further washing, 200 μl tetramethylbenzidine substrate were added and the colour allowed to develop for 0·5 h at room temperature in complete darkness. The reaction was stopped with 50 μl 2M H_2SO_4 and the A_{450} measured. The sensitivity of this ELISA was 0·5 ng/ml at the 95% confidence level, with a working range up to 250 ng/ml of standard OA (Fig. 1).

The MAb was further characterised in relation to isotype, affinity dissociation constant (K_D) and specificity. The isotype was determined by a modified sandwich ELISA to be IgG_1 kappa. The K_D value determined by ELISA was $9{\cdot}55 \times 10^{-9}$ M ($r = 0{\cdot}99$). The specificity of the MAb determined by the 50% displacement method in the indirect competitive ELISA was OA = 100%, ochratoxin C = 8·24% and ochratoxin $\alpha = 0{\cdot}6\%$; no cross-

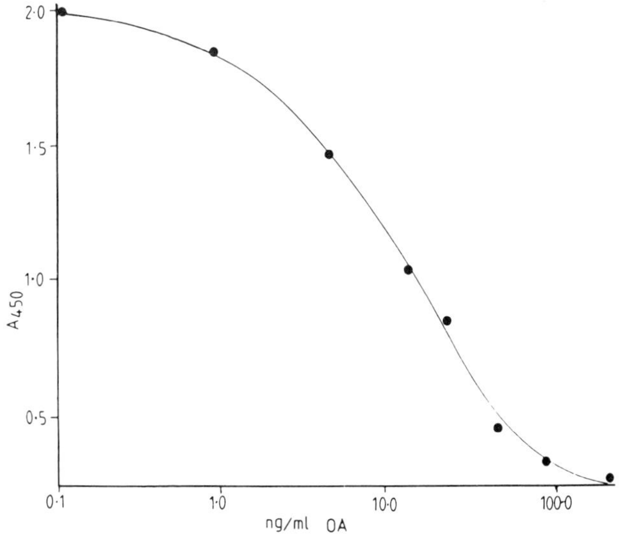

Fig. 1. Standard curve for OA by MAb-based competitive ELISA.

reaction was found with 4-OH coumarin, coumarin, phenylalanine, aflatoxin B_1, T-2 toxin or KLH.

CONCLUSIONS

It can be concluded that a highly sensitive and specific MAb-based ELISA has been developed for the quantitation of OA in standard solution. Furthermore, adequate amounts of this Ab can be produced by ascites tumours and the hybridoma cell line maintained for further use. The assay developed should prove most useful in the analysis of OA in natural substrates.

REFERENCES

CHU, F. S., CHANG, F. C. & HINSDILL, R. D. (1976) Production of antibody against ochratoxin A. *Applied and Environmental Microbiology*, **31**, 831–835.

HOWELL, M. V. & TAYLOR, P. W. (1981) Determination of aflatoxins, ochratoxin A, and zearalenone in mixed feeds with detection by thin layer chromatography or high performance liquid chromatography. *Journal of Association of Official Analytical Chemists*, **64**, 1356–1363.

KROGH, P., HALD, B., PLESTINA, R. & CEOVIC, S. (1977) Balkan (endemic) nephropathy and foodborne ochratoxin A: preliminary results of a survey of foodstuffs. *Acta Pathologia Microbiologia Scandinavica Section B*, **85**, 238–240.

KROGH, P., HALD, B. & PEDERSEN, E. J. (1973) Occurrence of ochratoxin A and citrinin in cereals associated with mycotoxic porcine nephropathy. *Acta Pathologia Microbiologia Scandinavica Section B*, **81**, 689.

MORGAN, R. A., MCNERNEY, R. & CHAN, H. W. S. (1983) Enzyme-linked immunosorbent assay of ochratoxin A in barley. *Journal of Association of Official Analytical Chemists*, **66**, 1481–1484.

ROUSSEAU, D. M., SLEGERS, G. A. & VAN PETEGHEM, C. (1985) Radioimmunoassay of ochratoxin A in barley. *Applied and Environmental Microbiology*, **50**, 529–531.

SHOTWELL, O. L., HESSELTINE, C. W. & GOULDEN, M. L. (1969) Ochratoxin A: occurrence as natural contaminant of a corn sample. *Applied and Environmental Microbiology*, **17**, 765–766.

STEYN, P. S. (1984) Ochratoxins and related dihydroisocoumarins. In: *Mycotoxins—Production, Isolation, Separation and Purification*, Betina, V. (ed.), Elsevier Science Publishers, Amsterdam, pp. 183–215.

A Monoclonal Antibody-based ELISA for T-2 Toxin

I. A. Goodbrand, W. H. Stimson and J. E. Smith

Department of Bioscience and Biotechnology, University of Strathclyde, Glasgow, UK

INTRODUCTION

The trichothecene mycotoxins are low molecular weight, toxic secondary metabolites, generally associated with the growth of *Fusarium* species on various grains and cereal crops (Joffe, 1978). The present methods of detection for these toxins, such as TLC and GC–MS, either lack sensitivity, specificity or both, while equipment costs can be prohibitively expensive for the routine screening of cash crops (Pathre & Mirocha, 1977). This problem has been a major contribution to a lack of knowledge regarding the passage of the trichothecenes through the food chain.

ELISAs using MAbs are becoming important methods of analysis for small molecules in many areas, including both medical and agricultural research. An ELISA for the detection of T-2 toxin, a trichothecene which has been implicated as the causal agent of various medical and veterinary conditions including alimentary toxic aleukia (Yagen *et al.*, 1977), has been developed using a MAb produced in this laboratory.

METHODS

Due to its low molecular weight, T-2 toxin has to be conjugated to a protein to make it immunogenic. However, the toxin contains no suitable reactive group to allow its direct linkage to a carrier protein. The hemisuccinate is therefore prepared by reacting T-2 toxin with succinic anhydride with subsequent linkage to KLH or BSA, utilising a water-soluble carbodiimide method (Chu *et al.*, 1979).

T-2–KLH was emulsified with an equal volume of Freund's complete adjuvant and used for primary immunisation of 8–12-week-old female NZB/BALB/c F_1 hybrid mice. A further immunisation followed using equal volumes of T-2–KLH and Freund's incomplete adjuvant. Three days prior to fusion the mice were given a final boost of T-2–BSA in saline.

Spleen cells from an immunised mouse (1×10^8) were used with myeloma cells in a ratio of 4:1 using 1 ml of polyethylene glycol 1500. Hybridoma supernatants were screened after 14 days by an indirect ELISA to identify hybridomas producing antibody specific for T-2 toxin. Positive cell lines were then cloned twice by limiting dilution in microtitration plates in the presence of murine peripheral blood feeder cells; they were then expanded into flasks. These positive clones (6×10^6/ml) were stored in liquid N_2 and also used to produce ascites tumours in histocompatible mice.

ELISA PROTOCOLS

Sensitised microtitration plates (Dynatech 'Micro ELISA') were coated with T-2-BSA in 0·02M Tris/HCl (pH 9·0, 0·2 ml) at 37°C overnight. Plates were washed four times with 0·2M Tris/HCl buffer (pH 7·4) containing 0·2M NaCl (wash buffer). An indirect ELISA was used to screen both the hybridoma supernatants and also to determine the titre of the ascites fluid. Aliquots (200 μl) of either medium were incubated on the T-2-coated plates at 37°C for 1 h. The plates were then washed five times with wash buffer containing 0·05% Tween 20. Wells were then incubated with 200 μl HRP-labelled sheep anti-mouse γ-globulin for 1 h at 37°C. This conjugate was diluted 1:2000 in 0·15M NaCl containing 25% normal sheep serum. After washing a further five times, enzyme activity was measured using a tetramethylbenzidine substrate at pH 5·5. The reaction was stopped after 30 min with 50 μl 2M H_2SO_4 and the A_{450} measured.

A competitive ELISA was performed as above using a 1:10 000 dilution of ascites fluid, incubated with an equal volume (100 μl each) of several concentrations of T-2 toxin or other trichothecene metabolites to determine the dynamic range of the assay and the sensitivity and specificity of the antibody. Cross-reactivity with metabolites was defined as the percentage ratio of the concentration of T-2 toxin, giving 50% of maximum absorbance to the concentration of test compound, also giving 50% of maximum absorbance.

The isotype of the antibody was determined using anti-mouse class- and subclass-specific antisera in a sandwich-type ELISA (Stimson & Sinclair, 1974).

RESULTS

Two positive hybridoma cell lines, directed to T-2 toxin, 15E7 and 16E3, were produced; 15E7 was chosen for further development on the strength of its good growth characteristics in tissue culture. It was therefore grown in large flasks, cloned by limiting dilution and used to produce ascites fluid in histocompatible mice. Some hybridoma cells were also frozen in liquid nitrogen for storage.

A batch of ascites fluid having a dilution titre of 1:500 000 was then used to develop an indirect competitive ELISA at a dilution of 1:10 000. This ELISA showed a detection limit of 5 ng/ml, with a dynamic range up to 1000 ng/ml (Fig. 1). The modified sandwich ELISA determined the isotype of the antibody to be IgG_1 (kappa); clone 15E7 was found to have a 25% cross-reactivity with HT-2 toxin. It did not, however, substantially react with any of the other trichothecenes tested.

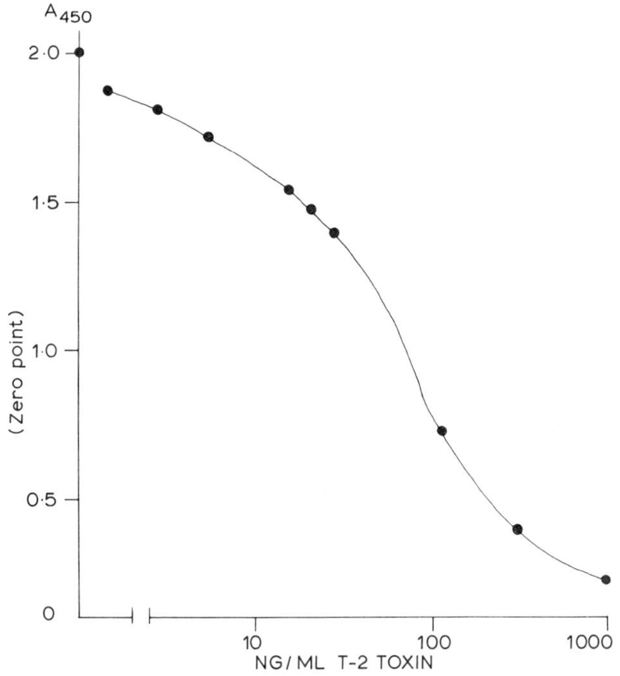

Fig. 1. Standard curve for T-2 toxin in buffer solution by competitive ELISA.

CONCLUSIONS

It has been shown that the MAb 15E7 has good sensitivity, a wide working dynamic range and is fairly specific for T-2 toxin. However, it may also be of use in the detection of HT-2 toxin. Further investigations will involve a study of the compatibility of the ELISA with existing grain extraction methods for T-2 toxin and the development of improved, quicker extraction protocols. In conclusion, the MAb-based ELISA may find application in the routine screening of various cereals and foodstuffs for the presence of low levels of T-2 toxin.

REFERENCES

CHU, F. S., GROSSMAN, S., RU-DONG, W. E. & MIROCHA, C. J. (1979) Production of antibody against T-2 toxin. *Applied and Environmental Microbiology*, **37**, 102–108.

JOFFE, A. Z. (1978) In: *Mycotoxic Fungi, Mycotoxins, Mycotoxicoses*, Volume 3, Wyllie, T. D. & Morehouse, L. G. (eds), Marcel Dekker, New York, pp. 21–86.

PATHRE, S. V. & MIROCHA, C. J. (1977) Assay methods for trichothecenes and review of their natural occurrence. In: *Mycotoxins in Human and Animal Health*, Rodricks, J. V., Hesseltine, C. W. & Mehlman, M. A. (eds), Pathotox, Park Forest South, IL, USA, pp. 229–253.

STIMSON, W. H. & SINCLAIR, J. (1974) An immunoassay for a pregnancy associated α-macroglobulin using antibody enzyme conjugate. *FEBS Letters*, **7**, 190–193.

YAGEN, B., JOFFE, A. Z., HORN, P., MOR, N. & LUTSKY, I. I. (1977) Toxins from a strain involved in ATA. In: *Mycotoxins in Human and Animal Health*, Rodricks, J. V., Hesseltine, C. W. & Mehlman, M. A. (eds), Pathotox, Park Forest South, IL, USA, pp. 329–336.

Comparison of RIA and ELISA for Analysis of the Food Additives Quinine, Quinidine and Quassin

S. Bramham and M. R. A. Morgan

AFRC Institute of Food Research, Norwich, UK

INTRODUCTION

Quinine and quinidine, isomeric cinchona alkaloids, and the secotriterpene quassin are important pharmaceuticals and food bittering agents. Their structures are illustrated in Fig. 1. The normal source of these compounds is the bark of mature trees; quinine and quinidine are extracted from *Cinchona ledgenaria* and *C. succirubra*; quassin from either *Quassia amara* L. or *Picrasma excelsa* (Swartz.) Planch, members of the pan-tropical family *Simaroubaceae*. For obvious reasons there is considerable interest in their biotechnological production by plant cell culture. Immunoassays have been developed for each of the three compounds to facilitate (i) analysis of plant material for screening as potential culture stock, (ii) rapid and simple screening of cultures for evidence of appropriate biosynthesis, (iii) monitoring of large-scale cultures for appropriate functions, and (iv) analysis of food, particularly soft drinks.

QUININE AND QUINIDINE IMMUNOASSAYS

Synthesis of Immunogens

Antisera to each alkaloid were raised in rabbits by coupling each alkaloid to BSA by the mixed anhydride method after alkaloid hemisuccinate formation.

Synthesis of Radio-labelled Tracers

To provide a labelled tracer for RIA, the hydroxyl groups of quinine and quinidine were acetylated using [^{3}H] acetic anhydride. Dextran-coated

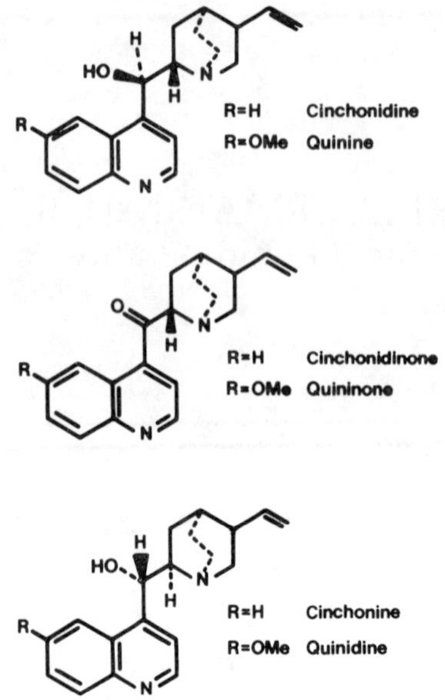

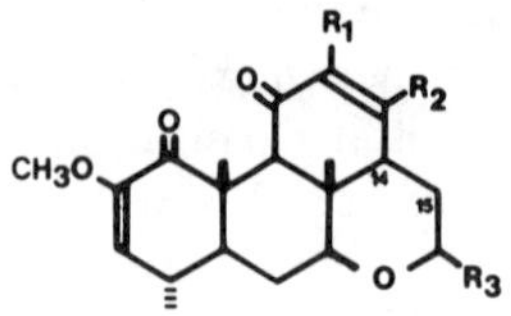

	R_1	R_2	R_3
Quassin	OCH_3	CH_3	=O
Neoquassin	OCH_3	CH_3	HOH
12-hydroxyquassin	OH	CH_3	=O
18-hydroxyquassin	OCH_3	CH_2OH	=O

Fig. 1. Structures of quinine, quinidine and quassin (and related compounds).

charcoal was used to separate the bound and free phases of the assay (Robins *et al.*, 1984*a*).

Synthesis of Immobilised ELISA Phases

Conjugates for use as ELISA solid phases were synthesised as described for immunogens, but with KLH as the carrier protein. Microtitration plates were coated with these conjugates by passive adsorption. ELISAs were carried out by the indirect method using alkaline phosphatase-labelled second antibody (Morgan *et al.*, 1985).

Comparison of RIA and ELISA

The antiserum dilution used in the quinine RIA was 1:10 000 whilst that in the quinine ELISA was 1:100 000. In the quinidine assays, the dilutions were 1:5000 and 1:50 000 for the RIA and ELISA respectively. For quinine, the assay limits of detection were 50 pg (by RIA) and 10 pg (by ELISA); for quinidine, the values were 1 ng (by RIA) and 100 pg (by ELISA).

The observed cross-reactions of the anti-quinine antiserum in the RIA showed that compounds with (8S) stereochemistry exhibited interaction dependent on their structural similarity to quinine. Thus 10,11-dihydroquinine exhibited 35% cross-reaction whereas cupreine and cinchonidine had values of 7 and 4% respectively. The compounds with a 9-keto group, which are intermediate between the (8S) and (8R) isomers, showed little or no interaction with the antibody. Alkaloids of the (8R) series showed no cross-reaction at all. Though the quinine RIA seemed to be very specific for quinine, the specificity was improved further by using the same antiserum in the ELISA. Cross-reactions, with the exception of that for quininone, were reduced by approximately 10-fold with the figures for cupreine, cinchonidine and 10,11-dihydroquinine being 0·75, 1·2 and 2·7% respectively. The major reason for the considerable difference in specificity of the two assays is likely to be due partly to the influence of the antibody being solid phased in the ELISA and partly due to the competing antigen being coupled to a protein carrier.

QUASSIN IMMUNOASSAYS

Synthesis of Immunogens and ELISA Coating Conjugates

Two anti-quassin antisera were raised; one, a broad specificity preparation capable of recognising neoquassin, 18-hydroxyquassin and 12-hydroxy-quassin as well as quassin. For broad specificity, the immunogen was synthesised after opening the lactone ring of quassin and coupling the resultant carboxylic acid group to protein (Robins *et al.*, 1984*b*). For specific antisera, the immunogen was produced by linking the hemi-succinate of 18-hydroxyquassin to protein by the mixed anhydride method (Robins *et al.*, 1984*c*). ELISA coating conjugates were synthesised in the same way as the immunogens but using a different protein.

Assay Characteristics

The two antisera demonstrated the required specificity characteristics. The limit of detection of quassin in the broad specificity assay was 5 ng, presumably because of the extensive modification of the hapten required for immunogen synthesis. In the specific quassin assay, as little as 5 pg quassin could be detected.

CONCLUSIONS

Many types of immunoassay are available. Comparison of the RIAs and ELISAs which have been developed in this Institute have shown the advantages of the ELISA procedure in alkaloid analysis. Where we have been able to compare the performance of the same antisera preparations in the two assay formats, the ELISAs were more sensitive and more specific.

ACKNOWLEDGEMENT

This work was partly funded by the Ministry of Agriculture, Fisheries and Food.

REFERENCES

MORGAN, M. R. A., BRAMHAM, S., WEBB, A. J., ROBINS, R. J. & RHODES, M. J. C. (1985) Specific immunoassays for quinine and quinidine: comparison of radioimmunoassays and enzyme-linked immunosorbent assay procedures. *Planta Medica*, **51**, 237–241.

ROBINS, R. J., WEBB, A. J., RHODES, M. J. C., PAYNE, J. & MORGAN, M. R. A. (1984*a*) Radioimmunoassay for the quantitative determination of quinine in cultured plant tissues. *Planta Medica*, **50**, 235–238.

ROBINS, R. J., MORGAN, M. R. A., RHODES, M. J. C. & FURZE, J. M. (1984*b*) An enzyme-linked immunosorbent assay for quassin and closely related metabolites. *Analytical Biochemistry*, **136**, 145–156.

ROBINS, R. J., MORGAN, M. R. A., RHODES, M. J. C. & FURZE, J. M. (1984*c*) Determination of quassin in picogram quantities by an enzyme-linked immunosorbent assay. *Phytochemistry*, **23**, 1119–1123.

Detection of Enzymes used as Food Additives by Immunoassay as Exemplified by an ELISA for *Mucor miehei* Rennet in Cheese

R. L. Darley, B. A. Morris, M. N. Clifford and B. J. Gould
Department of Biochemistry, University of Surrey, Guildford, UK

INTRODUCTION

Owing to the dwindling supply of calf rennet (chymosin EC 3.4.23.4) and the steady increase in cheese production, there has been an extensive search for other acid proteases suitable as milk coagulants in traditional cheese manufacture. A number of rennets of fungal and bacterial origin are now used in commercial cheese production (Scott, 1986) and one derived from the fungus *Mucor miehei* (EC 3.4.23.6) accounts for 40% of the rennet used in the United States (Harboe, 1985). In the United Kingdom, microbial rennets are mainly used in the production of vegetarian cheese.

The following is a preliminary report of an ELISA for the detection and quantitation of *M. miehei* rennet in mature cheese. This was achieved with minimal sample preparation using an indirect ELISA.

MATERIALS

Apparatus

Flat-bottomed PVC microtitration plates (M29), the plate washer (Miniwash) and the automatic spectrophotometric plate reader (MR 580) were obtained from Dynatech Laboratories Limited (Billingshurst, Sussex). Incubations were carried out in a LEEC incubator type K2 (LEEC Limited, Nottingham). The positive displacement pipette, M25 Microman, was supplied by Anachem (Luton, Bedfordshire).

Chemicals

All chemicals and buffer salts (analytical grade where possible) were purchased from BDH (Poole, Dorset). Purified acid protease from *M. miehei* (Novozyme 119) was obtained from Novo Industri A/S (Copenhagen). *Endothia parasitica* rennet was purified from a sample obtained from Pfizer Limited (Sandwich, Kent). *M. pusillus* rennet was purified from a sample supplied by Boehringer Ingelheim AG (Ingelheim-am-Rhein, West Germany). Purified chymosin (60 units/mg) was purchased from Sigma (Poole, Dorset).

Buffers

Plate-coating buffer was 0·1 M carbonate–bicarbonate buffer (pH 9·6). PBST, containing 0·05% Tween 20 and 0·1% gelatin (pH 7·4), was used both as the assay diluent and washing buffer.

Substrate Solution

o-Phenylenediamine (0·4 mg/ml) was dissolved in 0·024 M citrate–0·05 M phosphate buffer (pH 5·0); 0·04% hydrogen peroxide (30%) was then added.

Antisera

An antiserum to *M. miehei* protease was raised in a sheep by injection of the purified enzyme preparation emulsified in non-ulcerative Freund's adjuvant (Morris) (Guildhay Antisera Limited, University of Surrey, Guildford, Surrey). Affinity-purified HRP-labelled donkey anti-sheep IgG was also supplied by Guildhay Antisera.

Cheeses

Mature cheddar cheese, made with known rennet, was obtained direct from the Dairy Crest creamery at Sturminster Newton, Dorset. The cheese was grated and stored at −40°C prior to analysis.

METHODS

Sample Preparation

Cheese samples were homogenised in assay buffer (MSE Homogeniser) and insoluble material removed by centrifugation for 20 min at 3600*g* and 4°C (Beckman J6-B centrifuge). The supernatant was drawn off using a syringe and fine tubing. Extraneous material in the supernatant was removed by precipitation with ammonium sulphate (26·4 g/100 ml) at 0°C (pH 5·4). The precipitate was removed by re-centrifuging as previously. The clear supernatant was dialysed against three changes of assay buffer before being analysed.

Antigen-free Matrix

An extract of a mature cheddar cheese, made with chymosin, was prepared as described above. This was used as the antigen-free matrix, since the antiserum to *M. miehei* protease was found not to cross-react with this rennet.

ELISA Protocol

Microtitration plates were pre-washed by soaking with coating buffer for 15 min. All incubations were carried out in a humid environment within a closed sandwich box.

Pre-washed plates were coated overnight at 4°C with *M. miehei* antigen (1 μg/ml, 0·2 ml/well). At the same time, dilutions of standard and test extract were prepared and pre-incubated (16 h at 37°C in the LEEC incubator) with excess anti-*M. miehei* antiserum (1:50 000 dilution). After coating, the plates were washed four times and the pre-incubated standards and test extracts were added (0·2 ml/well). After incubation (90 min at 20°C), the plates were again washed four times and labelled second antibody (0·2 ml of 1:5000 dilution) added to each well. Following a further incubation (2 h at 37°C in the LEEC incubator), the plates were washed five times and substrate solution added (0·15 ml/well). After 30 min at 37°C, the reaction was stopped by the addition of 0·05 ml of 2·5 M H_2SO_4 and the absorbance of the individual wells read at 490 nm using the automatic plate reader.

RESULTS

Antiserum Production

Acid protease from *M. miehei* proved to be a potent immunogen, producing a titre of 1:100 000 in the immunised animal following the priming dose. After boosting, the most suitable bleed with respect to avidity and titre was selected for assay development. The cross-reactivity of the antiserum with other acid proteases using the assay described was determined on a weight basis. Chymosin and *E. parasitica* rennet showed no cross-reactivity (<0·01%). *M. pusillus* rennet showed partial cross-reactivity (1%).

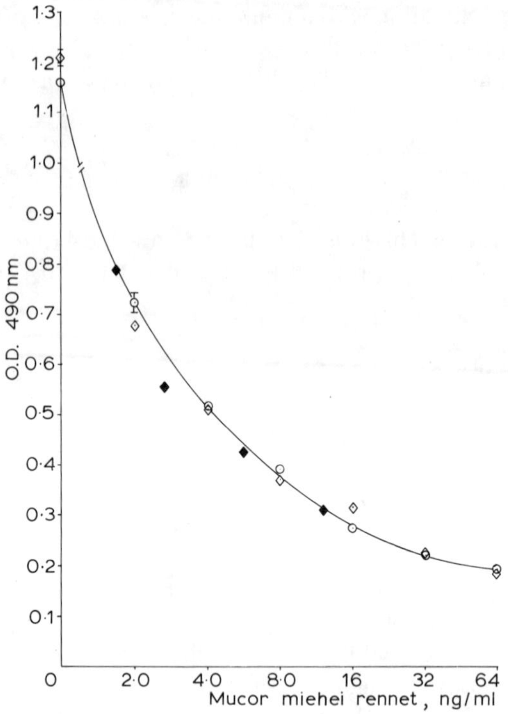

Fig. 1. Estimation of *M. miehei* rennet using indirect ELISA. Standard curve in buffer (○—○). Corresponding standards in antigen-free matrix (◇). Interpolated values for serial dilutions of an extract containing *M. miehei* rennet (◆): 1:2 = 23·7 ng/ml, 1:4 = 20·2 ng/ml, 1:8 = 29·2 ng/ml. Limits represent ranges given by duplicate determinations.

Analysis of Cheese Samples

A standard curve for the estimation of *M. miehei* rennet in cheese is shown in Fig. 1. Serial dilutions of a sample extract in antigen-free matrix were assayed for the presence of *M. miehei* rennet. The extract contained a mean content of 24·4 ng/ml *M. miehei* rennet, 1 ml of extract being derived from 0·33 g of cheese. The detection limit of the assay was 0·55 ng/ml, calculated as 2 SD from zero analyte.

DISCUSSION

The cross-reactivity with *M. pusillus* rennet was not surprising since it is very similar in structure to *M. miehei* rennet (Etoh *et al.*, 1979), and any common determinant will result in some cross-reaction. A more specific two-site (sandwich) assay is now being developed in an attempt to distinguish between these two enzymes.

The presence of extraneous material in the sample being analysed frequently interferes with the antigen–antibody reaction, constituting a matrix effect which is often a cause of considerable inaccuracy. Figure 1 demonstrates the absence of any matrix effect, since identical standard curves were obtained, when standards of *M. miehei* rennet were diluted in assay diluent and in antigen-free matrix. The figure also demonstrates that the dilutions of sample extract show parallelism with the standard curve, indicating that the same epitopes are being recognised in the sample extract as in the standard. This implies that the native structure of the enzyme has remained substantially unaltered throughout the manufacturing stages and subsequent extraction procedure.

CONCLUSION

The study so far has shown that it is possible to detect immunologically, even after all manufacturing stages including maturation, enzymes used as food additives.

ACKNOWLEDGEMENTS

The authors wish to acknowledge the generous financial support of the Ministry of Agriculture, Fisheries and Food, the gifts of enzyme samples from Novo Industri A/S, Pfizer Limited and Boehringer Ingelheim AG, and the provision by Dairy Crest of cheese samples made with known rennets, without all of which this work would not have been possible.

REFERENCES

ETOH, Y., SHOUN, H., BEPPU, T. & ARIMA, K. (1979) Physicochemical and immunological studies on similarities of acid proteases *Mucor pusillus* rennin and *Mucor miehei* rennin: Milk clotting enzymes from microorganisms Part XII. *Agricultural & Biological Chemistry*, **43**, 209–215.

HARBOE, M. K. (1985) Commercial aspects of aspartic proteases. In: *Aspartic Proteinases and Their Inhibitors*, Kostka, V. (ed.), Walter de Gruyter & Co., pp. 537–550.

SCOTT, R. (1986) Coagulants and precipitants. In: *Cheesemaking Practice*, Scott, R. (ed.), Elsevier, London, pp. 167–185.

The Measurement of Hypoxanthine (6-Hydroxypurine) in Meat and Fish Samples by RIA

B. ROBERTS, B. A. MORRIS and M. N. CLIFFORD

Department of Biochemistry, University of Surrey, Guildford, UK

INTRODUCTION

The hypoxanthine content in the flesh of fresh and processed fish is of interest as an index of eating quality and as a predictor of remaining storage life (Burt, 1977). It is produced shortly *post mortem*, by autolysis of ATP, and rather later by microbial activity. Hypoxanthine is normally accompanied by a range of structurally related nucleotides and nucleosides. Erlanger & Beiser (1964) have observed that antibodies can discriminate small structural differences in purines and pyrimidines. The aims of this investigation were as follows:

1. To develop a radioimmunoassay for hypoxanthine (MW = 136).
2. To develop an extraction procedure that would minimise any matrix effect.
3. To compare the RIA with an established enzyme–spectrophotometric assay for hypoxanthine in stored fish muscle and pigs' liver (Jones *et al.*, 1964).

CHOICE OF HAPTEN

The structures of hypoxanthine and other ATP catabolites that generally accompany it in flesh foods are shown in Fig. 1. Examination of the structural formulae indicated that in order to produce an antibody specific for hypoxanthine the region distal to the 6-oxo substituent of hypoxanthine must be exposed to the circulating lymphocytes.

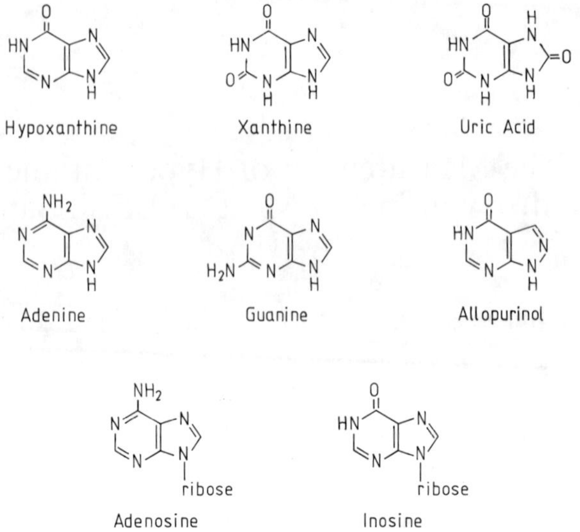

Fig. 1. The structures of hypoxanthine and ATP catabolites that generally accompany it in flesh foods.

PREPARATION OF IMMUNOGEN

Attempts to conjugate the 6-hydroxy enol tautomer to a carrier protein proved unsuccessful due to the unfavourable position of the keto–enol equilibrium. Conjugation of the 6-oxo keto tautomer was also unsuccessful due to its resistance to attack by nucleophiles. This is a feature of bicyclic systems where one ring (pyrimidine) is π-electron deficient, and the other (imidazole) has an excess of π-electrons. A more reactive analogue, 6-trichloromethylpurine (TCM-purine), was prepared from commercially available 6-methylpurine, by the procedure of Cohen *et al.* (1962). The 6-TCM-purine was conjugated to ovalbumin using a modification (Roberts, 1986) of the periodate conjugation method of Butler *et al.* (1962). The degree of derivatisation was 3:1, as judged by the resultant decrease in trinitrobenzenesulphonic acid-reactive lysine (Hall *et al.*, 1973).

ANTISERUM PRODUCTION

A female Suffolk cross sheep was immunised intramuscularly, at multiple sites, with the 6-TCM-purine–ovalbumen conjugate (6 mg) in non-ulcerative Freund's complete adjuvant (Morris) (2 ml). The animal was boosted after approximately four months and blood subsequently collected from the jugular vein.

Antibodies specific to hypoxanthine were isolated by affinity chromatography using a 6-TCM-purine–AH Sepharose 4B solid support and elution with 0·05 M sodium hydroxide. A RIA was developed using tritium-labelled hypoxanthine (Amersham) and ammonium sulphate phase separation. A calibration curve and precision dose profile were prepared. The nucleotides and nucleosides illustrated in Fig. 1, known to occur in flesh foods, were tested for cross-reaction in the assay. Adenine, which would only be present in traces, if at all, showed a 1·4% cross-reaction with the affinity-purified antibody. The other compounds tested had no cross-reactivity, even at levels which grossly exceeded their likely relative concentrations in food samples.

THE ANALYSIS OF FOOD SAMPLES

Analyses were performed on perchloric acid (protein-free) extracts prepared by homogenising 5 g samples of tissue that were free from skin and bone. Excess perchlorate was removed by precipitation of the sparingly soluble potassium salt at 0°C, as described by Jones *et al.* (1964). There was no detectable matrix effect, and standards were prepared in barbitone buffer (0·05 M, pH 8·6). The detection limit (the hypoxanthine concentration causing a 10% fall in binding compared to binding at zero concentration) was 12·2 μg/g sample (fresh weight basis).

Figure 2 illustrates the progressive accumulation of hypoxanthine *post mortem* in commercial samples of freshly killed rainbow trout and frozen whitebait, which were allowed to deteriorate at 4°C for 9 days. Traces of hypoxanthine were detected in the trout at about 1 h *post mortem*. The much higher level of hypoxanthine in the zero time whitebait sample reflects the accumulation that had occurred during handling and storage prior to purchase. After six days the hypoxanthine content of the whitebait began to fall, probably because of catabolism by microbes, since spoilage was extensive. These observations are consistent with previously published data (Burt, 1977, and references therein). In contrast, analyses of pigs' liver showed a progressive decline in hypoxanthine content during storage over 10 days, probably reflecting the activity of endogenous xanthine oxidase. No previous data on the hypoxanthine content of pigs' liver are available for comparison.

The results for hypoxanthine content of the fish samples obtained by the

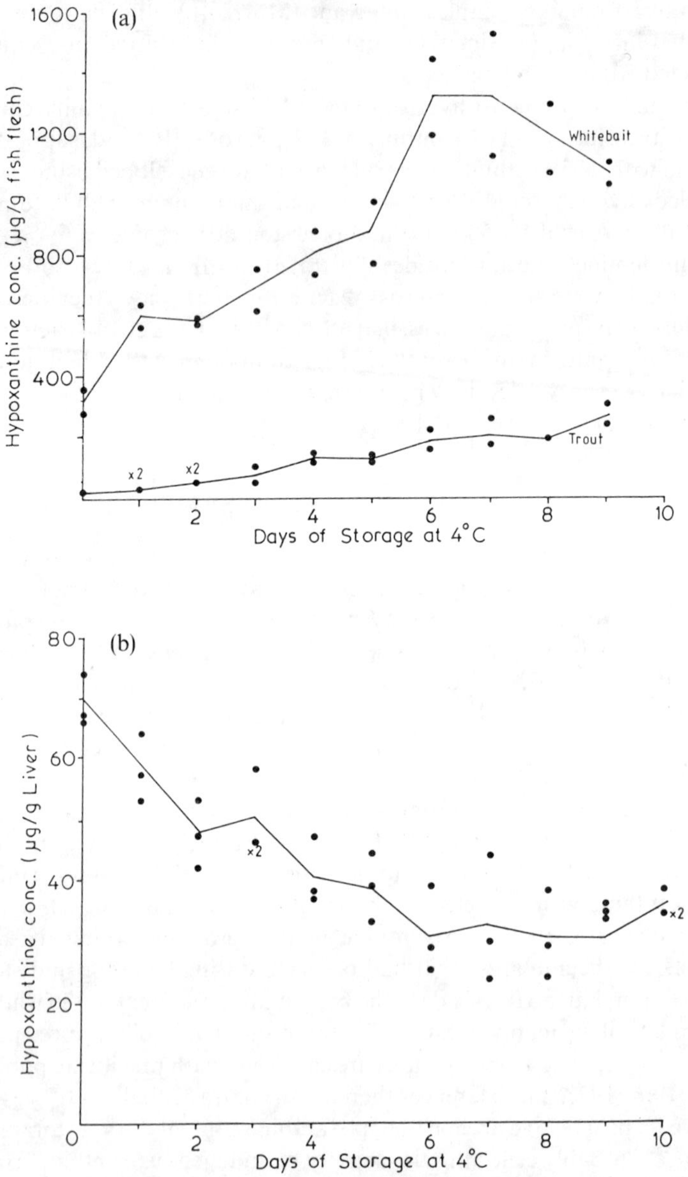

Fig. 2. Hypoxanthine concentrations *post mortem* in commercial samples of (a) freshly killed rainbow trout and frozen whitebait, and (b) pigs' liver, which were allowed to deteriorate at 4°C.

RIA correlated well with those obtained by the xanthine oxidase enzyme-spectrophotometric method of Jones *et al.* (1964). The statistical method was that of Brace (1977). The calculated relationships were $r = 0{\cdot}933$, $n = 33$, $P > 0{\cdot}001$ for the trout and $r = 0{\cdot}845$, $n = 45$, $P > 0{\cdot}001$ for the whitebait. Thus the RIA appears to be a realistic alternative. However, it must be noted that the xanthine oxidase method is known to be imprecise at high substrate concentrations (>125 nmol/ml) due to substrate inhibition; for example, in this study standards of 100 and 500 nmol/ml gave the same result. Furthermore, it does not discriminate between xanthine and hypoxanthine. Therefore, the greater dynamic range, greater specificity and potentially lower limit of detection together make RIA the method of choice for routine quantification of hypoxanthine. The potential of the perchloric acid method to provide extracts free from matrix effects is being evaluated in other immunoassays for small molecules.

ACKNOWLEDGEMENT

This work was funded by an SERC Case Award Studentship to BR.

REFERENCES

Brace, R. A. (1977) Fitting straight lines to experimental data. *American Journal of Physiology*, **233**, R94–R99.

Burt, J. R. (1977) Hypoxanthine: a biochemical index of fish quality. *Process Biochemistry*, **12**, 25–32.

Butler, V. P., Beiser, S. M., Erlanger, B. F., Tanenbaum, S. W., Cohen, S. & Bendich, A. (1962) Purine-specific antibodies which react with deoxyribonucleic acid (DNA). *Proceedings of the National Academy of Sciences, USA*, **48**, 1597–1602.

Cohen, S., Thom, E. & Bendich, A. (1962) The preparation and properties of 6-halomethylpurines. *Journal of Organic Chemistry*, **27**, 3545–3549.

Erlanger, B. F. & Beiser, S. M. (1964) Antibodies specific for ribonucleosides and ribonucleotides and their reaction with DNA. *Proceedings of the National Academy of Sciences, USA*, **52**, 68–74.

Hall, R. J., Trinder, N. & Givens, D. I. (1973) Observations on the use of 2,4,6-trinitrobenzenesulphonic acid for the determination of available lysine in animal protein concentrates. *Analyst*, **98**, 673–686.

Jones, N. R., Murray, J., Livingstone, E. I. & Murray, C. K. (1964) Rapid estimations of hypoxanthine concentrations as indices of the freshness of chill-stored fish. *Journal of the Science of Food and Agriculture*, **15**, 763–774.

Roberts, B. (1986) Development and critical evaluation of an immunoassay for hypoxanthine in biological matrices. PhD Thesis, University of Surrey, Guildford, UK.

Index